Language Disabilities in Children and Adolescents

Elisabeth H. Wiig

Boston University

Eleanor Messing Semel

Boston University

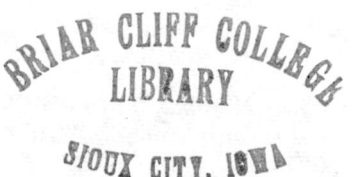

Charles E. Merrill Publishing Company
A Bell & Howell Company
Columbus, Ohio

To Charlotte, Erik, and Jack

Published by
Charles E. Merrill Publishing Company
A Bell & Howell Company
Columbus, Ohio 43216

The book was set in Caledonia.
The Production Editor was Linda Hillis.
The cover was designed by Will Chenoweth.
Cover photograph by Bernstein Photo.

International Standard Book Number: 0-675-08614-0
Library of Congress Catalog Card Number: 75-40978
1 2 3 4 5 6 7—81 80 79 78 77 76

LC
4704
.W54

Printed in the United States of America

Foreword

The most non-controversial evidence for the importance of language to reading is right before our eyes. For example, I have an intact nervous system, good memory, adequate sensory and perceptual systems; and I am able to recognize, sound out and name letters, organize them into larger units, make the appropriate eye tracking movements from left to right and back. Yet I cannot read a word of Russian. In order to learn to read Russian I would first have to learn the language.

In order to learn Russian or any other language one must know its sounds (phonology), its words (lexicon), and its sentence formation (syntax and semantics), each of which is crucially involved in the process of reading as well as speaking. Thus it seems apparent to me that one cannot separate reading from language itself.

Nor do I think one can clearly separate reading disabilities from language disabilities from learning disabilities.

When we examine the heterogenous group of children called learning disabled, excluding those who suffer from mild retardation, specific sensory defect or primary emotional problems, we can identify roughly two major categories. Those children whose school failure is in reading and spelling, and those whose school problems are more generalized and include arithmetic. Those with reading disability tend to score higher in performance items and the second group score higher in verbal items of intelligence tests. Those with reading disability tend to have specific problems with establishing verbal associations, while those with more generalized disabilities tend to demonstrate perceptual-motor deficits. Principles of remediation will vary according to the child's needs, of course. We seem to have an infinite variety of remedial materials and techniques designed to help the child with perceptual-motor problems in learning disability but there are relatively few remedial programs for children with language and reading disabilities. Yet it is this latter group which seems to rouse heated controversy among several disciplines, which is helpful neither to the advancement of knowledge nor, more importantly, to the child.

Several disciplines concern themselves with normally intelligent children who fail to learn reading in particular: professionals in the fields of reading, learning disabilities, speech and language, and even linguistics are all involved. Although these fields are already separated by basic differences in training curricula, theoretical constructs, views on etiological factors, methods of diagnosis and treatment, and general terminology, they overlap to varying degrees in their concern for and management of children with language/learning disabilities. Ultimately, if we hope to help the *child* instead of just tackle his problems, we will need to develop a framework that can accommodate each of these fields, that will enhance their systems of studying and treating language problems, and that will provide their students with insight, skills and competencies reflecting this broad framework.

Here is a volume which provides both breadth and depth of information on the nature, assessment and remediation of language deficits in learning disabilities. The authors provide a clear and comprehensive presentation of the complexities of the language processing and language production problems of children with learning disabilities. They draw chiefly from Guilford, Luria, Miller and Chomsky in introducing their models.

The authors have done a unique service in attempting to bring order out of chaos. They introduce a model for language processing which emphasizes (1) perceptual processing, (2) linguistic processing, (3) cognitive-semantic processing and (4) the relationships between the various aspects of these processes. The oral language production problems of learning disabled children and adolescents are reviewed with reference to models for: (1) convergent semantic production and (2) divergent semantic production, as introduced by Guilford. They also present with clarity the evidence of relationships between language processing and production deficits in learning disabilities.

Having established a firm foundation for their approach, the authors outline in detail their rationale for diagnosis and remediation, step by step, through each phase of language processing and production. This material is written predominantly for the educator-clinician and I believe it is the only volume in which the theoretical constructs of language clinicians and linguists are brought together in such a way that they can be utilized by reading and learning disabilities specialists.

The student is provided with extensive and detailed review of the methods for assessment of the various functions of language. But this is no cookbook. The authors in effect are teaching the educator-clinicians to *think* their way through assessment by asking specific questions about the child who is to be evaluated.

Similarly, the principles of remediation are presented systematically. These principles are based on the premise that remediation of language processing deficits should precede intervention for language production deficits, since language processing and comprehension involve recognition, while language production requires recall and retrieval. This premise is supported by the normal progression of developmental sequence in the child, which is so frequently overlooked in the usual cookbook approach to remediation.

Here at last is a book which provides the educator-clinician, the reading specialist, the learning disabilities specialist, the speech and language clinician, the audiologist, and student of linguistics a framework upon which they may all meet together and from which they can gain a deeper understanding of the nature and treatment of children with language/learning disabilities.

Sylvia O. Richardson, M.D.
University of Cincinnati

Preface

During the past decade, speech and language pathologists have received an increasing number of referrals of learning disabled children and adolescents. The purpose of these referrals has often been to provide an in-depth evaluation of the youngsters' speech and language status, discuss the implications of language deficits for achievement in specific academic areas, and prescribe a program of language intervention or therapy to meet the youngsters' needs. As professionals, we experienced the same frustrations as many others. The research of language abilities or disabilities of youngsters with learning disabilities was limited, discussions of language tests appropriate for a school-age population were practically nonexistent, and sources which discussed the rationale for or design of remedial strategies were limited.

In our search for answers and in preparation for this text, we designed and conducted research of the morphologic, syntactic, and cognitive-semantic abilities in language processing and production. We also reviewed and selected tests which we considered appropriate for a differential diagnosis of language disabilities in school-age children and adolescents and considered strategies for intervention. The tests and strategies we identified have been used by us and by our students during the past decade. This text presents our experiences, observations, and clinical-educational procedures in the management of language disabilities. It is intended for use by teachers, special educators, speech pathologists, psychologists, and other professionals involved in the process of educating language and learning disabled children and adolescents.

The organization of the text was dictated by the consideration that the reader should be introduced to the implications of language and communication deficits (chapter 1) and to underlying cognitive, neuropsychological, and psycholinguistic theories and models (chapter 2) before a detailed study of the characteristics and diagnoses of and the remediation strategies for language disabilities (chapters 3 through 10). Finally, we felt that a discussion of the language and communication deficits of school-age children and adolescents would be incomplete unless the significance of nonverbal communication and the implications of deficits on interpersonal communication were discussed (chapter 11). Since the text draws upon information from many disciplines, a glossary of specialized terms from the specific areas involved has been provided at the end of the book.

Although the discussions in the text focus on studies and observations of learning disabled youngsters, the discussions of the implications for the clinical–educational management may apply to youngsters with language disabilities caused by factors other than those associated with learning disabilities. We recognize that the current knowledge of the bases and nature of language disabilities associated with learning disabilities is limited and that several of the models and strategies presented deserve verification; however as clinician-educators we were concerned with ameliorating the frustrations of professionals responsible for the management of the language disabilities of school-age youngsters and the often neglected adolescents.

Acknowledgement

No work ever stands alone. To all who have con-
tributed to our lives and professional careers,
past and present, we express our gratitude.

Contents

Language Disabilities in
Children and Adolescents

1

Implications of Language and Communication Deficits on Academic Achievement and Interpersonal Interaction

Overview

Language and learning disabled youngsters may experience academic and psycho-social problems during preschool and school age, adolescence, and young adulthood. This chapter focuses on the implications of language and communication deficits on academic achievement and psycho-social development.

The nature of the academic and social problems observed in association with language and learning disabilities varies with educational level. Observations suggest that these disabilities may result in academic and social failure, social rejection, development of nonadaptive emotional reactions and psycho-social problems, as well as in problems of sexual identity and role development. It is suggested that early identification and intervention or adaptation of academic or vocational tasks may increase the potential for self-actualization.

Evidence is presented for the relationships among language abilities, reading, and mathematics. The consensus of investigations indicates that auditory-perceptual abilities and reading generally correlate at low but significant levels (Hammill & Larsen, 1974). Psycholinguistic abilities and reading appear more strongly related based on, among others, evidence that perception is determined by linguistic knowledge (Mehler, Bever, & Carey, 1967; Levin & Kaplan, 1971), that error patterns in reading reflect transformation of syntactic structure and semantic information (Clay, 1968, 1969, Goodman, 1967, 1969; Kolers, 1972), and that specific linguistic deficits relate to reading retardation (Semel & Wiig, 1975; Vogel, 1974; Wiig, Semel, & Crouse, 1973). Evidence is also presented that linguistic abilities may influence math problem solving (Linville, 1970; Rosenthal & Resnick, 1974; Sax & Ottina, 1958). This evidence concurs with preliminary findings that reductions in mathematics correlated significantly with specific deficits in linguistic processing (Semel & Wiig, 1975).

The Preschool Years

Learning disabled children are frequently born at a disadvantage. High-risk pregnancy and birth histories and early perceptual and motor deficits are common in this population (Clements, 1973; Denhoff, 1967; Johnson & Myklebust, 1967; Kass, 1962; Kawi & Pasamanick, 1958; Myklebust, 1964; Pasamanick, Rogers, & Lilienfeld, 1956). The learning disabled child is often recognized by his parents as being "different" (Brutten, Richardson, & Mangel, 1973). He may have allergies, colics, and other physical problems that require the parents to handle him differently from their other children during the early months of life. Later, the LD child may show delays in developmental milestones in motor development, in the acquisition of ability to localize environmental sounds, and in speech and language development. All of these deficits may result in subtle changes in the quantity and quality of the interaction between parents and child and significantly reduce the quality of the infant's upbringing.

Developmental delays in the area of language may become apparent when the child is late in acquiring his first word and slow in the subsequent acquisition of knowledge of linguistic rules and use of linguistic structures. The learning disabled child may use one- or two-word utterances for a longer period of time than his achieving peers. In a similar vein, the normal articulatory deviations and periods of nonfluency may be extended. The learning disabled child may reveal phoneme discrimination, sequencing, and word-finding problems during the early preschool years. He may consistently reverse phonemes and repeat *emeny* when he hears the word *enemy* and *aminals* when he hears *animals*. He may have severe problems in recalling proper and concept names, reflected in frequent word substitutions, circumlocutions, and use of stereotypes such as "That guy, he. . . ."

In response to the learning disabled child's receptive and expressive language problems, he may be judged to be slow to respond, confused, impulsive, inattentive, or even obstinate. Parents may react to their LD child's language and communication problems with guilt, overprotection, rejection, or concern. If parental and peer reactions are overwhelmingly negative or punishing, the learning disabled child may develop nonadaptive emotional reactions or secondary emotional problems that may cause present and future difficulty in interpersonal interaction and thus emphasize the specific learning disorder. The emotional reactions and problems which may be associated with learning disabilities have been eloquently discussed by Brutten, Richardson, and Mangel (1973).

It is unfortunate that learning disabled children who develop later language deficits frequently acquire a large vocabulary with ease. This facility often camouflages specific problems in language processing and oral language formulation and production. Learning disabled children may be given to excessive talking and fail to recognize the social cues to stop. This behavior may turn off overtures to verbal interactions by their achieving age peers and by concerned adults. In a similar fashion, by use of negative attitudes, overt criticisms, requests for perfection, or unrealistic demands, parents frequently sabotage listening and communication efforts by their LD children. They may also fail to facilitate auditory perception and comprehension by failing to organize the environmental and verbal stimuli for their children.

The Early Grades

Kindergarten

When the learning disabled child enters kindergarten he may not know colors and their names or be able to use scissors, tie shoelaces, color within lines, or arrange two or three objects according to size. In the language area, he may not be able to follow verbal directions, and he may not be able to tell the names of the days of the week, months of the year, or count. Other verbal skills may also be deficient. He may not be able to sit through listening to a story; learn the alphabet, word rhyming, finger plays, or songs; or make one-to-one correspondences between sounds and letters.

The kindergarten teacher is generally able to identify the children who are academically at risk but frequently finds attempts to obtain early assistance for the child's language problems futile. Several investigations have established that learning disabled children detected in the third and fourth grades were frequently identified in kindergarten. As a result of the language deficits and the lack of early intervention, preacademic skills necessary for first grade work may not have been acquired, leaving the LD child at an early disadvantage and open to academic and social failures and frustrations.

Learning disabled children with language deficits who are admitted to the first grade without having acquired preacademic skills frequently show limited ability to identify phonics sounds. They may have problems in same-different discriminations of sounds, in analyzing and synthesizing phonemes and phoneme sequences, in segmenting words into smaller grammatical units, and in forming stable sound-symbol associations. These deficits may result in limited or slow academic achievement in spelling, reading, and math, among others.

Language disabilities in learning disabled children can often be discerned by observing their verbal interactions with parents and teachers who frequently limit their verbal interactions and employ restricted verbal codes with these children. When giving them instructions, teachers and parents may be observed resorting to motor or gestural demonstrations rather than providing verbal directions. As a result they limit the LD child's opportunities to gain experiences in and obtain reinforcement for processing and producing increasingly complex language.

First Grade

During this academic year learning disabled children become increasingly aware of their academic and social failures and of being different, and emotional reactions may be registered with increasing frequency. These may take the form of aggression, anxiety, compulsiveness, frustration, rigidity, or withdrawal and may go unnoticed by parents and teachers until overt acts of aggression, pilfering, or severe nightmares reveal the LD child's emotional turmoil. The child may not be able to verbalize these reactions until the second through fourth grades. Generally, we find that intellectual ability determines the age when the emotional reactions will be verbalized. The higher the child's intellectual ability, the earlier he tends to gain insight into his problems and in his ability to verbalize frustrations. When LD children are provided with counseling, they often reveal the depth of their anguish. As an example, a seven-year-old language and learning disabled child expressed guilt toward his parents for being "dumb," a wish to "be dead so nobody will bug me," and a sense of "being ugly and a polluter." These are serious emotional reactions and deserve professional attention by providing counseling in association with intervention.

Second and Third Grades

The demands for auditory language processing, oral presentations, and verbal recall increase significantly in the second grade. Language problems which existed in the first grade tend to persist or increase in severity due to the increased demands. At the same time, less classroom time is spent with manipulative materials. New knowledge must be acquired rapidly from verbal presentations, and verbal directions must be followed accurately. There is a heavy emphasis on phonics and on the acquisition of more abstract words and concepts, for example, linguistic concepts such as *few, some, most, many, either-or,* and temporally and spatially based language concepts such as *before-after, second, third,* etc. The delays demonstrated by LD children in the acquisition of syntactic skills and linguistic concepts appear to limit their potential for achievement in reading comprehension, spelling, and mathematics (Aiken, 1972; Semel & Wiig, 1975).

Basic skills continue to be taught in the third grade, but specific learning disabilities now tend to become blatantly obvious. Oral language deficits, however, appear to decrease at this stage. Sentence length and syntactic complexity often seem to increase, and it seems as if the learning disabled child may be catching up with his peers. Word-finding problems seem to decrease as do incidences of nonfluency, and sentence intonation seems to improve.

Subtle, high level deficits in processing auditory language and in language formulation and production may, however, continue and influence reading comprehension and mathematical skills. Word substitutions may persist in reading, sentence repetition, copying, or writing from dictation. When the LD child is engaged in oral reading, he may substitute words such as *kitten* for *cat* or *knife* for *fork*. This type of oral reading error seems most prevalent when the difficulty level of the material is well below achievement level; it seems to decrease when the level of difficulty increases. Visual discrimination errors appear to increase in oral reading when the level of difficulty of the material is at or above the level of achievement.

The Middle Grades and Adolescence

The demands on the child change drastically when he enters the fourth grade. From now on there is generally no skill building in phonics, vocabulary, or number or language concepts, and specific deficits receive minimal attention in the regular classroom. As a result, learning disabled children tend to be lost in reading sessions and may retain limited language processing skills that affect achievement in all academic areas. It is notable in this context that texts in areas such as social studies contain reading vocabulary well above reading level, magnifying the problems for the child with a language deficit. Math problems also increase significantly in complexity at this grade level, placing greater demands on both linguistic and cognitive processing.

The Middle Grades

In the fourth grade and above, adequate cognition of semantic classes, relations, systems, transformations, and implications is a prerequisite for academic achievement. There is also an increasing emphasis on convergent and divergent semantic production abilities for academic performance. Processing the complex auditory-verbal and visual-symbolic materials requires parallel, simultaneous linguistic, semantic, and logical processing, areas of weakness that persist into adolescence in association with learning disabilities (Wiig & Roach, 1975; Wiig & Semel, 1974). The educational implications appear to be that language disabled youngsters may benefit from intervention from kindergarten through fourth grade to provide augmented opportunities for skill-building activities.

In the areas of nonverbal communication and social interaction, the learning disabled youngster in the middle grades seems to grow increasingly insensitive and clumsy. He may give inappropriate social responses, show delays in acquiring various social skills, and get into trouble because he is unable to interpret the emotions and predict the intentions of others. He is in turn liable to be rejected by his peers, and his emotional problems may increase.

Adolescence and Young Adulthood

During prepuberty and puberty and into adolescence and young adulthood, verbal and nonverbal language and communication deficits will negatively influence the quality of interpersonal interactions and the potential for self-realization. Deficits in social perception, that is, the ability to perceive and interpret nonverbal communication cues, are augmented by increasing social demands. Adult sexual identities and roles emerge and develop during this period and require adjustments of body image and self-concept. Sensitivity to nonverbal as well as to verbal communication cues may constitute an important avenue for external evaluations and facilitate the development of an appropriate sexual identity (Wiig & Harris, 1974). Attention to developing adequate nonverbal and verbal communication skills or adaptation of academic or vocational tasks may improve the language and learning disabled youngster's potential for self-actualization through vocational or professional pursuits or interpersonal interactions (Wiig, 1972). The subsequent sections will explore the current evidence of relationships between deficits in language processing in reading and mathematics.

Relating Language Processing and Reading Deficits

Reading is a complex skill that depends upon processing, among others, written, phonetic, syntactic, and semantic information in response to a visual-graphic display. Impaired reading in adults with acquired brain damage may result from a combination of specific oculo-motor and visual processing deficits (Luria, 1966; Schuell, Jenkins, & Jimenez-Pabon, 1964; Wepman, 1951). Several investigations have offered support for the view that form discrimination deficits may be basic factors in reading reductions in asphasic adults (Bender, 1938; Cohen & Edwards, 1964; Marshall & Newcombe, 1973; Rosenberg, 1965; Schuell & Jenkins, 1959). There is, however, also evidence that dyslexia in adults may result from difficulties in sound-letter association or from syntactic-semantic deficits (Marshall & Newcombe, 1973).

Historically, the literature concerned with reading deficits in learning disabilities has stressed underlying perceptual-motor deficits and has suggested perceptual-motor training as a means of improving reading (Hallahan & Cruickshank, 1973). This trend has been challenged by authorities, linking reading deficits to reductions in auditory processing (Calfee, Chapman, & Venezky, 1972; Chalfant & Flathouse, 1971; Chalfant & Scheffelin, 1969; Flower, 1965; Johnson & Myklebust, 1967; Klasen, 1972). Recent trends indicate an increasing awareness of the cognitive and linguistic processing deficits of youngsters with learning disabilities and of the relationship of these deficits to reading difficulties (Kolers, 1972; Liberman, 1971; Semel & Wiig, 1975; Vogel, 1974; Warrington & Kinsbourne, 1967). This trend has been supported by investigations of reading as a psycholinguistic process and by observations that the strategies utilized in the process of reading may change over time.

Kershner (1975) has distinguished two visual-spatial abilities involved in reading: perceptual and cognitive (operational). An investigation of the relationships between the two abilities and reading achievement in second graders indicated no significant correlation between perceptual-spatial ability and reading achievement. There was, however, a significant relationship between reading achievement and cognitive-spatial ability, suggesting that second graders with inadequate perceptual skills were able to compensate by using cognitive skills. Kershner introduces a theory of stage-related learning strategies in which, for example, the child's conceptual abilities may be considered of greater significance than the perceptual abilities during the concrete-operational stage. He also hypothesizes that learning strategies and relationships between visual-spatial perceptual skills and reading may not maintain similar significance at other stages. In a similar vein, Hallahan and Cruickshank (1973) have suggested that there is a shift in reading from visual to auditory and intersensory modes at about the fourth grade level.

Reading as a Psycholinguistic Process

With these theories and hypotheses as a background, the cognitive-semantic and psycholinguistic processes involved in skilled reading deserve further examination. Several authorities have stressed the dependency of reading upon knowledge of the structural and semantic (selectional) rules of the native language. This relationship has been expressed in various forms. Kavanagh (1968) has stated that reading is parasitic on language. These views have been supported by observations and investigations of the processes involved in reading by Goodman (1967, 1969), Kolers (1972), Levin and Kaplan

(1971), Mattingly (1972), Mehler, Bever, and Carey (1967), and Ryan and Semmel (1969), among others.

Mehler, Bever, and Carey (1967) evaluated whether phrase structure affected eye-fixation patterns in reading and whether surface- and deep-structure sentence levels shared an equal effect. The reading materials used were three types of ambiguous sentences in which the interpretations differed at (1) the level of surface structure, (2) the level of deep structure, and (3) both levels. The results indicated that visual scanning patterns interacted with the surface phrase-structure level. Thus, the eye was observed to fixate on the beginning or first half of a surface phrase-structure constituent, suggesting that perception was determined by linguistic knowledge.

In a related study, Levin and Kaplan (1971) investigated the relationship between linguistic structure and eye-voice span, that is, the distance that separates eye fixation and oral (voice) encoding in reading. Their findings indicated that efficient readers processed the graphic material in terms of phrase units based on structure and content and not word-by-word. The authors concluded that the efficient reader formulates tentative interpretations or hypotheses about the material and confirms or rejects the interpretations on the basis of additional information about grammatical structure and semantic context.

Mattingly (1972) has suggested that the efficient reader must possess two types of linguistic abilities: (1) primary linguistic activity and (2) linguistic awareness. Primary linguistic activity is viewed to comprise the ability to apply a set of internalized, unconscious rules to the processing, comprehension, and production of language. Linguistic awareness refers to the ability to talk about or reflect on language, to segment spoken language into phoneme sequences, and to handle written text in alphabetic form. Recent studies of the language processing and production abilities of learning disabled children and adolescents suggest reductions that may negatively affect primary linguistic activity (Rosenthal, 1970; Semel & Wiig, 1975; Vogel, 1974; Wiig & Roach, 1975; Wiig & Semel, 1973, 1974, 1975; Wiig, Semel, & Crouse, 1973).

Analyses of Error Patterns in Reading

Several analyses of error patterns in reading have supported the view that psycholinguistic processes are basic to reading (Clay, 1968, 1969; Goodman, 1967, 1969; Kolers, 1972; Shankweiler & Liberman, 1972). Goodman (1967, 1969) has presented a model for reading based on error analysis for proficient and beginning readers. Reading within the model is viewed as a selective, tentative, anticipatory process. The proficient reader decodes directly from the graphic stimuli and encodes from the deep structure. The verbal output in reading may therefore reflect transformations at the syntactic and semantic (vocabulary) levels even though the meaning (deep structure) is retained. The efficient reader is also considered to use three kinds of information simultaneously: (1) graphic input, (2) syntactic structure, and (3) semantic interpretation. Anticipatory, tentative hypotheses about the input are formulated on the basis of syntactic and semantic information. The graphic information is sampled to either confirm or reject the initial hypotheses. The beginning reader is more dependent on graphic information to decode than the skilled reader. As graphic-phonic cues are processed more effectively, the syntactic and semantic information assumes greater importance in the reading process.

Clay (1968, 1969) performed a linguistic analysis of 10,525 reading errors made by 100 beginning readers during their first year in school. Attempts at self-correction, occurring for 26% of the total errors, were also analyzed. Spontaneous corrections of errors were observed to result from semantic, syntactic, phonemic, or visual-perceptual dissonance. A significant proportion of the errors were reported as grammatically acceptable substitutions. If the reading errors had been analyzed using a generative grammar (Chomsky, 1957), the number of acceptable substitutions would have been larger since they reflected optional transformations from the same deep structure. Clay (1969) further observed distinguishing characteristics between good and poor readers; good readers learned to verify predictions in reading at the phoneme—grapheme level while poor readers did not verify their predictions. On this basis, Clay states that "motor, perceptual and language differences would perhaps be of greater significance than general intelligence" (p. 55). Children with language reductions are suggested to experience:

> difficulty in predicting constructions likely to occur and in noticing the redundant cues which signal that errors have occurred. There is a good reason to believe that the very complexity that provides rich cue sources for the child who is able to discover the regularities of the code may present confusion to the child of limited language skill. [p. 55]

Kolers (1972) analyzed the reading speed and errors made by skilled readers. Based on the analyses, he concluded that "the experiment . . . disproved the idea that ordinary reading proceeds by a sequential perception of the individual letters composing words." Shankweiler and Liberman (1972) have reported data based on reading error analysis indicating that grapheme and grapheme sequence reversals did not correlate with each other in children's reading errors. Furthermore, errors reflecting a visual-perceptual basis constituted only a small proportion of those made by poor readers.

Reading and Auditory Perception

Rees (1973, 1974) has challenged the notion that most reading disorders reflect deficits in auditory perception, involving, for example, auditory discrimination, auditory memory span, or auditory sequencing. A critical review of investigations of the relationship between specific auditory-perceptual abilities and reading by Hammill and Larsen (1974) supports this challenge. The consensus of the more than thirty studies reviewed suggested that auditory-perceptual abilities did not relate significantly to general reading ability. The correlation coefficients reported between specific auditory skills and three reading subskills (word recognition, reading comprehension, and composite reading [a combination of word recognition and reading comprehension]) were significant but generally lower than .35, the criterion selected to indicate useful prediction. On this basis, the authors concluded: "the auditory skills auditory-visual integration, sound blending, auditory memory, auditory discrimination-phonemic, and auditory discrimination—nonphonemic are not sufficiently related to reading to be particularly useful for school practice" (p. 40).

It would be easy to draw the conclusion that most reading disorders reflect syntactic and semantic deficits, that is, language disorders. Such a conclusion must, however, be checked by evidence that "dyslexic data [obtained from adults with acquired brain lesions] reveal very clearly that . . . linguistically distinct aspects of words [phonological, syntactic and semantic] are involved in functionally separable performance systems" (Marshall & Newcombe, 1973).

Marshall and Newcombe (1973) have introduced a model for normal reading which introduces (1) a *primary visual register* for the perception of visual information and (2) a *visual address* that feeds into (a) a *phonological address* and (b) a *semantic address*. They further postulate: "For word perception to occur the value of the combination of phonological and syntactico-semantic information must exceed a certain threshold." If the threshold is exceeded, an association is made with an *articulatory address*, and the word is read.

Based on data from adults with acquired brain lesions, they further support the existence of three distinct types of dyslexia: (1) *pure, visual dyslexia*, (2) *surface dyslexia*, and (3) *semantic (deep) dyslexia*. Pure, visual dyslexia, characterized by letter confusions (*b* for *d*), sequencing errors (*saw* for *was*), and other visually based errors, was reported in two adults with left occipital lobe lesions. Surface dyslexia, characterized by difficulties in establishing correct grapheme-phoneme associations, was observed in two adults with lesions in the left tempero-parietal region. Their errors indicated that these adults had difficulty especially with grapheme-phoneme relationships that were context sensitive. They experienced problems with ambiguous consonants (*s, f, c, g, p, r*) whose phonetic value depends upon the graphemic context in which they are placed. Similarly, markers such as the terminal *e* which have no inherent phonetic value but specify the realization of some other part of the word were confusing.

Semantic dyslexia, characterized by semantic (word) substitutions (*speak* for *talk*), derivational errors (*hot* for *heat*), and nominalization of base verbs (*entertainment* for *entertain*), was reported in two adults with lesions of the left tempero-parietal and occipital-parietal regions. The deficits were considered to reflect that "they cannot find a semantic address which corresponds with the presented stimulus." Marshall and Newcombe (1973) are cautious in inferring relationships between disorders of reading and language. They conclude their article by saying: "Our sole claim about the relationship of reading to other aspects of language has been that 'visual' d lexia *may* occur in isolation and that 'deep' dyslexia does *not* occur without other aphasic features being present" (p. 194).

In a similar vein, reading disorders in learning disabilities may have several bases as indicated by Bannatyne (1971), de Hirsch, Jansky, and Langford, (1966), Johnson and Myklebust (1967), and Money and Shiffman (1966), among others. The relationship reported by Marshall and Newcombe (1973) between acquired, semantic (deep) dyslexia and other aphasic features is significant in view of the aphasic features observed in both language processing and production by learning disabled youngsters (Denckla, 1974; Wiig & Semel, 1973, 1974, 1975).

Reading and Specific Morphological and Syntactic Abilities

Several studies have investigated the relationship between reading achievement and specific language processing and production abilities (Bougere, 1969; Brittain, 1970; Gibson & Guinet, 1971; Reddell, 1965). Bougere (1969) assessed the relationship between measures of expressive vocabulary (range and diversity) and syntactic complexity and reading achievement on the *Gray Oral Reading* and *Stanford Achievement Test, Primary 1*. The results indicated no significant relationships at the first grade level.

The relationships between the morphological abilities of first and second graders and reading achievement were evaluated by Brittain (1970). The findings indicated: "There is a significant relationship, independent of intelligence, between inflectional performance and reading achievement at both the first and second grade level" (p. 44). Furthermore, there was a greater degree of relationship between reading ability and inflectional performance (knowledge of word-formation rules) at the second than at the first grade level, suggesting the fact that second grade reading materials contain more changes in word forms.

Gibson and Guinet (1971) investigated the influence of morphological inflections and word length on reading performance when words were presented for a brief period of time. They observed that word length rather than number and type of morphological units was the significant variable in reading performance. They concluded that there was little evidence "for a simple carry-over of unit-forming principles from speech to writing" (p. 187). There was, however, evidence that when length was constant, inflected endings were being treated as units. Thus, inflectional suffixes were read more correctly than other word endings, and inflectional suffixes were subject to independent substitution errors. It was therefore hypothesized that "the base word and the morphological inflection are separate features of a word; that they are picked up independently; that each is a unit, but that the base, if it is meaningful, has some priority for the actively engaged reader" (p. 187).

Reddell (1965) studied the effects of similarity between structural patterns in oral and written language on the reading comprehension of fourth graders. The findings indicated that reading comprehension scores on written materials that used structural patterns of high frequency in the oral language of fourth graders were significantly higher than reading scores on materials using low frequency patterns. The author concluded that reading comprehension is a function of the similarity between language structure patterns in written materials and in the youngster's spontaneous oral language.

The seeming inconsistencies between the results of the investigations of specific oral language factors and reading achievement may be resolved by considering the differences in the grade levels of the subjects and in the rela-

tive complexity of the reading materials. Bougere (1969) investigated relationships between oral syntax and reading and found no relationships at first
grade level when reading materials are characterized by syntactic simplicity.
At fourth grade level, when reading materials have increased in syntactical
complexity, reading comprehension and oral syntax were related (Reddell,
1965). Knowledge of morphological rules was related to reading achievement
at both first and second grade levels when reading materials reflected increases in the variety and use of morphological structures (Brittain, 1970).
The combined findings suggest that the relationships between reading comprehension and knowledge of morphology and syntax increase with advances
in educational level.

Effects of Training Knowledge of Sentence Structure on Reading

Investigations of the effects of training knowledge of sentence structure on
reading comprehension have provided conflicting evidence of the relationship between language status and reading (Hetrick, 1958; Reed, 1967;
Rinne, 1967; Samuels, Dahl, & Archwamety, 1974). Hetrick (1958) matched
seventy-five pairs of seventh grade students on the basis of sex, IQ, and reading comprehension score. The experimental group was provided with
twenty-five instructional sessions designed to improve knowledge of sentence
structure. The instruction included: (1) identifying complete subjects and
predicates, complete and incomplete sentences, transitive and intransitive
verbs, prepositions and prepositional phrases, adjectives, and adverbial
clauses, (2) combining simple sentences to form compound and complex sentences, (3) inverting the word order of sentences, (4) conjugating verbs, and
(5) diagramming sentences. No significant gains in reading comprehension
were made by either poor or good readers. Rinne (1967) provided five
weeks of programmed instruction in sentence pattern awareness to randomly selected ninth grade students. The results indicated low correlations between sentence pattern awareness and literal comprehension in reading.

These negative findings conflict with observations by Samuels, Dahl, and
Archwamety (1974). They designed an instructional sequence that emphasized using visual, auditory, and linguistic cues alone or combined to make
predictions. Their results indicated that experimentally trained normal and
mentally retarded subjects performed significantly better than controls in
reading accuracy, comprehension, and speed, as measured by tachistoscopic
recognition and cloze procedures in which words have been deleted from
sentences or paragraphs.

Correlational Studies

Correlational studies of the relationship between knowledge of sentence
structure and reading comprehension have generally reported significant,
positive correlations. O'Donnell (1961) assessed the knowledge of grammatical structure on a fifty item, three option multiple-choice test, using 101 high
school seniors as subjects. The correlation obtained between measures of
knowledge of syntax and reading comprehension was low, albeit significant
(.44).

Sauer (1968) evaluated the ability of 153 fourth grade children to translate four basic sentence patterns which varied according to three levels of structural complexity and were constructed using a nonsense language. Knowledge of the four sentence patterns, in combination, correlated significantly (.67) with a measure of reading comprehension (*Stanford Reading Test: Intermediate, Form W: Paragraph Meaning* subtest).

The relationships between language abilities and knowledge of morphology, syntax, and reading achievement observed among normal readers would be expected to be shown in retarded readers, an assumption that has received support from predictive, comparative, and correlational studies (de Hirsch, Jansky, & Langford, 1966; Semel & Wiig, 1975; Vogel, 1974; Warrington & Kinsbourne, 1967; Wiig, Semel, & Crouse, 1973). De Hirsch, Jansky, & Langford (1967) have reported that two measures of receptive language (*Wepman Auditory Discrimination* and *Peabody Picture Vocabulary Test*) were significantly associated with end-of-second-grade measures of reading and/or spelling. Among the experimental measures of language expression, number of words used in a story and organization of a story correlated significantly with end-of-second-grade measures of reading and spelling ability.

Language Disabilities and Reading Retardation

The relationship between verbal disabilities and reading retardation has received further support in studies by Warrington and Kinsbourne (1967). They considered the frequency and magnitude of verbal and performance scale discrepancies on the Wechsler Intelligence Scale for Children (WISC) of seventy-six retarded readers, ranging in age from seven to fifteen. Their data indicated that the majority of youngsters with reading or spelling backwardness demonstrated verbal deficits on the WISC. Furthermore, the proportion of children with negative verbal-performance discrepancies of twenty or more points was significantly larger among retarded readers than in a normal distribution.

The positive relationship observed between the knowledge of morphology and the reading achievement of first and second graders (Brittain, 1970) has been supported by observations of significant morphological deficits in learning disabled, dyslexic children (Vogel, 1974; Wiig, Semel, & Crouse, 1973). Vogel (1974) reported that among the three tests which best differentiated dyslexics and achieving readers, two assessed knowledge of morphology: (1) the *Illinois Test of Psycholinguistic Abilities* (ITPA) *Grammatic Closure* subtest and (2) the Berry-Talbott adaptation of the *Berko Experimental Test of Morphology.*

Semel and Wiig (1975) have reported significant relationships between (1) a measure of comprehension and expression of syntactic structures (*Northwestern Syntax Screening Test*), (2) a measure of comprehension of critical verbal elements in sequence (*Assessment of Children's Language Comprehension*), and (3) measures of reading achievement (*Peabody Individual Achievement Test*) in children with learning disabilities. Performances on the *Receptive* subtest of the NSST, which measures comprehension of syntactic structures, correlated significantly with the *Reading Recognition* (r = .64), *Reading Comprehension* (r = .77), and *Spelling* (r = .60) subtests of the PIAT. Performances on the *Expressive* subtest of NSST, which measures delayed recall of syntactic structures, correlated only with *Reading Comprehension* (r = .53). The performances on the ACLC *four elements* subtest, which assesses the comprehension of four critical words in sequence, correlated with *Reading Recognition* (r = .55), *Reading Comprehension* (r = .64), and *Spelling* (r = .49). The combined findings suggest that measures of linguistic abilities relate most closely to measures of reading comprehension and that deficits in language processing may be associated with reductions in reading comprehension.

Relating Language Processing and Mathematical Deficits

The relationships between language processing and problem solving in mathematics have been emphasized in theoretical discussions as well as in educational research (Aiken, 1972; Dahmus, 1970; Kaliski, 1962; Linville 1970; Rosenthal & Resnick, 1974; Sax & Ottina, 1958; Vander Linde, 1964). Aiken (1972) has stressed two aspects in considering the relationship between language abilities and learning mathematics. They relate to (a) the influence of linguistic abilities on mathematical problem solving and (b) the consideration that mathematics is a specialized language form. The specialized language of mathematics differs from social English in that it has a high, conceptual density factor, reflected by limited, if any, redundancy. This factor requires that the exact meaning of every concept (word) and logical-syntactic relationship must be discerned accurately since interpretation is not facilitated by the presence of additional semantic-syntactic cues (redundancy). Aiken also stresses that adjectives are more important in mathematical than in regular English and that common words are used with a limited rather than a generalized meaning. These observations immediately suggest that youngsters with learning disabilities who experience difficulties in processing auditory language which is semantically compressed or contains adjective sequences may experience associated reductions in solving verbal mathematics problems (Rosenthal, 1970; Wiig & Roach, 1975).

Aiken (1972) has further described two possible processes involved in solving verbal problems in mathematics. He suggests that they may be approached as: (1) complex verbal stimuli with an extra arithmetical dimension or (2) English statements which require translation into equivalent mathematical statements. Each approach may require sequential processing by first reading the verbal math problem to discern the overall situation or pattern, followed by reading to identify difficult vocabulary or concepts, and finally by rereading to discern the semantic system and plan the solution.

Dahmus (1970) has described a similar sequential approach to verbal math problems termed the DPPC (direct, pure, piecemeal, complete). This approach involves a translation of the words and concepts used in regular English statements into their equivalent mathematical statements followed by translation into an equation and/or systems of equations. This approach moves from the concrete level into hierarchial levels of abstraction. Learning disabled youngsters with deficits in abstraction and generalization (de Hirsch, 1957; Johnson & Myklebust, 1967; Lerner, 1971) may be expected to demonstrate deficits in performing the symbolic-conceptual processes required in the translation from regular to mathematical statements.

Linguistic Complexity and Math Problem Solving

The relationship between syntactic and semantic complexity and ability to solve verbal math problems has been further supported by Linville (1970), Kaliski (1962), Rosenthal and Resnick (1974), Sax and Ottina (1958), and Vander Linde (1964). Linville (1970) presented verbal math problems to fourth graders that differed only in the levels and combinations of syntactic complexity and difficulty of vocabulary. Four arithmetic word-problem tests were designed to reflect the characteristics of: (1) easy syntax and easy vocabulary, (2) easy syntax and difficult vocabulary, (3) difficult syntax and easy vocabulary, and (4) difficult syntax and difficult vocabulary. The results indicated significant performance differences in favor of easier syntax and vocabulary, with vocabulary level perhaps being more crucial than syntax. In a related study, Sax and Ottina (1958) established that specific training in syntax can improve verbal math problem solving in seventh graders.

Rosenthal and Resnick (1974) studied the effects of differences in three dimensions of math problem solving. The dimensions investigated were (1) order of mention (chronological or reverse), (2) identity of unknown set (starting or ending), and (3) type of verb (associated with gain or loss). They reported more errors in reverse order problems and longer response time for correct answers than for verbal problems mentioned in chronological order. The most significant variable was an unknown starting set as in $? + y = z$, particularly when associated with gain verbs. They concluded that higher level linguistic and cognitive abilities were required to perform the necessary mental operations.

The evidence suggests that solving verbal math problems requires abilities similar to those involved in processing complex verbal stimuli. In addition, adequate knowledge of mathematical vocabulary and concepts (spatial and temporal) seems required. Vander Linde (1964) has reported that fifth grade classes that received comprehension training for quantitative terms made significantly greater gains in mathematical problem solving than control classes matched for IQs and achievement scores in vocabulary, reading comprehension, arithmetic concepts, and problem solving. In a similar vein, Kaliski (1962) stresses the need to establish the concepts involved in mathematics using cognitive-linguistic training methods. Among concepts that need to be established are those related to size, number, space, and inclusion-exclusion, such as *fewer, less than, none, all,* etc.

Language Disabilities and Deficits in Mathematics

Johnson and Myklebust (1967) have emphasized the relationship between receptive language disorders and difficulties in mathematics in learning disabled youngsters. They have observed that "some children with auditory receptive language disorders learn to calculate but do poorly in mathematical reasoning because they do not comprehend the words" (p. 84). They further suggest that there are inner, receptive, and expressive aspects of mathematical language similar to other forms of symbolic behavior. The hierarchical acquisition of mathematical language is considered to progress from (1) assimilation and integration of nonverbal experiences to (2) association between experiences and numerical symbols to (3) expression of quantity, space, and order using mathematical language (p. 245).

Similar views of the relationships between learning disabilities, language deficits, and difficulties in mathematical problem solving have been expressed by Chon (1971) and Kaliski (1962). Kaliski (1962) suggests that the difficulties are related to deficits in abstract thinking and reductions in organizational abilities. The difficulties in math are related to receptive and expressive language in the following statements:

> First of all, "casual" language must never be used because of the brain-injured child's deficient ability to focus visually and/or auditorily. Second, the child's receptive language capacity is often inadequate in regard to symbols. Third, the child's ability to express himself accurately and to the point with mathematically correct answers is limited. [Kaliski, 1962, p. 247]

In direct agreement with these views of the interfacing between language and mathematical abilities, Kaliski (1962) suggests remedial strategies that emphasize concreteness and facilitate the development of language and reasoning. Similar suggestions have been introduced by Euphemia (1970) and Horowitz (1970). Chon (1971) views the relationship between mathematics and language deficits as follows:

> as numbers and their generalized algebraic forms are used as a specific language to establish logical relations for mathematics, the individual with general difficulties in operating with symbols can do math with no more facility than he can handle other elementary language functions. [p. 326]

Semel and Wiig (1975) have reported significant positive correlations between measures of achievement in mathematics and measures of language comprehension in thirty-four learning disabled children, ranging in age from 7 to 11½ years. Academic achievement was assessed using the *Peabody Individual Achievement Test* (PIAT) (Dunn & Markwardt, 1970). Receptive language skills were evaluated using the *Northwestern Syntax Screening Test* (NSST) (Lee, 1969, 1971), which requires comprehension of syntactic structures, and the *Assessment of Children's Language Comprehension* (ACLC) (Foster, Giddan, & Stark, 1972), which requires comprehension of critical verbal elements in sequence.

The results indicated that the performances on the PIAT *Math* subtest correlated with performances on the NSST *Receptive* subtest (r = .57) and on the ACLC *4 elements* subtest (r = .60). When the performances on the PIAT *Math* and *Reading Comprehension* subtests were combined, the correlation with performances on the NSST *Receptive* subtest (r = .78) and on the ACLC *4 elements* subtest (r = .70) increased, suggesting that some processes involved in the tasks were shared. The common features may relate to syntactic processing, simultaneous analysis, and synthesis and memory, among others.

References

Aiken, L. R., Jr. Language factors in learning mathematics. *Review of Educational Research*, 1972, **42**, 359-85.

Bannatyne, A. *Language, reading and learning disabilities*. Springfield, Ill.: Charles C Thomas, 1971.

Bender, L. A. *A visual-motor Gestalt test and its clinical use*. New York: American Orthopsychiatric Association, 1938.

Bougere, M. Selected factors in oral language related to first grade achievement. *Reading Research Quarterly*, 1969, **4**, 31-57.

Brittain, M. M. Inflection performance and early reading achievement. *Reading Research Quarterly*, 1970, **5**, 34-48.

Brutten, M., Richardson, S. O., & Mangel, C. *Something is wrong with my child*. New York: Harcourt Brace Jovanovich, 1973.

Calfee, R., Chapman, R., & Venezky, R. How a child needs to think to learn to read. In L. W. Gregg (Ed.), *Cognition in learning and memory*. New York: John Wiley & Sons, 1972. Pp. 139-82.

Chalfant, J. C., & Flathouse, V. E. Auditory and visual learning. In H. R. Myklebust (Ed.), *Progress in learning disabilities*. Vol. 2. New York: Grune & Stratton, 1971.

Chalfant, J. C., & Scheffelin, M. *Central processing dysfunctions in children: a review of research*. U.S. Dept. Health, Education, and Welfare, National Institute of Neurological Diseases and Stroke, 1969.

Chomsky, N. *Syntactic structures*. The Hague: Mouton, 1957.

Chon, R. Arithmetic and learning disabilities. In H. R. Myklebust (Ed.), *Progress in learning disabilities*. Vol. 2. New York: Grune & Stratton, 1971. Pp. 322-89.

Clay, M. M. A syntactic analysis of reading errors. *Journal of Verbal Learning and Verbal Behavior*, 1968, **7**, 434-38.

Clay, M. M. Reading errors and self-correction behavior. *British Journal of Educational Psychology*, 1969, **39**, 47-56.

Clements, S. D. Minimal brain dysfunction. In S. G. Sapir & A. C. Nitzburg (Eds.), *Children with learning problems*. New York: Brunner/Mazel, 1973. Pp. 159-72.

Cohen, J., & Edwards, A. E. Word length and discrimination behavior of aphasics. *Journal of Speech and Hearing Research*, 1964, **8**, 39-42.

Dahmus, M. E. How to teach verbal problems. *School Science and Mathematics*, 1970, **70**, 121-38.

de Hirsch, K. Tests designed to discover potential reading difficulties at the six-year-old level. *American Journal of Orthopsychiatry*, 1957, **27**, 566-76.

de Hirsch. K., Jansky, J. J., & Langford, W. S. *Predicting reading failure*. New York: Harper & Row, 1966.

Denckla, M. B. Naming of pictured objects by dyslexic and non-dyslexic "MBD" children. Paper presented at the Academy of Aphasia, 1974.

Denhoff, E. *Cerebral palsy in preschool years*. Springfield, Ill.: Charles C Thomas, 1967.

Dunn, L. M., & Markwardt, F. C. *Peabody individual achievement test*. Circle Pines, Minn.: American Guidance Service, 1970.

Euphemia, R. Mathematics for the special child. *Academic Therapy*, Fall 1970, 13-15.

Flower, R. M. Auditory disorders and reading disorders. In R. M. Flower, H. F. Gofman, & L. I. Lawson (Eds.), *Reading disorders: a multi-disciplinary symposium*. Philadelphia: F. A. Davis, 1965. Pp. 81-102.

Foster, R., Giddan, J. J., & Stark, J. *Assessment of children's language comprehension*. Palo Alto, Calif.: Consulting Psychologists Press, 1972.

Gibson, E. J., & Guinet, L. Perception of inflections in brief visual presentations of words. *Journal of Verbal Learning and Verbal Behavior*, 1971, **10**, 182-89.

Goodman, K. Reading a psycholinguistic guessing game. *Journal of the Reading Specialist*, 1967, **4**, 126-35.

Goodman, K. Analysis of oral reading miscues: applied psycholinguistics. *Reading Research Quarterly*, 1969, **4**, 9-30.

Hallahan, D. P., & Cruickshank, W. M. *Psychoeducational foundations of learning disabilities*. Englewood Cliffs, N.J.: Prentice-Hall, 1973.

Hammill, D. D., & Larsen, S. C. The relationship of selected auditory perceptual skills and reading ability. *Journal of Learning Disabilities*, 1974, **7**, 40-46.

Hetrick, J. An experimental study of the effect of training in sentence structure and reading comprehnsion. Doctoral dissertation, University of Pittsburgh, 1958.

Horowitz, R. Teaching mathematics to students with learning disabilities. *Academic Therapy*, Fall 1970, 17-35.

Johnson, D. J., & Myklebust, H. R. *Learning disabilities: educational principles and practices*. New York: Grune & Stratton, 1967.

Kaliski, L. Arithmetic and the brain-injured child. *The Arithmetic Teacher*, 1962, **9**, 245-51.

Kass, C. Some psychological correlates of severe reading disabilities (dyslexia). Doctoral dissertation. University of Illinois, 1962.

Kavanagh, J. F. (Ed.) *Communicating by language: the reading process*. Bethesda, Md.: National Institute of Child Health and Human Development, 1968.

Kawi, A. A., & Pasamanick, B. Association of factors of pregnancy with reading disorders in children. *JAMA*, 1958, **166**, 1420.

Kershner, J. R. Visual-spatial organization and reading: support for a cognitive-developmental interpretation. *Journal of Learning Disabilities*, 1975, **8**, 30-36.

Klasen, E. *The syndrome of specific dyslexia*. Baltimore: University Park Press, 1972.

Kolers, P. A. Experiments in reading. *Scientific American*, 1972, **227**, 84-91.

Lee, L. L. *Northwestern syntax screening test*. Evanston, Ill.: Northwestern University, 1969, 1971.

Lerner, J. *Children with learning disabilities*. Boston: Houghton Mifflin Co., 1971.

Levin, H., & Kaplan, E. L. Listening, reading and grammatical structure. In D. L. Horton & J. J. Perkins (Eds.), *Perception of language*. Columbus, Ohio: Charles E. Merrill, 1971. Pp. 1-16.

Liberman, I. Y. Basic research in speech and lateralization of language: some implications for reading disability. In *Status report on speech research*, Haskins Laboratories, SR 25-26, 51-66, 1971.

Linville, W. J. The effects of syntax and vocabulary upon the difficulty of verbal arithmetic problems with fourth-grade students. Doctoral dissertation, State University of Iowa, 1970.

Luria, A. R. *Higher cortical functions in man*. New York: Basic Books, 1966.

Marshall, J. C., & Newcombe, F. Patterns of paralexia: a psycholinguistic approach. *Journal of Psycholinguistic Research*, 1973, **2**, 175-95.

Mattingly, I. G. Reading, the linguistic process, and linguistic awareness. In J. F. Kavanagh & I. G. Mattingly (Eds.), *Language by ear and by eye*. Cambridge, Mass.: M.I.T. Press, 1972. Pp. 133-47.

Mehler, J., Bever, T. G., & Carey, P. What we look at when we read. *Perception and Psychophysics*, 1967, **2**, 213-18.

Money, J., & Shiffman, G. *The disabled reader: education of the dyslexic child*. Baltimore: Johns Hopkins Press, 1966.

Myklebust, H. R. Learning disorders: psychoneurological disturbances in childhood. *Rehabilitation Literature*, 1964, **25**, 354-60.

O'Donnell, R. C. The relationship between awareness of structural relationships in English and ability in reading comprehension. Doctoral dissertation, George Peabody College for Teachers, 1961.

Pasamanick, B., Rogers, M. E., & Lilienfeld, A. M. Pregnancy experience and the development of behavior disorders in children. *American Journal of Psychiatry*, 1956, **112**, 613-18.

Reddell, R. B. The effect of oral and written patterns of language structure on reading comprehension. *Reading Teacher*, 1965, **18**, 270-75.

Reed, E. E. Improving comprehension through study of syntax and paragraph structure in seventh grade English classes. *Proceedings of the I.R.A.*, Newark, Del.: International Reading Association, 1967.

Rees, N. S. Auditory processing factors in language disorders: the view from Procrustes' bed. *Journal of Speech and Hearing Disorders*, 1973, **38**, 304-15.

Rees, N. S. The speech pathologist and the reading process. *ASHA*, 1974, **16**, 255-58.

Rinne, C. H., III. Improvement in reading comprehension through increasing awareness of written syntactic patterns. Doctoral dissertation, Stanford University, 1967.

Rosenberg, B. The performance of aphasics on automated visuo-perceptual discrimination, training, and transfer tasks. *Journal of Speech and Hearing Research*, 1965, **8**, 165-81.

Rosenthal, D. J. & Resnick, L. B. Children's solution processes in arithmetic word problems. *Journal of Educational Psychology*, 1974, **66**, 817-25.

Rosenthal, J. H. A preliminary psycholinguistic study of children with learning disabilities. *Journal of Learning Disabilities*, 1970, **3**, 391-95.

Ryan, E., & Semmel, M. Reading as a constructive language process. *Reading Research Quarterly,* 1969, **4,** 59-83.

Samuels, S. J., Dahl, P., & Archwamety, T. Effect of hypothesis/test training on reading skill. *Journal of Educational Psychology,* 1974, **66,** 835-44.

Sauer, L. E. Fourth grade children's knowledge of grammatical structure and its relationship to reading comprehension. Doctoral dissertation, University of Wisconsin, 1968.

Sax, G., & Ottina, J. R. The arithmetic achievement of pupils differing in school experience. *California Journal of Educational Research,* 1958, **9,** 15-19.

Schuell, H., & Jenkins, J. J. The nature of language deficit in aphasia. *Journal of Speech and Hearing Research,* 1959, **66,** 45-67.

Schuell, H., Jenkins, J. J., & Jimenez-Pabon, E. *Aphasia in adults.* New York: Harper & Row, 1964.

Semel, E. M., & Wiig, E. H. Comprehension of syntactic structures and critical verbal elements by children with learning disabilities. *Journal of Learning Disabilities,* 1975, **8,** 53-58.

Shankweiler, D., & Liberman, I. Y. Misreading: a search for cues. In J. F. Kavanagh & I. G. Mattingly (Eds.), *Language by ear and by eye.* Cambridge, Mass.: M.I.T. Press, 1972. Pp. 293-317.

Vander Linde, L. F. Does the study of quantitative vocabulary improve problem solving? *Elementary School Journal,* 1964, **65,** 143-52.

Vogel, S. A. Syntactic abilities in normal and dyslexic children. *Journal of Learning Disabilities,* 1974, **7,** 47-53.

Warrington, E. K., & Kinsbourne, M. The incidence of verbal disability associated with reading retardation. *Neuropsychologia,* 1967, **5,** 175-80.

Wepman, J. *Recovery from aphasia.* New York: Ronald Press, 1951.

Wiig, E. H. The emerging LD crisis. *Journal of Rehabilitation,* May–June 1972, 15-17.

Wiig, E. H., & Harris, S. P. Perception and interpretation of nonverbally expressed emotions by adolescents with learning disabilities. *Perceptual and Motor Skills,* 1974, **38,** 239-45.

Wiig, E. H., & Roach, M. A. Immediate recall of semantically varied "sentences" by learning-disabled adolescents. *Perceptual and Motor Skills,* 1975, **40,** 119-25.

Wiig, E. H., & Semel, E. M. Comprehension of linguistic concepts requiring logical operations. *Journal of Speech and Hearing Research,* 1973, **16,** 627-36.

Wiig, E. H., & Semel, E. M. Logico-grammatical sentence comprehension by learning disabled adolescents. *Perceptual and Motor Skills,* 1974, **38,** 1331-34.

Wiig, E. H., & Semel, E. M. Productive language abilities in learning disabled adolescents. *Journal of Learning Disabilities,* 1975, **8,** 578-86.

Wiig, E. H., Semel, E. M., & Crouse, M. A. The use of English morphology by high-risk and learning disabled children. *Journal of Learning Disabilities,* 1973, **6,** 457-65.

2 The Nature of Language Deficits in Learning Disabilities

Overview

This chapter illustrates the multi-faceted nature, complexity and subtlety of the language processing and production problems of youngsters with learning disabilities. A model is introduced for language processing that emphasizes (1) perceptual processing, (2) linguistic processing, (3) cognitive-semantic processing, and (4) the relationships among the various aspects of these processes.

This model reflects a heavy emphasis on the Structure-of-Intellect model introduced by Guilford (1967), one which has provided the background for discussions of deficits in learning disabilities, testing, and curriculum design by Lerner (1971) and Meeker (1969). In addition, the neuropsychological model for language processing discussed by Luria (1973) is introduced to form a background for the interpretation of various language processing deficits observed in learning disabilities. The relationships among memory, evaluation, and language processing and production are discussed and stressed with reference to work by, among others, Guilford (1967), Miller (1956), Miller and Chomsky (1963), and Simon and Chase (1973).

The oral language production problems of learning disabled children and adolescents are reviewed with reference to models for convergent and divergent semantic production introduced by Guilford (1967). Observations of problems in the productive control of linguistic structure are also introduced, and the current evidence of relationships between language processing and production deficits in learning disabilities is presented. The characteristics and nature, assessment, and remediation of the language processing and production problems of learning disabled children and adolescents will be discussed in greater detail in succeeding chapters. The models introduced in the present chapter will serve as the basis for both the organization of and the interpretations in subsequent discussions. Although the discussions focus on the problems of school-age children and adolescents with diagnosed learning disabilities, similar problems may be encountered in youngsters who fall within other clinical-diagnostic categories.

Language Deficits in Learning Disabilities:
A Multi-faceted Problem

Language and communication deficits associated with learning disabilities were recognized early in the history of the field by Borel-Maisonny (1951), Cruickshank et al. (1961), Myklebust (1954), Orton (1937), and Strauss and Kephart (1955), among others. These deficits have been reported to extend through the domains of verbal and nonverbal communication. Recent literature has supported that children and adolescents with learning disabilities may exhibit a variety of language and communication deficits, reflecting problems in, among others, language processing and production, and social perception (Bannatyne, 1971; Johnson, 1968; Johnson & Myklebust, 1967; Lerner, 1971; McGrady & Olson, 1970; Meier, 1971; Rosenthal, 1970; Vogel, 1974; Wigg & Harris, 1974; Wiig & Semel, 1973; Wiig, Semel, & Crouse, 1973). Clinical observations and research suggest that the language and communication problems exhibited by learning disabled youngsters are multi-faceted, defying unitary description.

A discussion of the diverse nature of the problems demonstrated by language impaired, learning disabled youngsters seems appropriate against the background of definitions of learning disabilities that describe multi-faceted syndromes. Among these definitions, the following, formulated at the Learning Disabilities Division Formulational Meeting, National Council on Exceptional Children (CEC), St. Louis, April 1967, has been widely accepted. It states:

> A child with learning disabilities is one with adequate mental abilities, sensory processes and emotional stability who has a limited number of specific deficits in perceptive, integrative, or expressive processes which severely impair learning efficiency. This includes children who have central nervous dysfunction which is expressed primarily in impaired learning efficiency. [Chalfant & Scheffelin, 1969, p. 148]

Learning disabled children and adolescents may exhibit a variety of isolated or combined deficits in language processing or production. The problems of two randomly selected, learning disabled youngsters are rarely alike. One may have difficulties in both auditory language processing and oral language production, and the other may function at or above age level in these areas; both may demonstrate similar visual-motor deficits. The ability to predict the nature and degree of language processing and production deficits in a youngster with learning disabilities remains limited, suggesting a need for future research. In the following sections, the multi-faceted manifestations of language deficits associated with learning disabilities will be discussed in relation to perceptual, cognitive, linguistic, and productive aspects of the communication process.

Language Processing

The complex act of processing auditory language can be subdivided into three levels: (1) the perception of the sensory data, (2) linguistic processing of the phonological, morphological, and syntactic structure and semantic aspects, and (3) cognitive processing of auditory-symbolic (phoneme sequences) and semantic units (words and concepts), semantic classes (verbal associations), semantic relations (verbal analogies and linguistic concepts), semantic systems (verbal problems), semantic transformations (redefinition of concepts), and semantic implications (cause-effect, predictions, etc.) (Figure 1). Efficient processing of auditory language occurs simultaneously at all levels and it places demands upon auditory attention, short- and long-term memory, feedback, and evaluation.

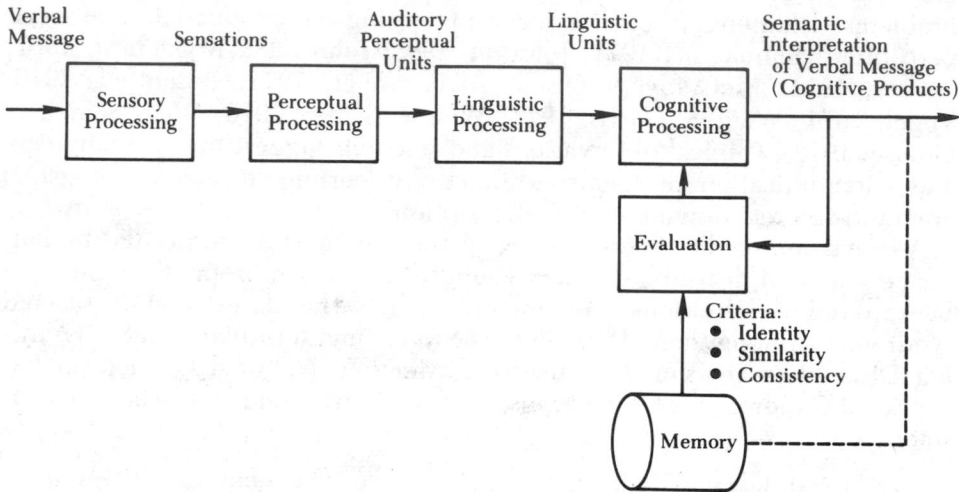

FIGURE 1. Illustration of the relationships between perceptual, linguistic, and cognitive processing in language comprehension.

Recent research has supported the position that normal language processing takes place simultaneously at all available levels (lexical, phonetic, semantic, and syntactic) of analysis. Marslen-Wilson (1975) introduced word and context anomalies in sentence pairs. These anomalies occurred at two levels: (1) the lexical (vocabulary) and phonetic (speech-sound) level, considered to provide lower-order analysis; and (2) the semantic (sentence meaning) and syntactic (sentence structure) level, providing higher-order information. At the first level, word anomalies were introduced by substituting nonsense words such as *tomorrane* for words such as *tomorrow*. At the second level, context anomalies were introduced by substituting semantically or syntactically inappropriate words for grammatically correct ones. As an example of a semantic substitution, a noun would be substituted for another which was inappropriate in the context as in "They call for the unconditional *universe* of all the enemy forces." In a syntactic substitution, a word (noun, verb, etc.) would be replaced by another which did not belong to the same grammatical class (adjective, adverb, etc.) as in "He's afraid he forgot to put a stamp on the *already* before he went to post it." The anomalies were designed to evaluate the effects of changes in sentence meaning and structure on sentence repetition while shadowing each word as it was heard.

Analysis of the restorations of the disrupted or substituted words to their original forms indicated that 88% were word restorations (repeating *tommorrane* as *tomorrow*) while the remaining 12% were context restorations (restoring semantically and syntactically deviant words). On the basis of this finding, in conjunction with corroborating observations of shadowing latencies, Marslen-Wilson concludes:

> sentence perception is most plausibly modeled as a fully interactive parallel process: that each word, as it is heard on the context of normal discourse, is immediately entered into the processing system at *all* levels of description, and is simultaneously analyzed at all these levels in the light of whatever information is available at each level at that point in the processing of the sentence. [p. 226]

Marslen-Wilson stresses that this view contrasts with recent psycholinguistic theories of sentence processing which imply a serial processing model (Fodor, Bever, & Garrett, 1974). The serial processing model proposes that higher-level analyses occur toward the end of a clause; in contrast, the parallel processing model implies that "information at each level can constrain and guide simultaneous processing at other levels" (Marslen-Wilson, 1975, p. 227).

Luria (1973) has introduced three principal, neuropsychological processes considered to be necessary for processing and interpreting language with any degree of complexity. They are (1) retention of elements of sentences, (2) simultaneous analysis and synthesis of the elements, and (3) active analysis of the significant elements to detect the hidden, underlying meaning or problem. Each of these processes is considered to be dependent upon different parts of the brain. In processing complex language, it is first considered necessary to retain the various elements of each sentence, a process involving the temporal region of the left hemisphere. Secondly, these elements must be simultaneously analyzed and synthesized, a process involving the parieto-occipital zones of the left hemisphere. Finally, the product must be subjected to active analysis of the most significant elements and relationships to detect the implied meaning or structure of the problem. This process involves the frontal lobes of the brain which are responsible for planning and organizing intellectual activity as a whole. Although Luria's model differs from the one presented here (Figure 1), it does not conflict. It will serve as an alternative basis for interpretations of the nature and bases of language processing deficits in children and adolescents.

Auditory Perception

Auditory perception has been broken down into seven distinct tasks by Chalfant and Scheffelin (1969). These tasks are considered to be (1) attention to auditory stimuli, (2) differentiation of sound versus no sound, (3) sound localization, (4) discrimination of phonemes, (5) discrimination of sound sequences, (6) auditory figure-ground selection, and (7) association of sound with sound sources. To these can be added the tasks of segmentation and synthesis.

The process involved in segmentation requires ability to divide perceived words into their smallest grammatical units, called morphemes. As an example, the word *steamboat* contains two morphemes, *steam* and *boat*. The word *unacceptable* may be segmented into three morphemes, *un, accept,* and *able*. The meaning of the individual morphemes contained in the two words *steamboat* and *unacceptable* should be fairly evident to a person competent in English. There are, however, morphemes in the English language with more elusive meanings.

Some English morphemes have no meaning in isolation, but acquire meaning when they are combined with other morphemes. As examples, the morpheme *s* as in *boys* has no meaning in isolation, but signifies plurality in the morpheme combination. Similarly, the morpheme *est* as in *tallest* signifies superlative and the morpheme *ly* in *friendly* signifies an adverb in the respective morpheme combinations.

There are numerous words in English such as *truthfulness, belongings, inadvertently,* and *secured* that can only be interpreted correctly if the segmentation process is adequate and efficient. It can be argued that segmentation is primarily not a perceptual process since it depends heavily upon linguistic knowledge and cognitive abilities (awareness of semantic [meaning] aspects). The segmentation process is, however, equally dependent upon adequate phoneme discrimination and sequencing and must therefore be considered a process in which auditory perception interfaces with linguistic and cognitive processing.

Synthesis requires ability to combine sounds and sound sequences into larger units. It encompasses, among others, the abilities to perform sound blending and closure. Sound blending is the process of synthesizing sounds and sound sequences which are separated in time into meaningful units. Closure, a related process, requires prediction of sounds or sound sequences which were inaudible or inadequately perceived in order to form a meaningful whole.

Auditory-perceptual problems may constitute one of the bases for the auditory language processing deficits observed in learning disabled youngsters. The auditory-perceptual deficits associated with specific learning disabilities sometimes reflect impaired, sustained, or selective attention to auditory stimuli. Learning disabled children with auditory attention problems may appear distractable and susceptible to interferences from random, unpredictable auditory or meaningful, linguistic stimuli in the environment. They may also experience auditory figure-ground selection problems. The auditory perceptual deficits associated with learning disabilities may also reflect problems in sound localization, phoneme discrimination, discrimination of phoneme sequences, segmentation, or synthesis (Aten & Davis, 1968; Flowers & Costello, 1970; Lasky & Tobin, 1973; Orton, 1937; Zigmond, 1969).

Linguistic Processing

Within a linguistic framework, the language deficits demonstrated by learning disabled children and adolescents span a wide range. These deficits may be observed at the phonological (speech-sound), morphological (word formation), syntactic (sentence structure), and semantic (meaning) levels. Thus, delays have been noted in the acquisition of morphological and syntactic rules, suggesting deficits in linguistic competence (knowledge of linguistic structure) (Rosenthal, 1970; Semel & Wiig, 1975; Vogel, 1974; Wiig, Semel, & Crouse, 1973).

Other observations suggest that learning disabled youngsters may experience problems in interfacing surface structure, relating to the structural properties of sentences, and deep structure, relating to the semantic or meaning properties of sentences. On a sentence repetition task, learning disabled adolescents showed limited ability to code syntax and heavy dependence on semantic aspects for language processing and were deficient in recalling sentences which violated semantic (selectional) rules (Wiig & Roach, 1975).

Some learning disabled youngsters appear to easily abstract and interpret the concepts expressed in sentences, but fail to extract relationships implied by sentence structure; that is, they appear to process at the deep structure level with minimal reference to the surface structure. They may abstract the concepts *cat, dog,* and *bite* correctly in a sentence such as "The cat was bitten by the dog," but may fail to identify the animal that did the biting because the passive sentence structure was not processed correctly.

Other LD youngsters appear to process the surface and deep structures in sequence and may need extended time to comprehend the meaning of a sentence. As an example, it may take a long time before a learning disabled youngster responds to a relatively simple question such as "Did you go to school today?" if he first has to process the question transformation and then attend to the meaning (deep structure). Sequential processing usually results in accurate comprehension by the learning disabled child if the sentence length is within short-term memory capacity. Longer and complex sentences with embedding such as "John who was the boy who had the birthday party opened the presents over there" may be lost in the process due to limitations in auditory memory, reauditorization, or temporal sequencing ability.

Linguistic processing deficits may also result in problems in interpreting ambiguous sentences, idioms, and puns, all of which lack a one-to-one relationship between surface and deep structure. Typically, learning disabled youngsters misinterpret ambiguous sentences such as "Jane saw Tom walking across the street," "John found a book on Broadway," or "Mary saw the skyscrapers flying across New York," and alternate interpretations are not perceived.

Cognitive Processing

The Structure-of-Intellect model (Guilford, 1967) may be used to characterize deficits associated with learning disabilities in the cognitive processing of semantic aspects of auditory language. This model has three dimensions: operation, content, and product. The mental operations which may be performed on various stimuli are (1) cognition, (2) memory, (3) divergent production, (4) convergent production, and (5) evaluation. The content or form of the information transmitted by stimuli may be (1) figural, (2) symbolic, (3) semantic, or (4) behavioral. The product which results from structuring the information transmitted by the stimuli may be (1) units, (2) classes, (3) relations, (4) systems, (5) transformations, or (6) implications. In the discussion of cognitive processing of language, the focus will be on the semantic content of cognition, the information transmitted (Figure 2).

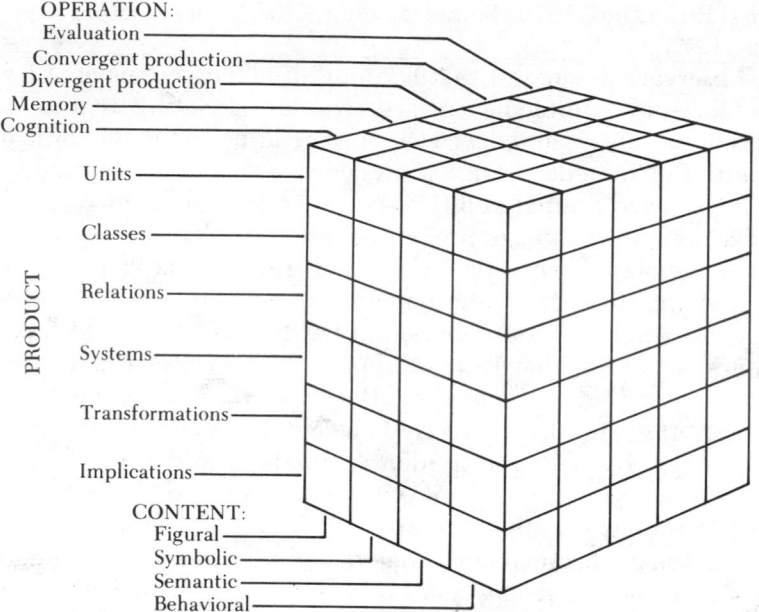

OPERATION:
Evaluation
Convergent production
Divergent production
Memory
Cognition

Units
Classes
Relations
Systems
Transformations
Implications

PRODUCT

CONTENT:
Figural
Symbolic
Semantic
Behavioral

FIGURE 2. The Structure-of-Intellect model, with three parameters.

SOURCE: From "The nature of human intelligence" by J. P. Guilford. Copyright 1967 by McGraw-Hill, Inc. Used with permission of McGraw-Hill Book Co.

Deficits in the Cognition of Auditory-Symbolic Units

The ability to derive word structure from auditory stimuli constitutes the cognition of auditory-symbolic units. Deriving word structure requires the ability to "code" speech phonologically and morphologically. Deficits at any level of auditory perception may be reflected by reductions in the cognition of auditory-symbolic units. As earlier indicated, learning disabled children frequently experience problems in auditory perception. Cognitive problems in abstracting and categorizing the distinctive features that constitute the English phonemes (significant speech sounds) may combine with problems in synthesis and result in phoneme discrimination deficits. Reduced abstraction and classification abilities (Goldstein, 1948; Johnson & Myklebust, 1967) may also contribute to deficiencies in phoneme sequencing, segmentation, and discrimination of the suprasegmental phonemes (pitch, intensity, and duration), all of which may be observed in association with learning disabilities.

Deficits in the Cognition of Semantic Units

Cognition of semantic units implies knowledge of the precise meaning of familiar words as well as broad knowledge of the meaning of less familiar words. This cognition is based on adequate concept formation and is reflected on tests of vocabulary comprehension, following oral directions, general information, verbal relations, and comprehension of verbal analogies. Adequate concept formation depends upon abstraction and generalization, categorization, symbolization (establishing a relationship between symbol and referent), perceptual effectiveness, and memory, as well as other factors.

Learning disabled youngsters frequently exhibit problems in concept formation and in the cognition of semantic units. They may not possess precise and comprehensive knowledge of the meaning of familiar words. They may have focused on one of the attributes implicit in a word meaning but may have failed to synthesize other attributes to form a precise and comprehensive meaning. For example, the word *ball* may be interpreted to refer to an object (ball). The basic functions of a ball may be adequately demonstrated, but the child may have failed to abstract and synthesize other qualities of the object such as form, size or color variations, and alternative functions, resulting in narrow word meaning. On vocabulary comprehension tests, LD children frequently show spotty knowledge of words which are well *above* age level. At higher age levels, concrete words used in the vernacular may be readily understood although abstract words at lower age levels may not be comprehended. Learning disabled children may also experience problems in following oral directions, which may reflect deficits in comprehending the semantic aspects of the verbal directions or in sequencing the steps involved.

Deficits in the Cognition of Semantic Classes

Individual semantic units (words) may be classified into larger groups or semantic classes, according to a variety of criteria. Consider the concepts *cat, dog, lion,* and *zebra*. They may be classified as *animals*, or they may be further categorized as being either *pets* or *wild animals*. The ability to name the superordinate (class name) when given names of class members constitutes one aspect of the cognition of semantic classes. The ability to name subordinates (class members) when given a superordinate such as *fruit* comprises another aspect. Either aspect of the verbal classification process may be impaired in children with learning disabilities. They may not be able to identify a word that does not belong to a given semantic class or to classify new vocabulary items (semantic units) into appropriate semantic classes. The achieving child may easily classify the word *peach* as the name of a fruit if it is presented in a sentence such as "Oranges and peaches grow on trees."

The learning disabled child with word classification problems may need to see or eat a peach before he can codify the word *peach* as a subordinate of the class *fruit*. The normal child also utilizes his classification abilities to interpret the meaning of ambiguous sentences such as "John saw the mountains driving through Wyoming." He may classify the word *mountain* as a member of the semantic class *immovable objects* and solve the structural ambiguity easily. The learning disabled child may ponder whether John or the mountains were driving and may fail to process other verbal input while he solves the problem.

Deficits in the Cognition of Semantic Relations

Semantic units or classes may be juxtaposed according to logical sequencing principles to form a semantic relation. For example, the concepts *flour, dough, bread, toast,* and *crumbs* form a semantic relation with respect to an underlying logical sequence, which reflects seriation in time. Verbal analogies contain logical sequence and seriation in time and space and constitute a specific type of semantic relation. Linguistic concepts such as sentences expressing comparative, passive, spatial, temporal, or familial relationships also reflect a logical sequence and seriation in time and space.

Learning disabled youngsters may not discern the underlying logical sequence when presented with semantic relations; as a consequence, they may not comprehend linguistic concepts requiring logical processing such as comparative, temporal, spatial, passive, and familial relationships (Wiig & Semel, 1973, 1974). As an example, they may not be able to tell who came first when hearing a sentence such as "Ted came before Mary." The problems in comprehending these statements may reflect that the underlying temporal sequence relating to the concept of *before-after* was not well established.

Within Luria's model (1973), the deficits in the cognition of semantic relations can be considered to reflect reductions in the simultaneous analysis and synthesis of the elements and problems in handling quasi-spatial concepts, a function of the left parieto-occipital zones. Similarly, the learning disabled child may not derive new meaning from previously understood semantic units or classes when they are presented in a verbal analogy, a frequently used strategy in teaching. The bright achieving child will generally derive new, expanded meaning for the word *brook* when it is presented in the verbal analogy "Rivers are to brooks as mountains are to hills." The equally gifted learning disabled child may not discern the underlying seriation in the semantic relation or may focus on only one of the verbal elements.

Deficits in the Cognition of Semantic Systems

In order to solve verbal problems it is necessary to first understand their nature, that is, to discern the inherent relations in the problem and the processes to be applied to arrive at a solution. The ability to analyze and understand the structure of a verbal problem involves the cognition of semantic systems and reflects general reasoning ability. It is basic to mathematical and spatial reasoning, reading comprehension, and planning (Guilford & Lacey, 1947). According to Piaget (1950), logico-mathematical knowledge requires classification, seriation, and conservation of number. Others have emphasized that an active search is involved to discern relations and associations, synthesize isolated experiences, and reorganize the material (Russell, 1956).

Observations of LD children indicate that they may experience problems in reading comprehension and in mathematical, spatial, and temporal reasoning. The cognitive problems underlying these deficits may also be reflected in the processing of auditory language. The following example illustrates the problems encountered by a group of learning disabled children when they were asked to analyze the structure of a verbal problem. The task was as follows:

> "At four o'clock Joe rode on a merry-go-round eight times. Each ride cost him
> five cents. It took him fifteen minutes to finish the rides. How much did he pay
> for all the rides? What should we do to get the correct answer?"

A few of the learning disabled children said they multiplied because they
heard the word *times*. Some said they would add because there were lots of
numbers. One child said: "If there were just two numbers, I would subtract.
If they come out even, I would divide. If they don't, I'd multiply," showing
his inability to comprehend the structure or the semantic system involved in
the problem.

It may be argued that the problems experienced by these children were in
handling the numbers involved or in knowing number facts; however, this
was not the case for this group of youngsters. In conclusion, their inability to
analyze and understand the structure of the semantic system reflects problems in classification, seriation, synthesis, or reorganization.

Deficits in the Cognition of Semantic Transformations

The information transmitted by a word or word sequence may vary depending upon the attributes stressed or the context, role, or significance of
the utterance. The command *Go!* in a dangerous situation conveys significantly different information from the word *go* in the sentence "Go to
school." The word *soft* may describe volume or texture depending upon
the attribute stressed, as a pillow and a quiet tone can be described as sharing the attribute *soft*. All of these changes in meaning involve a semantic
transformation. The awareness and recognition of changes in word meaning
(redefinitions) reflect the cognition of semantic transformations.

Learning disabled children may fail to grasp semantic transformations.
They may have limited knowledge of attributes, be unable to discern subtle
qualities, or they may fail to generalize attributes from one object or situation
to another; as a result, they may demonstrate problems in processing multiple—meaning words, idioms, metaphors, and puns. These problems may
be expected to interfere with academic achievement and social adequacy.

Deficits in the Cognition of Semantic Implications

The highest level of comprehension of auditory language involves the ability to discern information that was implied, but not provided, that is, cognition of semantic implications. It reflects awareness of possible causes, effects,
and concomitant conditions, and results in logical conclusions, anticipations,
expectations, and predictions. Youngsters with learning disabilities frequently have impaired cognition of semantic implications.

After hearing part of a story such as *The Little Red Hen*, the learning disabled youngster may not be able to predict the outcome, and he may not be
aware of the reasons why the hen denied the cookies to the other animals. He
may not understand the moral of the story and may be unable to generalize
the implications to past and future personal interactions. Many LD children
experience similar problems in understanding fables, myths, parables, and
proverbs. These deficits may be interpreted to reflect reductions in the active

analysis of the significant verbal elements and relationships, a process involving the frontal lobes (Luria, 1973). Paradoxically, as adults they often use proverbs and sayings in stereotyped expressions. Deficits in the cognition of semantic implications may have vast impact on reading comprehension, problem solving, discrimination between fact and fiction and fact and opinion, and moral judgment.

Memory

Children with learning disabilities frequently exhibit limitations in auditory memory (Chalfant & Scheffelin, 1969). Investigations of memory have resulted in a variety of conclusions regarding specific memory abilities. Nonverbal has been distinguished from verbal memory and visual from auditory. In the area of verbal memory, two separate abilities have been recognized, associative-memory and span-memory (French, 1951). Within the verbal domain, Guilford (1967) has identified memory factors for semantic units, classes, relations, systems, transformations, and implications. Guilford's model, however, combines short- and long-term memory.

Other models (Miller, 1956; Miller & Chomsky, 1963; Simon & Chase, 1973; Slobin, 1971) distinguish between short- and long-term memory abilities in processing verbal and visual input. Linguistic processing is considered to depend heavily upon short-term memory; cognitive-semantic (deep structure) processing upon long-term memory (Miller & Chomsky, 1963). Since memory (short- and long-term) interfaces with perceptual, linguistic, and cognitive processing it is viewed as an integral part of auditory language processing as indicated in Figure 1. Memory for auditory verbal input, semantic information, and linguistic structure is also considered to provide a link between auditory language processing and oral language formulation and production.

Learning disabled children may exhibit memory deficits that may influence various perceptual, linguistic, and cognitive aspects of auditory language processing as well as oral language production. They may experience specific deficits in recalling phoneme sequences, problems that may reduce their perceptual effectiveness. They frequently demonstrate long-term memory and retrieval deficits for semantic units within selected categories, such as proper names, adjectives, and prepositions. Within semantic classes, long-term memory and retrieval deficits are frequently encountered for verbal associations such as antonyms, synonyms, and subordinates or superordinates. They may also show deficient recall of semantic relations, such as verbal analogies, cause-and-effect relationships, and linguistic concepts that require logical operations.

Their short-term auditory memory is generally better for structurally simple sentences such as simple active declarative sentences than for structurally complex semantic systems such as complex or ambiguous sentences, limericks, and poems. Sentence recall tends to be facilitated by semantic aspects (deep structure) and therefore long-term memory (Wiig & Roach, 1975). When semantic aspects are altered by structural complexity, ambiguity, or by the presence of implied meaning, learning disabled youngsters may experience significant problems. They may also demonstrate long-term memory problems for semantic transformations, such as multiple-meaning words, synonyms, riddles, and puns and for semantic implications (cause-effect relationships, etc.).

Evaluation

Accurate auditory language processing and oral language production is considered to depend upon efficient evaluation of the structural and semantic aspects of the information transmitted (Guilford, 1967). Critical judgment of verbal information requires logical comparison of the product of information with previously stored, known information. Among the criteria for logical comparison and evaluation are identity, similarity, and consistency. Guilford (1967) stresses the difficulty in differentiating the semantic evaluative abilities from their cognitive counterparts. The process of evaluation is considered to be an integral part of auditory language processing (Figure 1) and provides a link between auditory language processing and oral language formulation and production.

Learning disabled children with adequate perceptual abilities are generally able to evaluate auditory verbal information according to the criteria of identity and similarity. Problems appear to occur when they are asked to evaluate the consistency of semantic aspects against information stored in long-term memory, or on the basis of the internal consistency in structure or meaning. Their problems may be reflected at the level of auditory-symbolic and semantic units, as reductions in the critical judgment of the use of morphology and the selection of vocabulary. As examples, learning disabled children may accept the incorrect past tense in the sentence "Yesterday he hitted the ball" or the incorrect preposition in the phrase *in the table* for *on the table*. At the sentence level, they may exhibit deficits in the critical judgment of syntactic consistency. Learning disabled youngsters frequently do not recognize the lack of subject-verb agreement in sentences such as "The men goes home" and may fail to detect an incorrect auxiliary verb in sentences such as "I cannot be able to leave."

At the level of semantic implications, they may not be able to evaluate cause-effect consistency and accept statements such as "Chocolate fudge is made with orange flavoring." Inconsistencies between premise and conclusion may also elude them, and they may accept a statement such as "She needed her mittens because it was hot outside." It should be recognized that deficits in evaluation may not always reflect inability to judge critically. Habitually lax criteria for the evaluation of internal consistency may result in similar misjudgments.

Language Production

The production of language has been suggested to be facilitated by cognitive storage and retrieval as well as by affective behaviors (ideas, practices, standards, values) and psychomotor behaviors (sensory perception, mental, physical and emotional set, etc.) (Ahmann & Glock, 1971). The formulation and production of oral language may be considered to involve four aspects: selectional, semantic, linguistic, and expressive (verbal encoding) (Figure 3). Retrieval from long-term memory and evaluation are considered integral aspects of the selectional process.

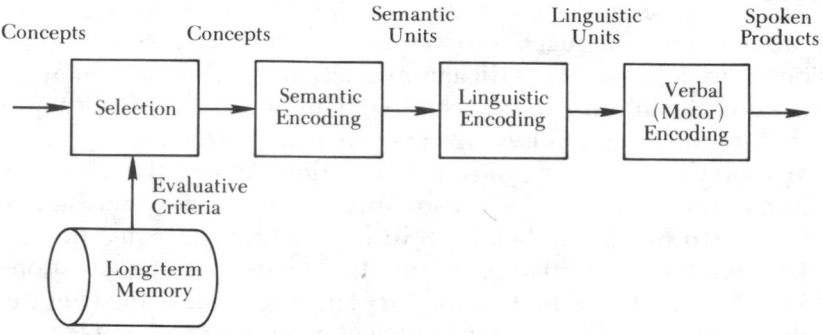

FIGURE 3. Illustration of the relationships between cognitive, linguistic, and expressive aspects in language production.

The selectional and semantic aspects of language production relate to the accuracy of retrieval and production of (1) auditory-symbolic units (phonemes and phoneme sequences), (2) semantic units (words and concepts), (3) classes (verbal associations), (4) relations (verbal analogies and linguistic concepts), (5) systems (verbal problems), (6) transformations (redefinitions of concepts), and (7) implications (cause-effect, conclusions, predictions, etc.). The linguistic aspects relate to the productive control of (1) phonology, (2) morphology, (3) vocabulary, (4) syntax, and (5) semantics. The expressive (verbal encoding) aspects relevant to oral language production are (1) articulatory agility (ease of articulation), (2) prosody (intonation), (3) sequencing, and (4) verbal fluency (speed of retrieval of words, concepts, and linguistic structures).

Convergent Production Abilities

Language formulation and production must often occur under imposed semantic, linguistic, or social restrictions. Only one word may satisfy the semantic restrictions imposed by a given context. This would be the case in naming the opposite of *night* or in completing a verbal analogy such as "Sons are to fathers as daughters are to _____." The ability to draw a logical conclusion from given verbal information and to produce a unique semantic response (word, concept, sentence, etc.) reflects a person's convergent semantic production ability. Guilford (1967) distinguishes between convergent production abilities for symbolic and semantic units, semantic classes, relations, systems, transformations, and implications.

Learning disabled children may exhibit deficits in several of these areas. They often demonstrate reduced accuracy and speed in naming pictured objects or events and verbal opposites, completing verbal analogies, completing sentences, and redefining words and concepts. Their errors in convergent semantic production are relatively more frequent when the restrictions are so narrow that only one response is satisfactory. The errors made by learning disabled youngsters on convergent language production tasks are frequently associative and perseverative (Wiig & Semel, 1975). Deficits in convergent semantic production may limit the learning disabled child's performance on verbal academic tasks and therefore demand the professional attention of educators and specialists responsible for the educational and clinical management of youngsters with learning disabilities.

Divergent Production Abilities

The fluency, flexibility, originality, and elaboration with which language is produced reflect a person's divergent semantic production abilities. According to Guilford (1967), divergent production abilities can be distinguished for word and concept naming, verbal associations and analogies, formulation of ideas and verbal problems, reformulation of concepts and ideas, and formulation of alternatives and solutions.

Divergent production abilities relate to aspects of creative potential, but show low relationships with IQ which depends heavily upon cognition.

Divergent production abilities usually constitute an area of relative strength in the learning disabled youngster. Specific deficits may, however, be observed in the fluency, that is, the speed and accuracy, with which semantic units, classes, relations, and transformations are retrieved and produced. Associative errors (paraphasias) and perseverations (repetition of a previous word or phrase) frequently interfere with the accuracy of production. The reductions in verbal fluency (speed and accuracy of oral language production) observed in association with learning disabilities have been described by Bannatyne (1971), Johnson and Myklebust (1967), Lerner (1971), Orton (1937), Wiig and Semel, (1975), among others.

Learning disabled youngsters may also demonstrate limited flexibility in the formulation of sentences. They tend to express themselves in simple declarative sentences, and verbal stereotypes abundantly appear. There is, however, frequent evidence of originality and elaboration at several levels of production such as in vocabulary selection, a factor which may serve to camouflage limitations in divergent language production.

Productive Control of Linguistic Structure

The formulation of a large variety of grammatically acceptable English sentences requires adequate knowledge of English morphology and syntax (linguistic competence) and ability to retrieve and control linguistic structures in spontaneous language production. Investigations of the knowledge and productive control of English morphology and syntax by learning disabled children have indicated significant reductions (Rosenthal, 1970; Semel & Wiig, 1975; Vogel, 1974; Wiig & Semel, 1975; Wiig, Semel, & Crouse, 1973).

At first glance, the spontaneous language of learning disabled youngsters may seem grammatically appropriate. Some LD children may, however, show significant deficits in the control of both morphology and syntax on structured linguistic tasks such as sentence repetition, completion, or transformation tasks (Rosenthal, 1970; Semel & Wiig, 1975; Vogel, 1974; Wiig, Semel, & Crouse, 1973). The syntactic problems observed in learning disabled children may persist into adolescence (Wiig & Roach, 1975; Wiig & Semel, 1975). For example, learning disabled children may demonstrate delays in acquiring productive control of the irregular past tense of verbs or of the comparative and superlative of adjectives; as a result, they may formulate and accept agrammatical sentences such as "John hitted the dog" or "Jane was more happy than Bill."

Similarly, some learning disabled youngsters may tell a story using a series of simple active declarative sentences of relatively short length. Their sentences may lack descriptive adjectives or prepositional phrases which delineate the events described in time and space. They may produce compound sentences conjoined by *and* or *but*. Complex sentences with embedding such as "Paul gave the book that he got last year to his best friend" may, however, be completely lacking, and the range of sentence transformations used may be very limited, indicating delays in syntactic maturation (Hass & Wepman, 1974).

Learning disabled adolescents may show similar difficulties in controlling linguistic structure in spontaneous language production as well as on structured linguistic tasks. They may express themselves in relatively short sentences of simple linguistic structure. They may produce and accept incomplete sentences such as *After the ballgame* when they are asked to formulate sentences that incorporate specific words such as *after* (Wiig & Semel, 1975). Their overall performances on both spontaneous and structured expressive language tasks suggest deficits in retrieving and formulating complex sentence transformations.

The spoken language of learning disabled youngsters seems characterized by a preponderance of interjections, such as *well it is . . .*, indefinite pronouns such as *somebody* and *something*, conjunctions, filled pauses and word repetitions while descriptive adjectives seem lacking. All of these features have been described to be characteristic of factors reflecting hesitancy and effort to maintain conversation (Jones & Wepman, 1961).

Some of the productive language deficits observed in learning disabled children and adolescents may be related to deficits in language processing. The process of storing information (semantic and linguistic) may be subdivided into three parts: (1) the act of storing, (2) the holding of information in storage, and (3) the retrieval of information. Each of the parts of this process may provide a source of impairment or error. Reductions or deficits in processing and interpreting language (linguistic structures, linguistic concepts, etc.) may interfere with the act of storing and consequently with the availability of semantic or syntactic information for retrieval.

Some of the problems observed in oral language production may reflect inadequate retrieval from long-term memory store. Observations suggest that this may be the case for some learning disabled adolescents (Wiig, Lapointe, & Semel, 1975). The deficits in language production observed among learning disabled adolescents appeared to constitute at least two distinct deficit syndromes: (1) cognitive-linguistic processing deficits characterized by reductions in morphology and syntax and in the comprehension of linguistic concepts, and (2) dysnomia characterized by verbal paraphasias (word substitutions) and word-finding and retrieval deficits.

The distinct deficit entity theory was supported by several findings. Measures of language processing abilities generally correlated positively with each other with the exception of measures obtained on a test of immediate recall of sentences. The related measures shared requirements for adequate cognition of semantic units, classes, and relations and adequate seriation (Guilford, 1967; Inhelder & Piaget, 1964; Piaget & Inhelder, 1969). There were few significant correlations between performances on language processing and production tasks. In a similar vein, measures of accuracy of retrieval and formulation in language production generally correlated positively with each other and negatively with speed of retrieval, indicating that accurate responses were produced with less delay than inaccurate responses.

References

Ahmann, F. S., & Glock, M. D. Evaluating pupil growth. Boston: Allyn & Bacon, 1971.

Aten, J., & Davis, J. Disturbances in the perception of auditory sequence in children with minimal cerebral dysfunction. *Journal of Speech and Hearing Research*, 1968, **11**, 236-45.

Bannatyne, A. *Language, reading and learning disabilities*. Springfield, Ill.: Charles C Thomas, 1971.

Borel-Maisonny, S. Les troubles du langage dans les dyslexies et les dysorthographies. *Enfance*, 1951, **4**, 400-444.

Chalfant, J. C., & Scheffelin, M. A. *Central processing dysfunctions in children*. Bethesda: National Institute of Neurological Diseases and Stroke, Monograph No. 9, 1969.

Cruickshank, W., Bentzen, F., Ratzeburg, F., & Tannhauser, M. *Teaching method for brain-injured and hyperactive children*. Syracuse: Syracuse University Press, 1961.

Flowers, A., & Costello, M. R. *Tests of central auditory abilities*. Dearborn, Mich.: Perceptual Learning Systems, 1970.

Fodor, J. A., Bever, T. G., & Garrett, M. F. *The psychology of language*. New York: McGraw-Hill, 1974.

French, J. W. The description of aptitude and achievement tests in terms of rotated factors. *Psychometric Monograph* No. 5, 1951.

Goldstein, K. *Language and language disorders*. New York: Grune & Stratton, 1948.

Guilford, J. P. *The nature of human intelligence*. New York: McGraw-Hill, 1967.

Guilford, J. P., & Lacey, J. I. (Eds.) *Report No. 5. Printed classification tests: army air forces aviation psychology research program reports*. Washington, D.C.: GPO, 1947.

Hass, W. A., & Wepman, J. M. Dimensions of individual difference in the spoken syntax of school children. *Journal of Speech and Hearing Research*, 1974, **17**, 455-69.

Inhelder, B., & Piaget, J. *The early growth of logic in the child*. New York: Norton, 1964.

Johnson, D. J. The language continuum. *Bulletin of the Orton Society*, 1968, **28**, 1-11.

Johnson, D. J., & Myklebust, H. R. *Learning disabilities: educational principles and practices*. New York: Grune & Stratton, 1967.

Jones, L. V., & Wepman, J. M. Dimensions of language performance in aphasia. *Journal of Speech and Hearing Research*, 1961, **4**, 220-32.

Lasky, E. Z., & Tobin, H. Linguistic and nonlinguistic competing message effects. *Journal of Learning Disabilities*, 1973, **6**, 243-50.

Lerner, J. *Children with learning disabilities*. Boston: Houghton Mifflin Co., 1971.

Luria, A. R. *The working brain*. New York: Basic Books, 1973.

McGrady, H. J., & Olson, D. A. Visual and auditory learning processes in normal children and children with learning disabilities. *Exceptional Children*, 1970, **36**, 581-89.

Marslen-Wilson, W. D. Sentence perception as an interactive parallel process. *Science*, 1975, **189**, 226-28.

Meeker, M. N. *The structure of intellect: its interpretation and use*. Columbus, Ohio: Charles E. Merrill, 1969.

Meier, J. H. Prevalence and characteristics of learning disabilities found in second grade children. *Journal of Learning Disabilities*, 1971, **4**, 1-16.

Miller, G. A. The magical number seven, plus or minus two. *Psychological Review*, 1956, **63**, 81-97.

Miller, G. A., & Chomsky, N. Finitary models of language users. In R. D. Luce, R. R. Bush, & E. Galanter (Eds.), *Handbook of mathematical psychology*. Vol. 2. New York: John Wiley & Sons, 1963. Pp. 419-91.

Myklebust, H. R. *Auditory disorders in children*. New York: Grune & Stratton, 1954.

Orton, S. T. *Reading, writing and speech problems in children*. New York: Norton, 1937.

Piaget, J. *The psychology of intelligence*. New York: Harcourt Brace Jovanovich, 1950.

Piaget, J., & Inhelder, B. *The psychology of the child*. New York: Basic Books, 1969.

Rosenthal, J. H. A preliminary psycholinguistic study of children with learning disabilities. *Journal of Learning Disabilities*, 1970, **3**, 391-95.

Russell, D. H. *Childrens Thinking*. New York: Ginn, 1956.

Semel, E. M., & Wiig, E. H. Comprehension of syntactic structures and critical verbal elements by children with learning disabilities. *Journal of Learning Disabilities*, 1975, **8**, 53-58.

Simon, H. A., & Chase, W. G. Skill in chess. *American Scientist*, 1973, **61**, 394-403.

Slobin, D. I. *Psycholinguistics*. Glenview, Ill.: Scott Foresman & Co., 1971.

Strauss, A. A., & Kephart, N. C. *Psychopathology and the education of the brain-injured child*. New York: Grune & Stratton, 1955.

Vogel, S. A. Syntactic abilities in normal and dyslexic children. *Journal of Learning Disabilities*, 1974, **7**, 47-53.

Wiig, E. H., & Harris, S. Perception and interpretation of nonverbally expressed emotions by adolescents with learning disabilities. *Perceptual and Motor Skills*, 1974, **38**, 239-45.

Wiig, E. H., Lapointe, C., & Semel, E. M. Relationships among language processing and production abilities of learning-disabled adolescents. Paper presented at the Annual Convention of the American Speech and Hearing Association, Washington, D.C., 1975.

Wiig, E. H., & Roach, M. A. Immediate recall of semantically varied "sentences" by learning disabled adolescents. *Perceptual and Motor Skills*, 1975, **40**, 119-25.

Wiig, E. H., & Semel, E. M. Comprehension of linguistic concepts requiring logical operations by learning disabled children. *Journal of Speech and Hearing Research*, 1973, **16**, 627-36.

Wiig, E. H., & Semel, E. M. Logico-grammatical sentence comprehension by learning disabled adolescents. *Perceptual and Motor Skills*, 1974, **38**, 1331-34.

Wiig, E. H., & Semel, E. M. Productive language abilities in learning disabled adolescents. *Journal of Learning Disabilities*, 1975, **8**, 578-86.

Wiig, E. H., Semel, E. M., & Crouse, M. A. The use of English morphology by high-risk and learning disabled children. *Journal of Learning Disabilities*, 1973, **6**, 457-65.

Zigmond, N. K. Auditory processes in children with learning disabilities. In L. Tarnapol (Ed.), *Learning disabilities: introduction to educational and medical management*. Springfield, Ill.: Charles C Thomas, 1969. Pp. 196-216.

3 Deficits in Language Processing

Overview

The present chapter provides a review of research of language processing deficits associated with learning disabilities. In this review, the current limitations of formal knowledge are emphasized. Clinical observations are also discussed to provide additional information about the characteristics of language deficits in learning disabilities.

Current research indicates that learning disabled youngsters may exhibit a variety of deficits in processing spoken language. Among possible bases for these problems are (1) reductions in auditory memory, temporal, sequencing, auditory figure-ground, reauditorization, and auditory-visual integration, (2) limitations in symbolization, abstraction, and conceptualization, (3) deficits in linguistic processing and in the conceptual synthesis underlying adult syntax, and (4) delays in cognitive and logical processing.

Clinical observations are presented which suggest that the phoneme discrimination errors of learning disabled children are predictable and consistent. Common error patterns are presented for consonants, consonant blends, and vowels. Frequently observed comprehension problems for semantic units (nouns, pronouns, verbs, adjectives, adverbs, and prepositions) are also introduced.

Recent investigations of linguistic processing deficits in learning disabilities are reviewed with regard to their characteristics and bases. They indicate that learning disabled children may experience significant reductions in the knowledge of morphology and syntax and that these problems may persist into adolescence. The literature further indicates that cognitive and logical processing deficits may be present among both learning disabled children and adolescents.

Characteristics and Bases

The ability to process, interpret, and respond to complex verbal input and information influences the potential for academic achievement, the quality of interpersonal interaction, and the potential for social and professional growth. Deficits in verbal comprehension may limit growth in all of these areas. Observations indicate that auditory language processing may be grossly inadequate in learning disabled school-age children (Bannatyne, 1971; Bender, 1968, 1973; Birch,1964; Chalfant & Scheffelin,1969; de Hirsch, Jansky, & Langford, 1966; Hammill & Bartel, 1975; Johnson & Myklebust, 1967; McGrady & Olson, 1970; Myers & Hammill, 1969; Orton, 1937).

The complexity and subtlety of the auditory processing deficits of learning disabled youngsters may explain why they have not been extensively explored. The relatively limited understanding of the bases of these problems may also explain why they have frequently resisted clinical management. The subtlety of the receptive language problems which may be associated with learning disabilities is best understood when it is realized that specific, isolated, or combined deficits may occur at various levels of perceptual, linguistic, and/or cognitive-semantic processing.

The perceptual, linguistic, and cognitive-semantic processes basic to language comprehension interrelate, and they may be applied simultaneously or successively during processing. Lenneberg (1973) describes the processes involved in language comprehension as follows:

> Understanding language involves two separate sets of computations, each one designed to extract a separate kind of relationship. It involves the extraction of relationships between objects and energies of the physical world; and it involves the extraction of relationships that are implied in sentences. [p. 55]

Efficient processing of auditory language requires ability to process simultaneously at several levels as well as ability to shift between simultaneous and successive processing. At the same time, different aspects of the process must be able to take the lead, depending upon the complexity of the auditory input. Consider as an example the task of discerning the differences between the two sentences "Sherry can't go, but Terry can" and "Terry can't go, but Sherry can." At the phonetic-phonemic level, it is necessary for the listener to discriminate between the initial sounds in the minimal pair *Sherry* and *Terry*. At the syntactic level, the two sentences are similar and interpretation depends upon retention of the sequence in which the proper names occurred. The youngster with auditory processing deficits may have problems dealing with one or more of these aspects, causing a total breakdown in comprehension.

In general, problems at the level of phoneme discrimination are more blatant and less likely to be overlooked than problems at the higher levels of processing. Deficits at the cognitive-semantic and logical processing levels are least likely to be detected early since inconsistencies at those levels may not be a cause for early concern. Parents, physicians, and educators appear prone to attribute higher level processing deficits to developmental lags and to expect spontaneous improvement with age. This expectation seems unwarranted in view of findings that many learning disabled adolescents exhibit significant reductions in auditory memory, syntactic processing, and comprehension of linguistic concepts requiring logical operations (Wiig & Roach, 1975; Wiig & Semel, 1974b).

The literature suggests several bases for the auditory language processing deficits observed in association with learning disabilities. Learning disabled youngsters have been reported to exhibit:

1. Auditory memory deficits (de Hirsch, Jansky, & Langford, 1966; Masland & Case, 1965; Spencer, 1959).
2. Temporal sequencing deficits (Aten & Davis, 1968; Orton, 1937).
3. Auditory figure-ground problems (Flowers & Costello, 1970; Lasky & Tobin, 1973).
4. Reauditorization deficits (Johnson & Myklebust, 1967).
5. Auditory-visual integration deficits (Birch & Belmont, 1964, 1965; Birch & Lefford, 1963; Stamback, 1951).
6. Limitations in symbolization, abstraction, and conceptualization (Johnson, 1968; Johnson & Myklebust, 1967; Myklebust, 1964; Strauss & Kephart, 1955).
7. Deficits in linguistic processing and in the conceptual synthesis underlying adult syntax (Farnham-Diggory, 1967; Menyuk & Looney, 1972a; Semel & Wiig, 1975; Wiig & Roach, 1975).
8. Deficits in cognitive and logical processing (Wiig & Semel, 1973, 1974b).

Cognition of Auditory-Symbolic Units

Comprehension of auditory language, that is, assigning meaning to heard phonemic, morphemic, and linguistic units, depends on accurate analysis and synthesis at all levels of processing. The process of assigning meaning to a sentence may break down at a relatively low level, the level of phoneme discrimination. Deficient analysis and synthesis of the distinctive features contained in a single phoneme may cause a child to misinterpret the location described in the sentence "It is on the bottom of the *page*" as "on the bottom of the *cage*."

Deficits in the analysis and synthesis of a phoneme's distinctive features do not always result in misinterpretation of sentence meaning. Semantic constraints generally assist in categorizing a phoneme even though the features were initially discriminated incorrectly. As an example, initial uncertainties in discriminating between the features contained in /m/ and /n/ rarely result in misinterpreting a sentence such as "I ate lunch at *noon*" to mean "I ate lunch at *moon*."

Discrimination between the various English phonemes in isolation depends upon adequate analysis and synthesis of their respective features. Each phoneme can be characterized by a number of significant acoustic and articulatory features which differentiate it from all other phonemes in the language (Jakobson, Fant, & Halle, 1952; Saporta, 1955). Phonemes such as /p/ and /b/ which are differentiated by two features (Saporta, 1955) tend to be more similar in articulation and in acoustic features than phonemes differentiated by several features.

Phoneme discrimination errors of children with learning disabilities appear remarkably predictable and consistent. The number of errors varies, however, from one learning disabled child to the next. Analysis of their misperceptions of linguistic units, sequences, and structures reveals that the perceptual confusions can be predicted based on the phoneme classification system devised by Miller and Nicely (1955). Phonemes separated by only one perceptual feature, for example, voicing, nasality, duration, or place of articulation, are more frequently confused than phonemes separated by two or more perceptual features. As an example, the voiced /d/ is frequently misperceived as /t/, and a word such as *dime* may be interpreted as *time*. Semantic constraints and redundant contextual cues may, however, facilitate correct categorization of the original phoneme in the presence of initially incorrect analysis and synthesis.

Discrimination of Consonants and Blends

Consonants

Observations of the frequency of confusions between the various initial consonants suggest that the voiced and unvoiced cognates are often interchanged. Learning disabled youngsters frequently seem to misperceive the voiced cognates as their unvoiced counterparts and vice versa. This pattern may result in misperceptions of /b/ as /p/, /d/ as /t/, /g/ as /k/, /v/ as /f/, /z/ as /s/, and / ð / as /θ/ or vice versa. The second most frequent pattern seems to reflect confusion among voiced phonemes that are differentiated by place and manner of articulation. Confusions within this pattern may occur among the phonemes /b/, /d/, /g/, /v/, / ð /, /z/, / ʒ /. Prevalent misperceptions seem to result in misinterpretations of /g/ as /d/ and /z/ as either /b/ or /v/, suggesting that a posterior point of articulation is substituted perceptually by an anterior point.

Blends

The discrimination and differentiation of initial blends may present another set of problems to the learning disabled child. The most common confusions between these blends appear for blends with /l/, /w/, or /r/ in the second position. Consonant blends such as /pr/, /fr/, and /kr/ are often perceived as /pl/, /fl/, and /kl/, respectively. Similarly, the blends /tr/ and /dr/ may be perceived as /tw/ and /dw/. A less frequent, but more persistent set of confusions may occur between the initial consonants of /-r/ blends such as /pr/, /tr/, /kr/, /dr/, /gr/, and /fr/.

When consonant blends are perceived as single sounds by children with learning disabilities, the severity of the problem seems to relate directly and positively to the distance in perceptual features between the intended and the perceived phonemes. For example, the problem may be considered less severe if *train* is misperceived as *rain* than if it is misperceived as *pain*. Although the foregoing examples illustrate only the confusions that may occur for /-r/ blends, the same principles appear to hold for /-l/ and /-w/ blends.

Consonant blends with /s/ in the initial position follow some of the same patterns of confusion as for /-r/, /-l/, and /-w/ blends. A frequently observed pattern of confusion exists when the second consonant of /s/ blends is misperceived. Consonant blends such as /sp/, /st/, /sk/, /sm/, /sn/, /sl/, and /sw/ are commonly and randomly substituted for each other. The confusions between /s/ blends are frequently predictable based on similarities in the place or manner of articulation of the second consonant. Typically, confusions occur between (1) /sp/, /st/, and /sk/; (2) /sp/ and /sm/; and/or (3) /st/ and /sl/.

When /s/ occurs initially in triple blends, it is often retained perceptually while the other consonants may be misperceived. As a consequence, the word *split* may be interpreted as *slit, spit,* or *sit,* and *scream* may be misperceived as *scheme* or *seam.* In a similar fashion, words beginning with initial /s/ may be interpreted to contain an initial double or triple blend by children with learning disabilities. As a result, *side* may be interpreted as *slide, soak* as *spoke,* and *sit* as either *slit* or *split.*

Facilitating Factors

Deficits in the cognition of auditory-symbolic units may result in misinterpretations of words in which the spoken and the perceived word belong to either the same or a different grammatical class. Observations suggest that when the intended and the interpreted words belong to the same grammatical class (noun, verb, adjective, etc.), the problem is least severe and least resistant to intervention. In remediation, accurate discrimination and categorization of phonemes may be facilitated by redundancy in the semantic aspects of the message. As an example, a youngster with phoneme discrimination problems may misperceive the sentence "The rain is gone," which has little semantic redundancy, as "The pain is gone" or "The stain is gone." A sentence such as "Put your money in your pocket," which has several cues to the meaning of the message, would rarely, if ever, be misperceived as "Put your money in your socket." When the intended and the perceived words do not belong to the same grammatical class, the problem appears more stubborn and resistant to intervention. This may indicate that the child does not use available semantic constraints and contextual cues effectively to facilitate accurate phoneme discrimination and categorization.

While efficient use of semantic constraints and contextual cues may facilitate accurate phoneme discrimination and categorization, constant dependence on such a strategy occurs at an expense. The rate with which auditory language can be processed decreases when inaccurate discrimination and categorization of phonemes has to be compensated for by cognitive-semantic processing and conceptualization. Accurate phoneme discrimination and categorization normally assist linguistic and semantic processing of language and facilitate simultaneous analysis and synthesis at various levels. Since conceptualization may be limited in some learning disabled children (Johnson, 1968; Johnson & Myklebust, 1967; Myklebust, 1964), it seems prudent to evaluate, in detail, phoneme discrimination and categorization abilities as part of the clinical-educational management of the language impaired, learning disabled child.

Vowel Discrimination

Vowels

Vowel discrimination and categorization may also present a significant problem to the learning disabled child and may interfere with auditory-visual integration basic to reading and writing. Confusions among vowels in auditory language processing appear to center around the "front" vowels

/i/, /e/, and /ae/ as in *bit, bet,* and *bat*. A frequently observed pattern of confusion occurs when the relatively low front vowel /ae/ (bat) is misperceived as one of the relatively higher front vowels /e/ and /i/ or vice versa. While confusions among these vowels appear to be the norm in kindergarten and first grade children, they frequently persist beyond the expected age levels in learning disabled children. These vowel discrimination problems are often reflected in spelling and writing.

Auditory-Visual Integration

Although the learning disabled child may discriminate accurately between the graphemes that represent vowel phonemes, the analysis and synthesis of distinctive features, reauditorization, encoding, and auditory-visual integration are frequently unstable. The implications of vowel confusions in auditory language processing for reading and writing are heightened by the fact that one phoneme may be represented by a number of graphemes. For example, the glide /ey/ can be represented by several graphemes as in the words *play, neighbor, race,* and *great*. Conversely, one grapheme may be used to represent a number of phonemes. For example, the graphemes *ea* represent several different phonemes in the written words, *bear, ear, Easter,* and *great*. Inaccurate or inconsistent analysis and synthesis of vowel features may impede the complex process of acquiring the necessary auditory-visual associations for reading, writing, and spelling.

Some of the problems experienced by learning disabled children in establishing auditory-visual integration for vowels may reflect difficulties in segmentation, that is, dividing words into their smaller grammatical units, and word classification. As an example, the graphemes *en* in *written* and *on* in *cotton* sound the same and are often spelled phonetically by learning disabled youngsters. Categorization of *written* as a verb form with subsequent identification of the verb ending *-en* as in *given, stolen,* and *taken* may assist in accurate auditory-visual integration. (Similarly, classification of *cotton* as a noun patterned similarly to the nouns *glutton* and *mutton* facilitates auditory-visual integration.) As another example, the derivational suffixes in the words *teacher* and *moderator* sound alike, but classification of *teacher* as a derivation of a verb of Anglo-Saxon origin and *moderator* as a verb derivation of Latin origin facilitate accurate auditory-visual integration. The achieving child seems to acquire and apply word categorization and segmentation rules with relative ease; in contrast, the learning disabled child must often be assisted to acquire alternative strategies to compensate for his deficits.

Cognition of Semantic Units

Comprehension of Nouns and Verbs

Observations of language impaired, learning disabled children indicate that their vocabulary may be as large as that of achieving age peers (Wiig & Semel, 1973; Wiig, Semel, & Crouse, 1973). It has been suggested that learning disabled children may compensate for sentence formulation problems by increasing the amount of available vocabulary items. It is also possible to interpret this finding to suggest that the cognition of semantic units may be adequate in these children.

Clinical evaluations generally reveal that learning disabled youngsters score within normal limits (above -6 months of CA [chronological age]) on tests of receptive vocabulary such as the *Peabody Picture Vocabulary Test* (Dunn, 1965) even though they may exhibit deficits in auditory memory and syntactic and logical processing (Semel & Wiig, 1975; Wiig & Semel, 1972, 1973, 1974b; Wiig, Semel, & Crouse, 1973). The comprehension of dual meaning words and specific word categories may, however, be inadequate even though overall vocabulary measures fall within normal limits (Johnson, 1968; Johnson & Myklebust, 1967; Myklebust, 1964). These problems have been attributed to retention of narrow word meanings and tendencies to remain concrete and limited in imagery, symbolization, and conceptualization. Deficits in the cognition of semantic units and retention of narrow and concrete word meanings may persist in learning disabled adolescents (Wiig & Semel, 1975).

Dual Meaning Words

Clinical examples of the learning disabled youngster's problems with dual meaning nouns and verbs are abundant. The learning disabled child may act confused when asked to point to *building* while being shown four action pictures, one of which shows a boy building a wagon. He may not be able to accommodate changes in word meaning which are contextually or syntactically determined and may fail to discern the contrast in word meaning when *building* is used in the sentences "He was in the building" and "He was building." In a similar vein, the learning disabled child may misinterpret a direction to "Go check it" and respond that he cannot write a check. The responses given by learning disabled youngsters to dual and multiple-meaning words suggest that they interpret these words according to their most frequent, concrete meaning.

Verbs

Verbs which cause problems in comprehension generally describe complex actions or movements for which the conceptual or semantic coding may not have been established. Among examples of problem verbs are *balancing, bouncing, crawling, crouching, evading, leaping, passing, punching, swaying, tossing, tumbling, twisting,* and *vaulting*.

The copula *to be* seems to present special problems for the LD child in both comprehension and expression. He may fail to grasp that the words *the tall man* and *the man is tall* express identical meaning. The semantically empty copula *to be* in sentences such as "The man is tall" and "Jane is pretty" is often interpreted to imply tense or change, leading to the interpretations that yesterday the man was not tall and Jane was not pretty.

Comprehension of Adjectives

The learning disabled child's difficulties in comprehending adjectives seem to reflect (1) inability to handle dual meaning or syntactic ambiguities, (2) problems in interpreting the temporal, spatial, or qualitative aspects expressed, and/or (3) memory deficits for sequentially presented adjectives (modifier strings).

There is abundant evidence from research that perceptual events are coded in an abstract, declarative sentence format. Differences in the interpretation of perceptual events, furthermore, appear to result in alternative linguistic descriptions and in differences in the ease with which linguistic descriptions of perceptual events are understood (Clark, Carpenter, & Just, 1973). The learning disabled youngster with visual-perceptual deficits may experience problems in interpreting and coding perceptual experiences. These problems are reflected in the comprehension and use of adjectives.

The comprehension of adjectives appears closely tied to the interpretation of spatial, temporal, tactile, kinesthetic, and affective events. Furthermore, perceptual confusions or deficits appear to result in deviations in the initial semantic coding and in the subsequent decoding and encoding of the aspects denoted by the various adjectives. Diagrams of the processes suggested for establishing adjective comprehension are presented in Figures 4 and 5. They illustrate the hypothesized relationship between sensory data, perceptual deficits, and symbol assignment (linguistic coding).

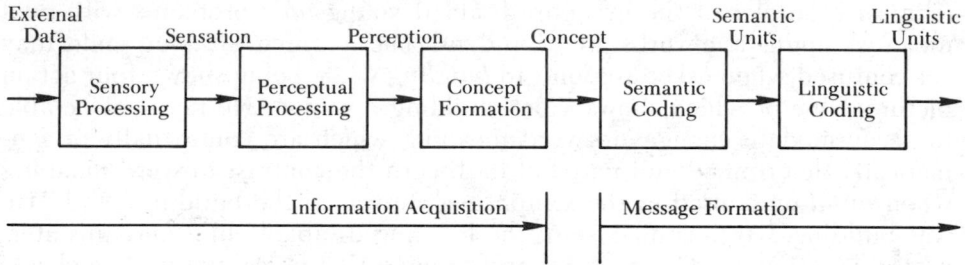

FIGURE 4. Illustration of the relationships between sensation and perception and linguistic coding.

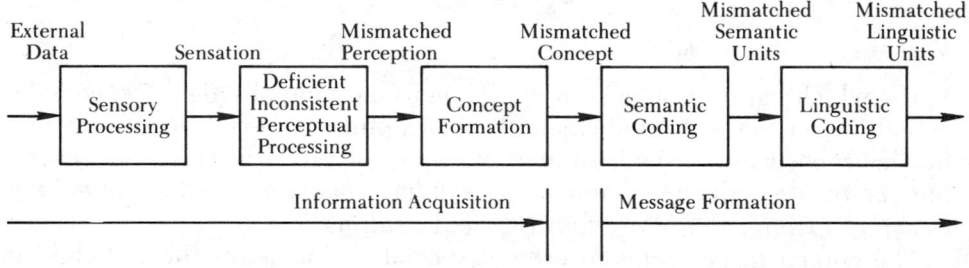

FIGURE 5. Illustration of the effects of perceptual deficits on linguistic coding.

Clinical observations suggest that adjectives that denote prominent dimensions such as color, size, and shape are more easily interpreted by the learning disabled child than adjectives that denote aspects of space, time, or seriation. Adjectives that denote affective, quantitative, or judgmental aspects appear even harder to grasp. A hierarchy of difficulty for adjectives seems to emerge when adjective confusions and misinterpretations by learning disabled youngsters are analyzed. The suggested hierarchy of difficulty for adjective comprehension is presented in Table 1.

TABLE 1

Suggested Hierarchy of Difficulty for Adjective Comprehension by Learning Disabled Children

Aspect	*Adjectives*
1. Color	red, blue, green
2. Size	big, small, large
3. Size-Color	big red, small blue, large green
4. Shape	round, square, oblong
5. Size-Color-Shape	big red round, small yellow square, large green oblong
6. Length	long, short
7. Height	tall, short
8. Width	wide, narrow, thin
9. Age	old, young, new
10. Taste	sweet, sour, bitter
11. Smell	sweet, pungent, stale
12. Attractiveness	pretty, ugly, beautiful
13. Speed	fast, slow
14. Temperature	hot, cold, tepid
15. Quality	rough, smooth, hard
16. Affect	happy, sad, angry
17. Distance	near, far, distant
18. Comparatives-Superlatives	bigger, hotter, nearer biggest, hottest, nearest

Variations in the order of difficulty do occur among LD children. They seem to reflect individual perceptual-motor deficits, deficits in logical processing and seriation, or reductions in simultaneous analysis and synthesis, among others. Deficits in spatial and temporal perception and seriation are commonly reflected in comprehension problems for concepts expressed by adjectives denoting length, height, width, distance, or age. Logical processing or seriation deficits commonly affect the interpretation of concepts expressed by adjectives denoting attractiveness and quality and by the comparative and superlative forms of various adjectives. Perceptual deficits may also result in problems in interpreting the concepts expressed by adjectives denoting taste, smell, temperature, and affect.

The comprehension and interpretation of adjective sequences such as *the big, heavy, shiny, grey* is particularly sensitive to deficits in short-term auditory memory, simultaneous analysis and synthesis, and rule learning for the constraints on adjective order. Learning disabled children have shown discrepancies in handling adjectives when compared with achieving peers on a variety of verbal tasks. Among poorly performed verbal tasks are (1) interpretation of critical verbal elements; for example, *Happy little boy sleeping*, (2) comprehension of linguistic concepts expressing comparative relationships, such as "Are apples bigger than watermelons?" and (3) repetition of sentences with varied syntactic and semantic constraints; for example, "He has sold the long heavy grey shiny car," and "She has washed plastic red small eight cups" (Semel & Wiig, 1975; Wiig & Roach, 1975; Wiig & Semel, 1973, 1974b).

Comprehension of Adverbs

Adverbs are often misinterpreted or not processed by learning disabled youngsters. The problems in interpreting the meaning of adverbs may relate to the heterogeneity of the aspects denoted by adverbs and of the functions of adverbs in relation to the deep structure of sentences. Traditional grammar defines the adverb as the part of speech which may serve to modify a verb, an adjective, or another adverb or adverbial phrase. Adverbs furthermore comprise a derived, highly complex category that is generally not assumed to have categorical identity in the deep structure of English (Lyons, 1971).

Clinical observations suggest that confusions and misinterpretations may occur for (1) adverbs derived from adjectives by adding -*ly* such as *quietly*, *quickly*, and *slowly*, (2) situationally-bound definite adverbs such as *here* and *there*, and (3) situationally-bound indefinite adverbs such as *somewhere*, *someplace*, and *anywhere*. Adverbs derived from adjectives by adding -*ly* (see foregoing examples) pose similar problems to the learning disabled youngster as do their adjective counterparts. The linguistic coding and interpretation of the derived adverbs may be deficient as a result of perceptual-motor deficits or problems in logical processing and seriation as discussed in the section on adjective comprehension.

The problems observed in interpreting situationally-bound definite and indefinite adverbs (see earlier examples) appear to reflect difficulty in the linguistic coding and interpretation of the reference points in space. Investigations have substantiated that the adverbs pose problems in both sentence repetition and in the comprehension of syntactic structures (Menyuk & Looney, 1972a, 1972b; Semel & Wiig, 1975; Wiig & Roach, 1975). Both learning disabled children and adolescents show significant deficits in recalling adverbs that occur in the final position in sentences, a position in which the recency effect generally results in relative ease of recall. On this basis their problems cannot be attributed to memory deficits alone, but must be considered to reflect semantic coding problems.

Comprehension of Prepositions

The comprehension of prepositions and prepositional phrases appears particularly sensitive to deficits in spatial perception and in the coding of visual-spatial events. Learning disabled children demonstrate problems in interpreting prepositions which vary from one child to the next. Prepositions denoting a position (locative) appear easier to comprehend for many learning disabled children than prepositions denoting changes in space or time. The locative prepositions are neutral with respect to fine distinctions of space and time and may for this reason be least sensitive to visual-spatial deficits. They may be classified with regard to space according to whether the location is definite or indefinite as illustrated in Table 2.

Locative Prepositions

Within this category, those prepositions denoting a definite, static position or state, with respect to location, quality, condition, or possession appear easiest for the learning disabled child to interpret. Those naming an indefinite, but static position in space are more frequently misinterpreted. Re-

TABLE 2

Classification of Selected Locative Prepositions

Locative Prepositions

Definite	Indefinite
in	over
on	at
under	by
above	beside
below	next to
on top of	
underneath	
beneath	
in front of	
behind	
between	

gardless of type, one-syllable prepositions tend to be easier to comprehend than two-syllable ones. Clinical observations further suggest that semantic confusions are prevalent between the opposites in the following pairs: (1) *over—under*, (2) *above—below*, and (3) *in front of—behind.*

Directional Prepositions

Prepositions noting a change in direction or condition (directional prepositions) are generally harder to code linguistically and interpret semantically for the learning disabled child. They imply movement or change in space and time and require fine distinctions of space and time which may render them sensitive to visual-spatial deficits. Directional prepositions may also be classified with regard to space according to whether the location is definite or indefinite (Table 3).

TABLE 3

Classification of Selected Directional Prepositions

Directional Prepositions

Definite	Indefinite
over	around
under	to
into	from
out of	toward
up	away from
down	
to the left	
to the right	

As can be seen from a comparison of the tables of locative and the directional prepositions, the meaning of several locative prepositions may change to imply directional change as a function of the context. As an example, a prior selection of a verb which implies movement changes the meaning of a locative preposition to denote a change in space as in the sentence "He went behind the building."

The LD child may react to commands containing directional prepositions as if they indicated a static condition or location. As an example, a learning disabled child directed to "crawl under the table and then over to the door" may remain under the table rather than emerge on the other side if he does not perceive the alternatives in meaning. The directional prepositions noting a specific, definite change in direction, condition, or possession appear easier to comprehend for the learning disabled child than ones that are indefinite with regard to either direction, condition, or possession.

Temporal Prepositions

Prepositions that usually denote spatial orientation (static or active) may also be used to denote a point or period in time and cause severe problems for the learning disabled youngster. As examples, the spatial prepositions *on, from,* and *around* describe temporal aspects in the phrases *on Sunday, from Monday to Friday,* and *around two o'clock.* It is no wonder that prepositions and prepositional phrases pose a multitude of problems for a child or adolescent with learning disabilities.

Semel and Wiig (1975) have reported that learning disabled children demonstrate significant deficits in interpreting the prepositions *over, under,* and *behind* in isolation and when presented as a part of a sequence of four critical verbal elements as in "Monkey sitting on fence." Learning disabled children and adolescents also show significant reductions in the comprehension of linguistic concepts that express spatial relationships such as "The dog fell on the cat. Who was on top?" (Wiig & Semel, 1973, 1974b).

Grammatical Conditioning

The learning disabled child seems to have particular problems in comprehension when the use of a specific preposition is grammatically determined. In answer to the question "Where did he go?" the sentences "He *went to* school" and "He *is at* school" share the same meaning and deep structure. The use of *to* and *at* is determined only by differences in the surface structure, that is, the selection of the predicates *to go* or *to be,* respectively. Comprehension problems are also prevalent for prepositions that indicate indefinite space, aspects of time, or instrumental functions. As a result, the following prepositions may be confused:

Space: at, beside, around, by . . .
Time: about, before, after, on . . .
Instrument: with, without . . .

Perceptual Confusions

Some prepositions may be confused by LD youngsters due to their phonemic similarities. The minimal pair *in* and *on* is frequently confused by learning disabled children; among achieving children the distinctions between *in* and *on* are usually developed by age two (Turton, 1966). Prepositions that share a

prefix may also be confused, causing comprehension problems for prepositions such as *beside, behind, beneath*, and *before*. Perceptual confusions can
also be observed for prepositions sharing the same consonants or vowel combinations, resulting in confusions among the prepositions be*f*ore, a*f*ter, and
in *f*ront of, and ab*ou*t, ar*ou*nd, and with*ou*t.

Unusual Uses

Special semantic problems can be observed in understanding unusual uses of
prepositions. As an example, the preposition *with* is generally used to denote
the instrument such as in "I write with a pen." When *with* is used to denote
the concept *together with* as in the sentence "He drove with his aunt," it
may cause utter confusion among learning disabled children. Instructions
such as "With the red pencil mark the square" or "With the blue pencil mark
the small circle" may not be understood by learning disabled children due to
the unusual sentence construction.

Comprehension of Pronouns

The comprehension of pronouns depends heavily upon ability to abstract and
categorize their functions in relation to events in time and space. Personal
pronouns contain an orientational (deictic) feature which orients an utterance specifically in time and space. The center of orientation is the speaker
and the typical situation of the utterance is egocentric. In interpersonal verbal interactions speakers and listeners constantly change roles; therefore, the
center of orientation changes constantly. As a result, the personal pronoun *I*
is interchanged between speakers, and the pronoun *you* is interchanged between listeners. All pronouns may be characterized similarly in relation to
spatial-temporal features even though the various subclasses of pronouns do
not constitute a homogeneous group. Pronouns can be grouped into the following subclasses: (1) personal, (2) indefinte, (3) demonstrative, (4) interrogative, (5) relative, (6) negative, and (7) inclusive.

   The normal developmental sequence for pronouns has been discussed by
Brown (1973). Longitudinal studies of language acquisition patterns indicated that the pronouns *I, you, it/that*, and *my* were developed during
stage I English in which semantic roles and grammatical relations emerge.
During this stage, *I* and *you* were used as the agents, *it* or *that* as the object of
actions, and *my* as the possessor. In stages IV and V, Brown reported that the
control of distinctions between definite and indefinite references for pronouns was still developing.

Comprehension of Personal Pronouns

Personal pronouns have among their features *person, number, gender*, and
case. The feature *person* is definable with reference to the notion of participant roles (Lyons, 1971). The first person singular *I* refers to the speaker as a
participant in the spatial-temporal event. The second person singular *you* refers to the listener, and the third person singular *he, she, it* to human beings
other than the speaker or listener, or animals, objects, or ideas. The third per-

son pronouns *he* and *she* differ from the first and second person pronouns in that they are not used to refer to participants in the conversation. Gender is only a distinguishing feature of the third person singular pronouns.

Some learning disabled children demonstrate problems in distinguishing between the differences in *gender* for *he* and *she*. Confusions between these words may persist into the fourth grade and may be observed in LD adolescents under duress. In rapid conversation, learning disabled youngsters may also confuse *I* and *you*. As an example, the question "Do you want ice cream?" may be interpreted as a request by the speaker for ice cream. The misinterpretation suggests problems in performing a shift in the referential basis of the conversation.

The plural forms of the personal pronouns *we, you*, and *they* do not contain a one-to-one relationship to the singular forms. The first person plural pronoun *we* includes persons in addition to the speaker. The second person plural pronoun *you* may or may not include the listeners. *We* is inclusive when it refers only to the speakers and listeners present and exclusive when it refers to a person or persons in addition to the participants. The feature *gender* is neutralized in the third person plural pronoun *they*.

Children with learning disabilities appear to experience fewer problems in handling the third person pronouns *it* and *they* than in handling the remaining personal pronouns. They often misinterpret the exclusive use of *you* to refer to only the speakers and listeners present. As an example, the statement "You have made a terrible mess, so you will have to stay after school" may refer to a single child or to a class. The learning disabled child with pronoun reversal for *you* and *I* and problems of a referential basis for the plural pronoun *you* typically considers the accusation to be personal. Some learning disabled children also demonstrate problems in distinguishing between the egocentric *I* and the social *we*, in that the meaning of the social *we* may not have been established or may have been classified as a form of *I*. As an example, the LD child may report "I built the castle" when the sand castle was in reality built by him and his friends.

The feature *case* becomes primary in the distinction between the personal pronouns *I, you, he, she, it, we, you, they* (nominative) and *me, you, him, her, it, us, you, them* (accusative). Learning disabled children may not be able to handle the distinction between the two cases, or they may not have formed firm associations between the corresponding nominative and accusative forms. Their problems seem compounded by the fact that the syntactic relationships within sentences may determine a change in the case of a pronoun from nominative to accusative. A sentence such as "The time for her to leave arrived too fast" may be incomprehensible for the learning disabled child or adolescent if *her* is interpreted as the object of the sentence. Similarly, the learning disabled youngster may experience difficulties in identifying the referent for a pronoun in the accusative case. Consider the statements: "The boy and his father went to the store. The man bought a hat for him to wear." When hearing these statements, learning disabled youngsters may show confusion in locating the referent for the pronoun *him* in the second sentence.

The comprehension and use of possessive pronouns implies that the concepts of belonging or ownership are established. LD children have demonstrated problems in the comprehension and use of noun possessives, suggesting that the concepts of belonging and ownership may be delayed (Vogel, 1974; Wiig, Semel, & Crouse, 1973). They seem to experience similar problems in understanding pronoun substitutions for noun possessives. They may not be able to discern the respective referents for *mine* and *yours*. The concept of inclusion of ownership expressed by *ours* seems to be acquired relatively late, causing problems in comprehending that pronoun. Learning disabled youngsters may also experience problems in discerning the similarities in the meaning of the sentences "It is my hat" and "This hat is mine."

Some of the confusions among personal pronouns demonstrated by learning disabled children appear to reflect difficulties in resolving phonological similarities. As a result, learning disabled youngsters may accept a sentence such as "He walked so far that her feet got tired" as grammatically correct. They may also interpret a sentence such as "He showed him the shoes" to mean "He showed her the shoes."

The reflexive pronouns *myself, yourself, himself, herself, itself, yourselves, ourselves,* and *themselves* present comprehension problems that relate to difficulties in identifying the referent and in categorizing the gender and number. Reflexive pronouns are used in constructions in which the subject and object refer to the same person or animal. Learning disabled children seem to have difficulty in understanding the concept that the subject and object of a sentence can share the same referent. They may therefore interpret the reflexive pronoun to indicate a second, implied person and may fabricate a second person to fit the context. As an example, the sentence "Mary washed herself before she came downstairs" may result in fantasies that Mary washed someone other than herself, for example, her sister, before she went downstairs.

Problems in comprehending and using personal pronouns may also reflect the learning disabled child's difficulty in associating one referent with a variety of pronouns. He may not understand that the pronouns *I, me, my, myself,* and *mine* all refer to him depending upon the syntactic constraints of the utterance.

Comprehension of Demonstrative Pronouns

The demonstrative pronouns *this, these,* and *those* are frequently confused by children with learning disabilities, presumably due to the relative similarities in phonemic structure. Confusions are prevalent between the minimal pairs *this* and *these* and *these* and *those*. The demonstrative pronouns *this* and *these* (close to the speaker) and *that* and *those* (remote to the speaker) are also difficult for LD children to recognize, due to differences in either space or time.

Learning disabled children frequently misinterpret the spatial-temporal orientational features denoted by the demonstrative pronouns and seem to confuse the implied proximity to either the speaker or the listener, that is, the proximal-distal contrast. Their problems are further compounded by the facts that the spatial reference in dialogue shifts between the speaker and the listener and that the listener and the speaker may move in space during their conversation. As a result, the learning disabled child may not be able to discern any internal consistency in the conversation. He may ponder statements such as "This is the book that belongs over there" or "These books belong to those girls over there." Semel and Wiig (1975) have shown that the demonstrative pronouns *this* and *that* pose significant problems in learning disabled children's comprehension of syntactic structures.

Comprehension of Indefinite and Negative Pronouns

Learning disabled children may exhibit difficulties in processing and interpreting indefinite pronouns (*any, anybody, anyone, anything* and *some, somebody, someone, something*) and negative pronouns (*nobody, no one, nothing*). Their problems seem related to difficulties in handling concepts that express quantity. They may exhibit similar problems in handling other concepts for quantity such as *few, most,* and *several.* They may also confuse pronouns within a category such as *some, somebody, someone,* and *something* and may fail to grasp the fine distinctions between the various forms.

There may be other bases for the learning disabled child's problems in comprehending indefinite and negative pronouns. Learning disabled children may experience problems in establishing polarity between forms such as *somebody—anybody* and *nobody—everybody,* as suggested by findings that learning disabled adolescents exhibited significant delays in naming verbal opposites (Wiig & Semel, 1974b). The achieving child may establish polarity between the indefinite and the negative pronouns more easily than the learning disabled child. The strategy of forming contrasts is considered to facilitate comprehension as suggested by Deese (1965) in the following statement:

> The data on associative distributions suggest that the two fundamental operations we have for sorting out meaningful—that is, logical and syntactical relations among words—are contrast and grouping. We can establish the position of any given element in a language within the larger vocabulary of the language by contrasting it with some element or elements and/or by grouping it with respect to some other element or elements [p. 165].

Processing Morphology, Syntax, and Linguistic Concepts

Comprehension and Recall of Sentences

Learning disabled children characteristically exhibit a number of deficits in sentence processing and comprehension, suggesting that the language system has not been internalized. The problems may be demonstrated by inadequate comprehension of connected speech, grammatical confusions and errors, and omissions of plurals, inflections, and participles in language production as well as in problems in processing and producing verbal elements in proper sequence (Lerner, 1971; Meier, 1971; Rosenthal, 1970; Semel & Wiig, 1975; Wiig & Roach, 1975).

The morphological and syntactic deficts of learning disabled children have been suggested to reflect, among others: (1) limited auditory memory capacities, (2) inability to apply phonological, morphological, and syntactic rules in sentence processing, (3) limited attempts to code linguistically, and (4) difficulty with the conceptual synthesis underlying adult syntax (Farnham-Diggory, 1967; Lerner, 1971; Menyuk & Looney, 1972a, 1972b; Rosenthal, 1970; Semel & Wiig, 1975; Wiig & Roach, 1975; Wiig, Semel, & Crouse, 1973).

Memory and Sentence Recall

The relationship between memory and syntactic and semantic aspects of sentences has been discussed by Slobin (1971). He suggests that meaning and form can be stored independently and that meaning (deep structure) is more persistent in memory than form (surface structure). This view is supported by the observation that a heard sentence may be paraphrased long after the verbatim form has been forgotten. Miller and Chomsky (1963) suggest that the surface structure of a sentence is computed within short-term memory and that the limitations of this memory relate directly to the syntactic complexity of language. Deep structure and semantic interpretation are considered to be derived within a larger and longer term stored memory.

Several investigators have presented evidence for the relationships among memory, grammatical structure, and semantic aspects (Blumenthal, 1967; Blumenthal & Boakes, 1967; Miller & Isard, 1964; Savin and Perchonock, 1965). Based on data obtained by Savin & Perchonock, Slobin (1971) reports a hierarchy for the recall of sentence structure which progresses from the easiest to the most difficult as follows:

1. Active declarative (The boy has hit the ball.)
2. Wh- question (What has the boy hit?)
3. Question (Has the boy hit the ball?)
4. Passive (The ball has been hit by the boy.)
5. Negative (The boy has not hit the ball.)
6. Negative question (Has the boy not hit the ball?)
7. Emphatic (The boy *has* hit the ball.)
8. Negative passive (The ball has not been hit by the boy.)
9. Passive question (Has the ball been hit by the boy?)
10. Negative passive question (Has the ball not been hit by the boy?)
11. Emphatic passive (The ball *has* been hit by the boy.)

Sentence Comprehension Deficits

Investigations of sentence comprehension and repetition by LD children and adolescents have indicated that they may experience significant deficits in linguistic rule learning and memory (Menyuk & Looney, 1972a, 1972b; Rosenthal, 1970; Semel & Wiig, 1975; Wiig & Roach, 1975). Rosenthal (1970) observed that syntactic compression was a more significant variable in sentence comprehension than length for learning disabled children and that increasing syntactic compression as in possessive or relative clause transformations caused increased comprehension problems.

Using a sentence comprehension task, Semel and Wiig (1975) reported comprehension problems that supported previous observations by Menyuk and Looney (1972a). Their findings indicated that learning disabled school children experienced significant comprehension deficits for syntactic structures and critical verbal elements (Table 4). The greatest relative comprehension deficits for syntactic structures occurred for questions, sentences with demonstratives and *wh* forms, passive sentences, and sentences which expressed relationships between direct and indirect objects.

Learning disabled children also demonstrated significant deficits in the comprehension of sequences of four critical verbal elements such as "Monkey sitting on fence" (Table 4). They made fewer errors involving the first and last elements of the sequences; most of their errors reflected memory problems for the middle elements of the sequences. The findings suggested that learning disabled children have problems in understanding specific prepositions (*over, under, behind*) in simultaneous analysis and synthesis and in verbal memory.

TABLE 4

Summary of scores obtained by 34 children with learning disabilities and 17 achieving controls on the NSST and ACLC

Test	Mean		Standard Deviation		
	LD	Controls	LD	Controls	t
NSST:					
Receptive	31.38	37.71	5.87	1.20	1.72°
Expressive	29.47	38.59	9.85	1.23	2.07°
ACLC:					
Vocabulary	49.26	50.00	1.22	0	-
2 elements (%)	97.35	100.00	6.09	0	-
3 elements (%)	92.06	98.82	7.58	3.33	-
4 elements (%)	77.06	98.24	15.62	3.69	-

SOURCE: Reprinted with permission of publishers from: Semel, E. M., & Wiig, E. H. Comprehension of syntactic structures and critical verbal elements by children with learning disabilities. *Journal of Learning Disabilities*, 1975, **8**, 53-58.

Note: t = t score; p = probability.

*p < .05.

The comprehension of syntactic structures and critical verbal elements related significantly to measures of academic achievement (Tables 5 and 6). This finding supports the need to consider auditory language comprehension deficits in the educational management of learning disabilities.

Sentence Repetition Deficits

The effects of varying the semantic and syntactic constraints on the recall of sentences by LD adolescents were recently investigated by Wiig and Roach (1975). They administered Newcombe and Marshall's experimental sentence test (Newcombe & Marshall, 1967) to thirty learning disabled and thirty academically achieving adolescents. Learning disabled adolescents exhibited significant quantitative reductions in recalling the sentences. They experienced the most significant reductions in the immediate recall for sentences that (1) were syntactically consistent, but violated semantic (selectional)

TABLE 5

Matrix of significant correlation coefficients (p < .01) between measures of intelligence (WISC), achievement (PIAT), comprehension and expression of syntactic structures (NSST), and comprehension of vocabulary and 4 elements (ACLC)

Test	NSST Receptive	NSST Expressive	ACLC Vocabulary	ACLC 4 elements
WISC:				
MA (Full-scale)	.73	.67	.60	.62
PIAT:				
Math	.57	.50	-	.60
Reading recognition	.64	-	-	.55
Reading comprehension	.77	.53	.54	.64
Spelling	.60	-	-	.49
General information	.60	.60	-	.60
NSST:				
Receptive	-	.78	.74	.62
Expressive	-	-	.61	-

SOURCE: Reprinted with permission of publishers from: Semel, E. M., & Wiig, E. H. Comprehension of syntactic structures and critical verbal elements by children with learning disabilities. *Journal of Learning Disabilities*, 1975, **8**, 53-58.

TABLE 6

Multiple correlations (R) between MA (WISC), measures of achievement (PIAT), and measures of comprehension of syntactic structures (NSST) and 4 elements (ACLC) (p < .01)

Criterion	Predictors		
	MA and Reading Comprehension	Math and Reading Comprehension	Spelling and Reading Comprehension
NSST:			
Receptive	.80	.78	.78
ACLC:			
4 elements	.67	.70	.65

SOURCE: Reprinted with permission of publishers from: Semel, E. M., & Wiig, E. H. Comprehension of syntactic structures and critical verbal elements by children with learning disabilities. *Journal of Learning Disabilities*, 1975, **8**, 53-58.

TABLE 7

Comparison of Verbatim Repetitions by 30 Learning Disabled and 30 Academically Achieving Adolescents

"Sentence"	Learning Disabled		Achievers		χ^2
	No.	%	No.	%	
1. The team of workers built the bridge.	30	100.0	30	100.0	0
2. Colorless green ideas sleep furiously.	16	53.3	26	86.7	7.16°°
3. The man posted the letter.	30	100.0	30	100.0	0
4. The boy hit the girl.	30	100.0	30	100.0	0
5. The politician nearly lost the election.	27	90.0	30	100.0	2.19
6. The boy easily passed the examination.	28	93.3	30	100.0	1.16
7. Didn't the mechanic repair the van?	26	86.7	30	100.0	3.28
8. Didn't the lion chase the tiger?	30	100.0	30	100.0	0
9. Wasn't the stone wall built by the kind husband?	29	96.7	30	100.0	0.72
10. Wasn't the rich uncle advised by the nice manager?	16	53.3	23	76.7	3.09
11. She has bought five large brown leather cases.	13	43.3	24	80.0	7.77°°
12. He has sold the long heavy grey shiny car.	11	36.7	16	53.3	1.36
13. She has washed plastic red small eight cups.	5	16.7	15	50.0	6.77°°
14. Not in a tree to the lake ran with.	8	26.7	13	43.3	1.48
15. Walk some by hard of clearly table very.	5	16.7	13	43.3	4.46°
16. The sky that the dream thought jumped cheaply.	14	46.7	26	86.7	9.92°°
17. The burglar that the police found escaped easily.	24	80.0	30	100.0	5.60°
18. The chair roughly painted the fire.	27	90.0	30	100.0	2.19
19. Wasn't the fat ceiling robbed by the tired pen?	16	53.3	28	93.3	11.27°°°
20. The man that the book read was interesting.	25	83.3	30	100.0	4.42°

SOURCE: Reprinted with permission of publishers from: Wiig, E. H., & Roach, M. A. Immediate recall of semantically varied "sentences" by learning-disabled adolescents. *Perceptual and Motor Skills*, 1975, **40**, 119-25.

NOTE: χ^2 = chi square.

*p < .05; **p < .01; ***p < .001.

rules, (2) contained correctly or incorrectly sequenced modifier strings, (3) consisted of a random word string, and (4) were syntactically complex (Table 7).

The responses by the learning disabled adolescents to the most discriminating sentences (2, 11, 13, 16, 19) were characterized by word omissions and substitutions, indicating inadequate recall of specific words. They also normalized deviant syntactic structure less frequently than the academically achieving adolescents, suggesting that they did not attempt to code the material in terms of linguistic structure. When the learning disabled adolescents substituted words, they were within class and similar to the substitutions made by dyslexic children during oral reading (Kolers, 1972). The findings suggested that the significant variables in the recall of sentences by learning disabled adolescents were semantic consistency and syntactic complexity. Their difficulties seem to reflect limitations in short-term memory, and deep structure and semantic interpretation, represented in long-term memory, appeared to facilitate auditory processing and recall.

Knowledge and Use of Morphology and Syntax

Learning disabled children have demonstrated deficits in the knowledge and use of English morphology (Vogel, 1974; Wiig, Semel, & Crouse, 1973). Wiig, Semel, and Crouse (1973) adapted Berko's test of morphology (Berko, 1958) and found that high-risk and learning disabled children shared problems in applying morphological rules to nonsense and real words. They shared significant deficits in forming the third person of verbs, possessives, and adjectival inflections when compared with age peers. In research with adult aphasics, Goodglass & Hunt (1958) established that the severity of aphasia was predictive of deficits in forming noun possessives. The inference can therefore be made that the knowledge of morphology relates directly to the language processing ability of the learning disabled child.

Verb Tense and Aspect

Clinical observations suggest a variety of other problems in sentence processing and comprehension by learning disabled youngsters. These include confusions between verb tenses and aspects. Learning disabled youngsters frequently demonstrate problems in distinguishing between the temporal aspects denoted by verb tenses. They may experience difficulties in distinguishing the nonpast aspects in *I walk* from the past aspects in *I walked* and *I have been walking* and the nonfuture aspects in *I walk* from the future aspects in *I will walk* and *I may walk*. Since sentences are expressed within a domain of time and space, the reference points used by the speaker and the listener become significant. If the temporal and spatial reference points are not shared by the speaker and the listener, messages may be totally confused by the learning disabled youngster.

Observation of learning disabled children often leaves the impression that the zero point of reference for the time domain, that is the *now*, is fluid. At times, their responses suggest that their zero reference point exists somewhere in the past or somewhere in the future. Examples that suggest a fluid point of time reference were given by two learning disabled children in the following statements: "Last Sunday I builded a plane, and then I finished it tomorrow," and "When I get twelve, I bees a grown-up." It appears that the *now* and *here* may not have been firmly established as the points against which these children measured and described events in time and space.

Learning disabled children may experience similar problems in differentiating among the temporal aspects when auxiliaries are added to denote distinctions within the past or future, as in *He has jumped, He had jumped, He will jump*, and *He would jump*. The subtle durational features denoted with the progressive aspects in verb phrases such as *was jumping, had been jumping, would have been jumping, will be jumping*, and *will have been jumping* are frequently overlooked by these youngsters. As a result, the progressive aspects of a verb may be confused with the present tense counterpart and *She walks* may be assumed to express the same meaning as *She is walking*.

Mood

Failure to comprehend distinctions in mood, that is, habitual aspects, inferences, or obligations, expressed by the auxiliaries *must, have to*, and *ought*, is also prevalent among learning disabled children. As a consequence, this type youngster may respond similarly to the sentences "I have to go to New York," "I must go to New York," and "I ought to go to New York." He may have similar problems in distinguishing between sentences such as "You will get the ball" and "You shall get the ball," indicating a lack of perception of the subtle differences in mood.

Learning disabled children and adolescents may also experience difficulties in processing and interpreting sentences in which tense, aspect, and mood are combined in verbs or verb forms. They frequently demonstrate problems in interpreting direct and indirect quotes such as "He said: 'I am reading' " and "He said he was reading." They may also have difficulties in differentiating between sentences such as "I will go to Boston tomorrow" and "I am going to Boston tomorrow," the latter expressing intent. The potentials for sentence comprehension problems of a similar nature are numerous in the English language. To experience the potential difficulties, consider the subtle differences as well as the similarities among the following sentences:

1. I will go to Boston tomorrow.
2. I will be going to Boston tomorrow.
3. I will probably go to Boston tomorrow.
4. I may be going to Boston tomorrow.
5. I think I will be going to Boston tomorrow.
6. I think I may go to Boston tomorrow.
7. I think I might go to Boston tomorrow.
8. I might go to Boston tomorrow.

Comprehension of Passive Sentences

Passive sentences are often misinterpreted by the learning disabled child. The interpretation of passive sentences seems to involve at least two steps: (1) processing of the surface structure, and (2) performing the required logical operations, that is, identifying and comparing subject-object relationships for semantic interpretation.

Clinical observations suggest that learning disabled youngsters comprehend irreversible passive sentences better than reversible ones. In an irreversible passive sentence such as "The ball was kicked by the boy," experience tells us that *boy* must be the subject of the action and *ball* the object since the latter is inanimate. In a reversible passive sentence such as "The girl was kicked by the boy," both the subject (boy) and the object (girl) have the potential to perform the act. The semantic constraints are therefore minimal and cannot serve to facilitate the required logical operations. The interpretation of the sentence depends upon knowledge of the syntactic transformation and adequate linguistic processing.

Research has substantiated that reversible passive sentences which contain proper nouns, for example, "Mary was followed by Joe," are significantly harder to understand for LD children and adolescents than for their academically achieving age peers (Wiig & Semel, 1973, 1974b). The problems encountered by the learning disabled youngster in interpreting passive sentences with proper nouns are considered to reflect (1) reduced ability to perform simultaneous analysis and synthesis of subject-object relationships, and (2) delays in cognitive and logical growth (Goodglass & Kaplan, 1972; Inhelder & Piaget, 1964; Luria, 1966; Piaget & Inhelder, 1969).

The clinical and formal observations of the order of difficulty experienced by learning disabled youngsters for passive sentences agree with observations by Slobin (1963, 1966) and Turner and Rommetveit (1967a, 1967b, 1968). The fact that mention of the actor may be deleted in English passive sentences such as "Mail is delivered every day" appears to cause further confusions for the learning disabled child. Typically, passive sentences in which the actor is not mentioned are interpreted in a concrete fashion, and abstract, indefinite aspects are overlooked. As a result, a sentence such as "Mail is delivered every day" may be interpreted to mean "I get mail every day."

Comprehension of Negation

The comprehension of negatives frequently poses problems for learning disabled children. They appear to experience difficulties in processing the surface structure and in logical processing for semantic interpretation. In an explicit negative the presence of the word *not* signifies that one of the expressed aspects must be deducted in a logical operation. Consider the sentences "The ball is not red. It is pink." In the first, a true negative sentence, the quality of the color *redness* must be subtracted from the attributes of the ball in question. The second, a true affirmative sentence, reestablishes the quality of color by stating that the ball is pink. In this example, the logical operations required are relatively simple because the true negative sentence is followed immediately by a true affirmative sentence and because *not* appears immediately preceding the attribute to be subtracted in the surface structure.

Mental Operations in Analyzing Negation

The mental operations involved in analyzing the structure of negatives and arriving at correct judgments have been discussed extensively by Wason and Johnson-Laird (1972). They demonstrated that negatives take longer time to verify than affirmative sentences, the difference being longer than half a second. The mental operations (algorithms) involved in verifying negatives were further delineated by Clark and his associates (Clark, 1974; Clark & Chase, 1972; Just & Carpenter, 1971). They established that when presented with a visual stimulus such as a plus placed above a star, a true affirmative (The plus is above the star) was processed in, on the average, 1,810 milliseconds. A false affirmative (The star is above the plus) required, on the average, an additional 187 milliseconds. A false explicit negative (The plus is not above the star) required 2,498 milliseconds, on the average, to provide time for reconciliation of the disparity introduced by the negative *not*. A true explicit negative (The star is not above the plus) required even longer time for processing and verification, on the average, 2,682 milliseconds. Inherent negatives, that is, sentences in which the negative aspect is conveyed by a prefix as in *uncover* and *undiscovered* or by the word itself as in *absent* and *forget*, were harder to process than their affirmative counterparts *(cover, discovered, present,* and *remember)*. They were, however, easier to process than their explicit negative counterparts *(not covered, not discovered, not present,* and *not remember)*.

Development of Comprehension

Developmental studies have considered the acquisition of negatives (Bloom, 1970; Brown, 1973; McNeill & McNeill, 1968; Schlesinger, 1971). Bloom (1970) distinguishes between three primary negative meanings: (1) nonexistence, (2) rejection, and (3) denial. She observed that the child's expressions of negation proceeded from nonexistence to rejection and denial, and that nonexistence was expressed by a negative operator with a nominal or predicate form in two-word utterances such as *no shoe, no more, shoe all gone,* and *shoe bye-bye.*

McNeill and McNeill (1968) distinguish between two additional dimensions, internal-external and entailment-nonentailment. In internal negations there is internal evidence for the statement as in "I don't want ice cream"; in external negations the evidence exists in the environment as in "Look, the glass didn't break." The distinction between entailment and nonentailment relates to whether or not the truth of an alternative proposition is part of the negation as in "The apple is not red, it is pink." Brown (1973) notes that the meaning of nonexistence may exist in all Stage I languages when semantic roles and grammatical relations develop.

Comprehension of Explicit Negatives

The ease with which explicit negatives are comprehended by learning disabled youngsters seems to relate to the ease with which the negated aspect can be identified. It seems to depend upon (1) the proximity and sequential

relationship between *not* and the negated aspect, (2) the saliency of the negated aspect, (3) the ability to process prosodic, suprasegmental features to
assist in the identification of the negated aspect, and (4) the complexity of the
logical operations required. As an example, the sentence "The ball is not on
the table" may be interpreted to mean somewhere other than *on* the table or
on something other than the table, depending upon the characteristics of the
prosodic features (pitch, stress, and juncture).

When we consider that learning disabled children frequently experience
problems in processing prosodic features (Vogel, 1974), it follows that the
ambiguities that exist in some explicit negatives may be hard to resolve.
Based on relationships between (1) the saliency of the negated aspect, (2) the
proximity and sequential relationship between *not* and the negated aspects,
and (3) the complexity of the logical operation, a tentative hierarchy of difficulty is suggested for the comprehension of some explicit negative statements
and questions (Table 8).

TABLE 8

Suggested Hierarchy of Difficulty of Comprehension of Explicit Negatives as a
Function of (1) Saliency of the Negated Aspect, (2) Proximity and Sequence
of the Negated Aspect, and (3) Logical Complexity

I. SALIENCY OF NEGATED ASPECT

1. The ball is not *red*.
2. The ball is not *round*.
3. The ball is not *jumping*.
4. The ball was not *hit*.

II. PROXIMITY AND SEQUENCE OF NEGATED ASPECT

1. The ball is not *on* the table. / The boy is not *walking* to the store.
2. The ball is not on the *table*. / The boy is not walking *to* the store.
3. The *ball* is not on the table. / The *boy* is not walking to the store.
4.   The boy is not walking to the *store*.

III. LOGICAL COMPLEXITY

1. This ball is not the *biggest*.
2. This ball is not *bigger than* that ball.
3. This is not the *girl's ball*.
4. Which item would you not *eat* for breakfast?
5. Which food would you not want to eat in the *winter*?
6. Which of these foods would you not *be able to purchase at a fruit stand*?

Comprehension of Linguistic Concepts

Relationships between two or more critical verbal elements are often expressed in linguistic concepts or logico-grammatical sentences. As an example, the sentence "I am my mother's daughter" expresses a familial, possessive relationship. This relationship can only be understood if the two

critical verbal elements *mother's daughter* are analyzed and synthesized simultaneously and compared logically (Goodglass & Kaplan, 1972; Luria, 1966). The comprehension of linguistic concepts has been related to abstraction and categorization ability (Lerner, 1971; Mecham et al., 1966), ability to perform simultaneous analysis and synthesis (Goodglass & Kaplan, 1972; Luria, 1966), and logical growth (Inhelder & Piaget, 1964; Piaget & Inhelder, 1969).

Types and Complexity of Linguistic Concepts

The English language contains a variety of linguistic concepts that may be expressed in syntactically simple or complex sentences. Among the linguistic concepts are sentences that express:

1. Comparative relationships (A watermelon is bigger than an apple.)
2. Passive relationships (The boy was brought by the lady.)
3. Possessive and familial relationships (My cousin Joe is my uncle's son.)
4. Spatial relationships (The dog is running in front of the house.)
5. Temporal relationships (Mary arrived before her mother.)

Examples of other linguistic concepts are:

6. Constructions with *if/then, either/or,* and *some* and *any.*
7. Statements of exception such as *all except* and *except for.*
8. Compound commands such as "*When I . . ., you . . .*
9. Multiple actions such as "Don't eat till you wash your hands" and "Pick up your pajamas before you go out."

The syntactic structure of linguistic concepts may vary from simple to complex. The same comparative relationship may be expressed in a simple sentence structure such as "Mary is bigger than Joan" or in a complex sentence structure such as "Yesterday I heard Mary say that she was bigger than Joan." While the logical comparison between the critical elements *Mary* and *Joan* is the same in the two sentences, the syntactic complexity of the second sentence complicates the abstraction of the elements and the simultaneous analysis and synthesis of the concept.

The logical complexity of linguistic concepts seems to relate to, among others, (1) the number of critical verbal elements to be compared, (2) whether or not the concept is true or false, and (3) whether or not the relationship is expressed in positive or in negative terms. It is generally easier to interpret linguistic concepts with two critical verbal elements than with three or more critical verbal elements. As a result, the concept "Mary is bigger than Joan" is easier to interpret than the concept "Mary is bigger than Joan but smaller than Jane." Most of the linguistic concepts discussed above may contain two or more critical verbal elements. Illustrative examples are temporal, spatial, and familial relationships such as "Mary came before Joan but after Jane," "Mary was in front of Joan but behind Jane," and "She is Mary's sister's mother-in-law."

A linguistic concept that expresses a true relationship is generally easier to process and interpret than a concept that contains a false statement. As a consequence, the question "Are watermelons bigger than apples?" is easier to answer than the question "Are apples bigger than watermelons?" Both of these linguistic concepts require a logical comparison that involves the ability to seriate according to size. The question "Are watermelons bigger than apples?" presents the elements in the correct sequence according to size, a fact which facilitates immediate verification. In contrast, the question "Are apples bigger than watermelons?" cannot be easily verified without independent formulation of the correct logical sequence according to size and subsequent comparison with the input. The formulation of a series according to size may require revisualization of the objects, broad knowledge of the concepts, and conceptualization, all of which may be impaired in some children with learning disabilities.

Linguistic concepts that are expressed in positive terms (*bigger than, warmer than, taller than*) are usually easier to interpret than concepts expressed in negative terms (*smaller than, colder than, shorter than*), an observation that agrees with findings by Clark, Carpenter, and Just (1973). As a result, it is easier to interpret and verify the question "Is Florida warmer than Maine?" than "Is Maine colder than Florida?" The natural tendency for people to express events and perceptions in positive terms appears to facilitate comprehension of the former question.

Development of Comprehension

Developmental data obtained from 210 children in the first through the eighth grades, using the *Wiig-Semel Test of Linguistic Concepts*, indicated significant increases in the comprehension of selected linguistic concepts during the age range from seven to eleven years (Wiig & Semel, 1974a). Thus, grade school children demonstrated increasing ability to interpret logico-grammatical sentences expressing comparative, passive, spatial, temporal, and familial relationships until about age eleven. Between ages eleven and thirteen their comprehension of these linguistic concepts remained stable (Table 9).

In relation to models of logical growth, the comprehension of logico-grammatical sentences improved throughout the concrete operational level of development (Inhelder & Piaget, 1964; Piaget & Inhelder, 1969). The stabilization in the comprehension of the linguistic concepts occurred during an age period that concurs with the period of normal transition from the concrete operational to the more abstract formal operational level of development.

The developmental data also suggested a hierarchy of difficulty for the linguistic concepts, which agrees with Piaget's model for logical growth. In the early grades (one through three) comparative relationships were most easily comprehended, followed in order of difficulty by passive, temporal, spatial, and familial relationships. Inhelder and Piaget (1964) and Piaget and Inhelder (1969) report that comparative relationships involve logical operations normally acquired at the preoperational level. Spatial and temporal relationships are considered to be based on logical operations acquired at the concrete operational level.

The comprehension of spatial relationships was stabilized at age ten while the comprehension of temporal relationships was stabilized about a year

TABLE 9

Correct responses to logico-grammatical sentences by 210 grade school
children by grade (nS = 30)

Relationship		Grade						
		1	2	3	4	5	6	7−8
Total test	M	26.30	34.90	37.13	41.06	45.40	46.97	46.27
	SD	4.99	4.76	6.14	3.99	3.86	2.06	2.00
Comparative	M	7.70	8.10	8.50	8.67	9.47	9.60	9.40
	SD	1.55	1.33	1.28	1.38	0.72	0.61	0.55
Passive	M	6.60	7.80	7.83	8.37	8.67	9.17	9.00
	SD	1.43	1.64	2.03	1.28	1.47	0.90	1.03
Temporal	M	6.50	6.53	6.77	7.60	8.73	9.07	8.73
	SD	1.50	1.83	1.75	1.33	1.41	0.82	0.99
Spatial	M	4.73	7.23	8.13	8.60	9.17	9.43	9.27
	SD	2.06	1.52	1.43	0.99	1.10	0.92	0.73
Familial	M	1.43	5.23	5.97	7.83	9.07	9.70	9.87
	SD	1.50	2.92	2.98	2.68	2.21	0.74	0.43

SOURCE: Reprinted with permission of publishers from: Wiig, E. H., & Semel, E.M.
Development of comprehension of logico-grammatical sentences by grade school
children. *Perceptual and Motor Skills*, 1974, **38**, 1331-34.

NOTE: nS = number of subjects at each grade level.

later, suggesting that linguistic concepts expressing spatial relationships are
established earlier in a developmental sequence than temporal relationships.
The comprehension of comparative relationships increased significantly between ages ten and eleven. This increase reflected improved comprehension
of concepts containing *darker than* and *heavier than*. The change also agrees
with models of logical growth since gradations in shade and weight tend to
be established later than gradations in size (Piaget & Inhelder, 1969). On the
verbal level, Sinclair-de-Zwart (1969) has reported that operational children
use more differentiated terms such as *wider, taller,* and *fatter* than do preoperational children.

The comprehension of familial relationships improved significantly during
two age periods. Linguistic concepts that contained logico-grammatical relationships with mother and father, for example, "What is another name for
your father's brother?" developed early between ages six and eight. Linguistic concepts involving aunt and uncle, for example, "What is another name
for your aunt's daughter?" developed about a year later. This sequence
agrees with observations by Inhelder and Piaget (1964) and Piaget and Inhelder (1969).

Comprehension Deficits

Learning disabled children have been observed to follow the same developmental sequence as randomly selected grade school children but to exhibit

significant delays in the acquisition of comprehension of selected linguistic concepts (Wiig & Semel, 1973). They demonstrated most errors in comprehending familial relationships, followed in decreasing order of difficulty by spatial relationships, temporal relationships between sequential events, passive relationships, and comparative relationships (Table 10). Research has suggested that these comprehension deficits may persist in an adolescent population with learning disabilities (Wiig & Semel, 1974b). The problems experienced by both learning disabled children and adolescents are considered to reflect impairments of abstraction, generalization and of simultaneous analysis and synthesis, and delays in logical growth (Goodglass & Kaplan, 1972; Inhelder & Piaget, 1964; Johnson & Myklebust, 1967; Luria, 1966; Mecham et al., 1966; Piaget & Inhelder, 1969).

TABLE 10

Mean number of comprehension errors for the logico-grammatical sentence test by 32 learning disabled and 16 achieving children

Subtest	Learning Disabled	Achievers	t
Total test	16.66	5.81	8.82 *
Comparative relationships	1.50	0.50	-
Passive relationships	2.56	1.44	-
Temporal relationships	3.13	1.75	-
Spatial relationships	4.70	1.56	-
Familial relationships	5.00	0.56	-

SOURCE: Reprinted with permission of publishers from: Wiig, E. H., & Semel, E. M. Comprehension of linguistic concepts requiring logical operations by learning disabled children. *Journal of Speech and Hearing Research*, 1973, **16**, 627-36.

*p < .001.

Goodglass and Kaplan (1972) have noted that the discrimination and interpretation of familial relationships depend entirely upon word order. Error responses by learning disabled children to linguistic concepts expressing familial relationships have suggested that one aspect of the concept, the last noun, assumes primary importance and that simultaneous analysis and synthesis may not occur (Wiig & Semel, 1973).

Learning disabled children demonstrated evidence of comprehending familial relationships at sensorimotor or preoperational levels (Wiig & Semel, 1973). Some assigned only proper names for family members. Others gave stereotyped substitutions or indications that they did not know or understand what was required of them. Their achieving age peers did not respond with proper names, and errors occurred only when the intended family member was *cousin*. Accordingly, their responses were considered to reflect performance at the higher, concrete operational level.

It was also observed that learning disabled children gave the largest number of correct responses to the linguistic concepts expressing comparative relationships. This finding concurs with an observation by Piaget and Inhelder (1969) that seriation of two nonverbal elements occurs early at the sensorimotor level of development. Their responses to passive constructions suggested that they reacted to the sequence of the critical verbal elements rather than to the syntactic structure, a finding which agrees with other observations of linguistic processing deficits associated with learning disabilities (Kirk, McCarthy, & Kirk, 1968; Minskoff, 1974; Rosenthal, 1970; Semel & Wiig, 1975; Vogel, 1974; Wiig & Roach, 1975). Learning disabled children also exhibited quantitative reductions in the comprehension of linguistic concepts expressing spatial and temporal relationships. These deficits are considered to reflect persisting preoperational cognitive and logical processes (Piaget & Inhelder, 1969). The observations have significant implications for the educational management of learning disabilities and suggest a need for cognitive training in association with psycholinguistic training.

Future Research

It is evident from the present review of auditory language processing deficits associated with learning disabilities that several of the areas discussed need to be investigated further. As examples, the comprehension of prepositions, negations, interrogatives, adjectives, and modifier strings by learning disabled children and adolescents merit further investigation. We should also consider the channel capacity (the amount of information that can be handled at one time) available to the learning disabled youngster and the number and the size of "chunks" which can be held in short-term memory, (Miller, 1956; Newell & Simon, 1972; Simon & Chase, 1974) and the relationships of channel and chunking capacity to the perceptual, linguistic, and logical processing abilities in learning disabilities.

References

Aten, J., & Davis, J. Disturbances in the perception of auditory sequence in children with minimal cerebral dysfuntion. *Journal of Speech and Hearing Disorders*, 1968, **11**, 236-45.

Bannatyne, A. *Language, reading, and learning disability*. Springfield, Ill.: Charles C Thomas, 1971.

Bender, L. Neuropsychiatric disturbances in dyslexia. In A. H. Keeney & V. T. Kenney (Eds.), *Dyslexia*. St. Louis: C. V. Mosby, 1968. Pp. 42-48.

Bender, L. Problems in conceptualization and communication in children with developmental alexia. In S. G. Sapir & A. C. Nitzburg (Eds.), *Children with learning problems*. New York: Brunner/Mazel, 1973. Pp. 528-48.

Berko, J. The child's learning of English morphology. *Word*, 1958, **14**, 150-77.

Birch, H. G. *Brain damage in children*. Philadelphia: Williams & Wilkins, 1964.

Birch, H. G., & Belmont, L. Auditory-visual integration in normal and retarded readers. *American Journal of Orthopsychiatry*, 1964, **34**, 852-61.

Birch, H. G., & Belmont, L. Auditory-visual integration, intelligence and reading ability in school children. *Perceptual and Motor Skills*, 1965, **20**, 295-305.

Birch, H. G., & Lefford, A. Intersensory development in children. *Monograph of the Society for Research in Child Development*, 1963, **28**, No. 5, (Serial No. 89).

Bloom, L. *Language development: form and function in emerging grammar*. Cambridge: M.I.T. Press, 1970.

Blumenthal, A. L. Prompted recall of sentences. *Journal of Verbal Learning and Verbal Behavior*, 1967, **6**, 203-6.

Blumenthal, A. L., & Boakes, R. Prompted recall of sentences. *Journal of Verbal Learning and Verbal Behavior*, 1967, **6**, 674-76.

Brown, R. *A first language: the early stages*. Cambridge: Harvard University Press, 1973.

Chalfant, J. C., & Scheffelin, M. A. *Central processing dysfunctions in children*. Bethesda, Md.: National Institute of Neurological Diseases and Stroke, Monograph No. 9, 1969.

Clark, H. H. The power of positive speaking. *Psychology Today*, 1974, **8**, (4), 102-11.

Clark, H. H., Carpenter, P. A., & Just, M. A. On the meeting of semantics and perception. In W. G. Chase (Ed.), *Visual Information Processing*. New York: Academic Press, 1973. Pp. 311-81.

Clark, H. H., & Chase, W. G. On the process of comparing sentences against pictures. *Cognitive Psychology*, 1972, **3**, 472-517.

Deese, J. *The structure of associations in language and thought*. Baltimore: Johns Hopkins Press, 1965.

de Hirsch, K., Jansky, J., & Langford, W. *Predicting reading failure*. New York: Harper & Row, 1966.

Dunn, L. M. *Peabody picture vocabulary test*. Circle Pines, Minn.: American Guidance Service, 1965.

Farnham-Diggory, S. Symbol and synthesis in experimental reading. *Child Development*, 1967, **38**, 223-31.

Flowers, A., & Costello, M. R. *Tests of central auditory abilities*. Dearborn, Mich.: Perceptual Learning Systems, 1970.

Goodglass, H., & Hunt, J. Grammatical complexity and aphasic speech. *Word*, 1958, **14**, 197-207.

Goodglass, H., & Kaplan, E. *The assessment of aphasia and related disorders*. Philadelphia: Lea & Febiger, 1972.

Hammill, D. D., & Bartel, N. R. *Teaching children with learning and behavior problems*. Boston: Allyn & Bacon, 1975.

Inhelder, B., & Piaget, J. *The early growth of logic in the child*. New York: W. W. Norton, 1964.

Jakobson, R., Fant, G. M., & Halle, M. *Preliminaries to speech analysis*. Cambridge: Acoustics Laboratory, M. I. T., Technical Report No. 13, 1952.

Johnson, D. J. The language continuum. *Bulletin of the Orton Society*, 1968, **18**, 1-11.

Johnson, D. J., & Myklebust, H. R. *Learning disabilities: educational principles and practices*. New York: Grune & Stratton, 1967.

Just, M. A., & Carpenter, P. A. Comprehension of negation with quantification. *Journal of Verbal Learning and Verbal Behavior*, 1971, **10**, 244-53.

Kirk, S. A., McCarthy, J. J., & Kirk, W. D. *Illinois test of psycholinguistic ability*. (Rev. ed.) Urbana: University of Illinois Press, 1968.

Kolers, P. A. Experiments in reading. *Scientific American*, 1972, **227**, 84-91.

Lasky, E. Z., & Tobin, H. Linguistic and nonlinguistic competing messages effect. *Journal of Learning Disabilities*, 1973, **6**, 243-50.

Lenneberg, E. H. Biological aspects of language. In G. A. Miller (Ed.), *Communication, language and meaning*. New York: Basic Books, 1973. Pp. 49-60.

Lerner, J. *Children with learning disabilities*. Boston: Houghton Mifflin Co., 1971.

Luria, A. R. *Higher cortical functions in man*. New York: Basic Books, 1966.

Lyons, J. *Introduction to theoretical linguistics*. Cambridge: Cambridge University Press, 1971.

McGrady, H. J., & Olson, D. A. Visual and auditory learning processes in normal children and children with learning disabilities. *Exceptional Children*, 1970, **36**, 581-89.

McNeill, D., & McNeill, N. B. What does a child mean when he says 'no'? In E. M. Zale (Ed.), *Language and language behavior*. New York: Appleton-Century Crofts, 1968. Pp. 51-62.

Masland, M. W., & Case, L. Limitation of auditory memory as a factor in delayed language development. Paper presented at the International Association for Logopedics and Phoniatrics, Vienna, August, 1965.

Mecham, M. J., Berko, M. J., Berko, F. G., & Palmer, M. F. *Communication training in childhood brain damage*. Springfield, Ill.: Charles C Thomas, 1966.

Meier, J. H. Prevalence and characteristics of learning disabilities found in second grade children. *Journal of Learning Disabilities*, 1971, **4**, 1-16.

Menyuk, P., & Looney, P. A problem of language disorder: length versus structure. *Journal of Speech and Hearing Research,* 1972, **15**, 264-79. (a)

Menyuk, P., & Looney, P. Relationships between components of the grammar in language disorders. *Journal of Speech and Hearing Research,* 1972, **15**, 395-406. (b)

Miller, G. A. The magical number seven, plus or minus two. *Psychological Review,* 1956, **63**, 81-97.

Miller, G. A., & Chomsky, N. Finitary models of language users. In R. D. Luce, R. R. Bush, & E. Galatner (Eds.), *Handbook of mathematical psychology.* Vol. 2. New York: John Wiley & Sons, 1963. Pp. 419-91.

Miller, G. A., & Isard, S. Free recall of self-embedded English sentences. *Information and Control,* 1964, **7**, 292-303.

Miller, G. A., & Nicely, P. E. An analysis of perceptual confusions among some English consonants. *Journal of the Acoustical Society of America,* 1955, **27**, 338-52.

Minskoff, E. H. Remediating auditory-verbal learning disabilities: the role of questions in teacher-pupil interaction. *Journal of Learning Disabilities,* 1974, **7**, 406-13.

Myers, P. I., & Hammill, D. D. *Methods for learning disorders.* New York: John Wiley & Sons, 1969.

Myklebust, H. R. Learning disorders: psychoneurological disturbances in childhood. *Rehabilitation Literature,* 1964, **25**, 354-60.

Newcombe, F., & Marshall, J. C. Immediate recall of sentences by subjects with unilateral cerebral lesions. *Neuropsychologia,* 1967, **5**, 329-34.

Newell, A., & Simon, H. A. *Human problem solving.* Englewood Cliffs, N.J.: Prentice—Hall, 1972.

Orton, S. T. *Reading, writing, and speech problems in children.* New York: Norton, 1937.

Piaget, J., & Inhelder, B. *The psychology of the child.* New York: Basic Books, 1969.

Rosenthal, J. H. A preliminary psycholinguistic study of children with learning disabilities. *Journal of Learning Disabilities,* 1970, **3**, 391-95.

Saporta, S. Frequency of consonant clusters. *Language,* 1955, **31**, 25-30.

Savin, H., & Perchonock, E. Grammatical structure and the immediate recall of English sentences. *Journal of Verbal Learning and Verbal Behavior,* 1965, **4**, 348-53.

Schlesinger, I. M. Production of utterances and language acquisition. In D. I. Slobin (Ed.), *The ontogenesis of grammar.* New York: Academic Press, 1971. Pp. 63-101.

Semel, E. M., & Wiig, E. H. Comprehension of syntactic structures and critical verbal elements by children with learning disabilities. *Journal of Learning Disabilities,* 1975, **8**, 53-58.

Simon, H. A., & Chase, W. G. Skill in chess. *American Scientist,* 1973, **61**, 394-403.

Sinclair-de-Zwart, H. Developmental psycholinguistics. In D. Elkind & J. H. Flavell (Eds.), *Studies in cognitive development: essays in honor of Jean Piaget.* New York: Oxford University Press, 1969. Pp. 315-36.

Slobin, D. I. Grammatical transformations in childhood and adulthood. Doctoral dissertation, Harvard University, 1963.

Slobin, D. I. Grammatical transformations in childhood and adulthood. *Journal of Verbal Learning and Verbal Behavior*, 1966, **5**, 219-27.

Slobin, D. I. *Psycholinguistics*. Glenview, Ill.: Scott Foresman & Co., 1971.

Spencer, E. M. Investigations of the maturation of various facets of auditory perception in preschool children. Doctoral dissertation, Northwestern University, 1959.

Stamback, M. Le probleme du rhythme dans le development de l'enfant et dans les dyslexies d'evolution. *Enfance*, 1951, **4**, 480-502.

Strauss, A. A., & Kephart, N. C. *Psychopathology and the education of the brain—injured child*. New York: Grune & Stratton, 1955.

Turner, E. A., & Rommetveit, R. The acquisition of sentence voice and reversibility. *Child Development*, 1967, **38**, 649-60. (a)

Turner, E. A., & Rommetveit, R. Experimental manipulation of the production of active and passive voice in children. *Language and Speech*, 1967, **10**, 169-80. (b)

Turner, E. A., & Rommetveit, R. Focus of attention in recall of active and passive sentences. *Journal of Verbal Learning and Verbal Behavior*, 1968, **7**, 543-48.

Turton, L. Status of prepositions in the verbal and nonverbal response patterns of children during third and fourth years of life. Unpublished doctoral dissertation, University of Kansas, 1966.

Vogel, S. A. Syntactic abilities in normal and dyslexic children. *Journal of Learning Disabilities*, 1974, **7**, 47-53.

Wason, P. C., & Johnson-Laird, P. N. *Psychology of reasoning: structure and content*. London: Batsford, 1972.

Wiig, E. H., & Roach, M. A. Immediate recall of semantically varied "sentences" by learning-disabled adolescents. *Perceptual and Motor Skills*, 1975, **40**, 119-25.

Wiig, E. H., & Semel, E. M. Comparison and analysis of morphological patterns in children with learning disabilities: research setting and remediation. Paper presented at the Annual Convention of the American Speech & Hearing Association, San Francisco, 1972.

Wiig, E. H., & Semel, E. M. Comprehension of linguistic concepts requiring logical operations by learning disabled children. *Journal of Speech and Hearing Research*, 1973, **16**, 627-36.

Wiig, E. H., & Semel, E. M. Development of comprehension and logico—grammatical sentences by grade school children. *Perceptual and Motor Skills*, 1974, **38**, 171-76. (a)

Wiig, E. H., & Semel, E. M. Logico-grammatical sentence comprehension by learning disabled adolescents. *Perceptual and Motor Skills*, 1974, **38**, 1331-34. (b)

Wiig, E. H., & Semel, E. M. Productive language abilities in learning disabled adolescents. *Journal of Learning Disabilities*, 1975, **8**, 578-86.

Wiig, E. H., Semel, E. M., & Crouse, M. A. The use of morphology by high-risk and learning disabled children. *Journal of Learning Disabilities*, 1973, **6**, 457-65.

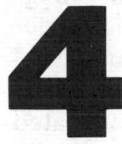

Assessing Auditory Sensation and Perception

Overview

This chapter presents a series of clinical questions designed to assist the educator-clinician in determining abilities and areas to be assessed and to aid the diagnostician in selecting tests for diagnosis. Test characteristics and factors relevant to the selection of a specific test or test battery are discussed to assist the educator-clinician in evaluating assets and limitations of the tests selected for review.

An overview of audiological procedures relevant to the assessment of sensation of auditory stimuli is presented to familiarize the educator-clinician with the variety and potential of assessment procedures available to the audiologist for differential diagnosis and with the scope of the competencies and responsibilities of the certified audiologist. Among audiological procedures reviewed are (1) standard measures of auditory acuity, (2) sound localization, and (3) speech reception and discrimination.

The chapter also presents an extensive review of clinical-educational methods for assessing auditory-perceptual abilities. The tests selected for review are categorized according to whether they evaluate primarily (1) attention, (2) figure-ground, (3) discrimination of nonverbal auditory stimuli, (4) discrimination of phonemes, (5) synthesis, or (6) segmentation and syllabication. Measures of auditory perception seem of limited value in predicting reading (Hammill & Larsen, 1974). The current practice of assessing auditory perception as part of the differential diagnosis of language disabilities is, however, supported strongly by recent evidence that sentence processing occurs simultaneously at all available levels of analysis and that "information at each level can constrain and guide simultaneous processing at other levels" (Marslen-Wilson, 1975).

A Brief View of Assessment Procedures

The previous chapters have described the interactions between language processing skills and the complexity of the auditory language processing deficits that may be encountered in learning disabilities. An appropriate

program for the clinical and educational management of language processing deficits depends upon identification of liabilities as well as assets.

In-depth analysis of the nature and extent of language deficits in youngsters with learning disabilities requires attention to the following major
areas: (1) sensory processing of auditory input, (2) perceptual processing, (3) linguistic processing, and (4) cognitive-semantic processing. Within each of these areas several component skills must be evaluated
in order to formulate a profile of assets and deficits, indicating the use of a
comprehensive test battery rather than a single instrument.

The examiner responsible for the diagnostic evaluation may find it helpful to formulate a set of general questions to be answered by the test results. These questions may assist in test selection as well as in generating
a remediation strategy. They should cover a broad range of characteristic
language processing problems and be applicable to a wide age range. This
implies that some questions would be relevant to children in the early
grades but not to adolescents. Others may be appropriate for children in
the middle grades but not for kindergarteners or preschoolers. With these
limitations in mind, the following suggested list of clinical questions is
organized to reflect various levels of language processing and their component skills. It is the examiner's responsibility to select those questions
that may assist him in designing an appropriate assessment battery for an
individual child or for a group of children. Page or chapter references to
discussions of relevant tests are indicated in parentheses.

I. Sensory processing (pp. 81-84)
   A. Are the auditory thresholds for hearing low-frequency and
      high-frequency pure tones adequate?
   B. Are the auditory thresholds for hearing speech adequate?

II. Auditory-perceptual processing (pp. 85-98; 82-83; chapter 9)
   A. Attention (pp. 87-88)
      1. Can the child sustain auditory attention over reasonable
         periods of time? If so, under what conditions?
      2. Is the child's auditory attention distracted by other stimuli
         (auditory or visual)?
      3. Do novel stimuli (auditory or visual) assist in focusing the
         child's attention?
   B. Localization (pp. 82-83)
      1. Does the child readily localize environmental sounds (turn
         his head in the direction of the sound source)?
      2. Does the child readily localize the source of speech sounds
         in the environment?
   C. Figure-ground (pp. 88-90)
      1. Can the child discern environmental sounds in the presence
         of competing auditory stimuli?
      2. Can the child distinguish a speaker in the presence of com-
         peting messages?

D. Discrimination of nonverbal stimuli (pp. 90-91)
   1. Can the child discriminate differences in the frequency (pitch), intensity (loudness), rhythm, duration, and timbre (the quality given to a sound by its overtones) of tonal pairs?
E. Discrimination of verbal stimuli (pp. 91-95)
   1. Can the child discriminate specific phonemes in words differing by only one speech sound, such as *cat* and *sat*?
   2. Does the child have difficulty discriminating between intial consonants, final consonants, medial consonants, vowels, and/or consonant blends?
   3. Can the child identify consonants, vowels, and blends in the initial, final, or medial positions of words?
   4. Can the child discriminate words against a background of noise or competing messages?
F. Sequencing (chapter 9)
   1. Does the child retain the sequence in a series of auditory stimuli consisting of digits, phonemes, words (related and unrelated), phrases and syntactic structures, and sentences?
   2. Can the child recall and repeat series of auditory stimuli consisting of the foregoing elements?
   3. Can the child follow a series of oral directions of increasing length and complexity?
G. Synthesis: resistance to distortion (pp. 96-98)
   1. Can the child form words out of separated, articulated phonemes?
   2. Can the child predict and formulate words when phonemes or syllables are missing?
H. Segmentation and syllabication (p. 98)
   1. Can the child identify the separate words that are parts of compound words?
   2. Can the child identify the number of syllables in words of increasing length?
   3. Can the child identify the position of a stressed syllable in multi-syllabic words?
   4. Can the child identify the initial and final syllables of multi-syllabic words?
   5. Can the child discriminate between stressed and unstressed syllables?
   6. Can the child identify and discriminate among meaningful prefixes and suffixes in complex words?
   7. Can the child discriminate among and identify inflectional suffixes? (Comparative -er; superlative -est; past tense -d, -t, -id, etc.)
   8. Can the child identify derivational suffixes? (Noun derivation -er, -or, -tion, -ion; adverb derivation -ly, -y, etc.)

III. Cognitive-semantic processing (pp. 104-18)
    A. Semantic units (pp. 105-9)
        1. Does the child comprehend selected vocabulary items such as verbs, adjectives, prepositions, pronouns, etc.?
        2. Does the child comprehend vocabulary items requiring classification such as multiple-meaning words, antonyms, synonyms, homonyms?
        3. Can the child grasp shades of meaning between selected vocabulary items such as laughing, smiling, giggling, etc.?
        4. Can the child comprehend selected vocabulary items in critical word sequences such as show me the kitten, show me the kitten on the mat, show me the kitten on the mat by the window?
    B. Semantic classes (pp. 109-10)
        1. Can the child classify selected vocabulary items (concepts) in appropriate semantic categories?
        2. Can the child identify vocabulary items (concepts) that do not belong to a given semantic category?
        3. Can the child comprehend linguistic concepts requiring logical operations such as comparative sentences, if-then constructions, etc.?
    C. Semantic relations (pp. 110-14)
        1. Can the child process and comprehend verbal analogies expressing logical relationships between words and concepts?
        2. Can the child process and comprehend sentences that express logical relationships (comparative, passive, spatial, temporal, or familial) between words or elements?
        3. Can the child process and comprehend sentences containing linguistic concepts of inclusion-exclusion (*some, none, all, any, all except,* etc.) or concepts such as if/then, either/or, because, or when/then?
    D. Semantic systems (pp. 114-15)
        1. Can the child discern the underlying structure of a verbal problem?
        2. Can the child detect errors, inconsistencies, absurdities, and ambiguities in sentences and stories?
    E. Semantic transformations (pp. 115-16)
        1. Can the child grasp and identify similarities and differences between the meanings of selected (words) concepts?
        2. Does the child have difficulty understanding idioms, metaphors, similes, and/or proverbs?
    F. Semantic implications (pp. 116-18)
        1. Can the child predict possible outcomes?
        2. Can the child identify expressed cause-effect relationships?
        3. Can the child identify cause-effect relationships by inference?
        4. Can the child identify fallacies in cause-effect and premise-conclusion arguments?

IV. Linguistic processing (pp. 119-26)
   A. Phonology (*See* Discrimination of verbal stimuli)
   B. Morphology (pp. 119-21)
      1. Can the child identify and differentiate morphological struc-
         tures? (*See* Segmentation and syllabication 1, 6, 7, 8)
   C. Syntax (pp. 121-25)
      1. Can the child differentiate grammatical phrases, clauses, and
         sentences from those that are grammatically incorrect or
         incomplete?
      2. Can the child discriminate among the various sentence trans-
         formations (active, declarative, interrogative, passive declar-
         ative, negative, etc.)?

Factors Relevant to Test Selection

The selection of a comprehensive test battery to answer a set of the clinical questions will depend upon a variety of factors such as (1) content
validity, (2) reliability, (3) efficiency and economy of administration and scoring, (4) task analysis, and (5) age level.

1. *Content validity.* A variety of tests designed to assess a general ability such as learning aptitude or psycholinguistic ability contain a
   variety of subtests. Each of these may assess a different component
   skill. The content of a test should focus on the specific skill that the
   examiner wishes to probe. The skill or skills evaluated by a specific
   test may or may not be reflected in the name of the test.
2. *Reliability.* The examiner of a child's language abilities is interested
   in obtaining reliable and consistent test results from one test to the
   next. When selecting a formal test, the examiner should therefore
   select the test with the highest reliability, all other things being
   equal. There are several types of reliability measures that reflect the
   consistency of test results. Measures of *test-retest reliability* indicate
   the consistency of the results when a child or a group of children are
   given the same test twice by the same or a different examiner over a
   period of time. *Split-half reliability* measures reflect the internal
   consistency of a test and compare the results obtained on one half of
   the test with those obtained on the other half.
      In evaluating the clinical significance of a test-retest reliability, the
   sample size, the level of significance, and the size of the correlation
   must be considered. For experimental tests using relatively small
   samples, reliability coefficients above .70 with significance levels at
   or smaller than .05 would indicate acceptable consistency.
3. *Efficiency and economy of administration and scoring.* The time
   demand of a test or subtest will influence its usefulness. Given a limited time period for assessment, the examiner may want to screen
   performances across various modalities and levels of processing.
   In-depth analysis using extensive and time consuming tests may be
   feasible only in already identified deficit areas. The time required for
   scoring similarly influences test utility. The efficiency and economy

of a test may also be determined by the level of training required to administer the test.

Most of the tests providing valuable information in assessing a child's language abilities should be administered by a trained examiner. Some tests may be administered only by psychologists, others only by speech pathologists, still others by the remedial reading specialist, and yet others only by the audiologist, the school counselor, or the occupational therapist. In order to adequately interact for the benefit of the child, the person directly responsible for the educational management of the child should, however, be familiar with the tests administered, their interpretation, and the implications of the results for the implementation of effective remedial strategies. Professional ethics should dictate that the person who is best trained in the administration and interpretation of a specific test be responsible for its administration.

4. *Task analysis.* The tasks required should be carefully analyzed to identify the modalities and processes involved, important aspects for planning intervention strategies. A task analysis should consider the following variables:
    a. Modality of input
    b. Response modality
    c. Level of processing required (sensation, perception, linguistic, cognitive-semantic, or combinations of these)
    d. Type of sensory integration (intersensory or intrasensory)

A comprehensive test battery should contain a proportionate number of subtests to tap intrasensory (within the same modality) as well as intersensory (across two modalities) functions. You should also consider the format of the items to determine whether they require recognition (alternate-choice, true-false, or multiple-choice responses) or recall (verbatim recall, completion, or recall of ideas or events). The format will determine the relative number of processes tapped and the probability of obtaining a correct response. As an example, verbatim recall of complex sentences taps perceptual processing, linguistic processing, and auditory memory, among others. Recognition of a spoken sentence in a written alternate-choice format reduces the influence of auditory memory and increases the probability of a correct response, provided there is adequate reading ability.

5. *Age level.* The age range for which a test may be appropriate for learning disabled children may not coincide with the age range for which it was standardized on normally developing children. Research suggests that certain language tests such as the *Assessment of Children's Language Comprehension* (Foster, Giddan, & Stark, 1972), the *Northwestern Syntax Screening Test* (Lee, 1969), and the *Wiig-Semel Test of Linguistic Concepts* (Wiig & Semel, 1974a) may reveal deficits in learning disabled children at age levels above that for which they were standardized (Semel & Wiig, 1975; Wiig & Semel, 1974a, 1974b). It may also be difficult to locate tests that

evaluate desired skills and are standardized for the appropriate age levels.

Diagnostic tests that differentiate performances within a relatively narrow age range (from three to eight years) within the normal population may be expected to cover a similarly narrow or only slightly wider age range (from three to eleven years) in a learning disabled population. Similarly, tests that do not differentiate between performances at relatively short time intervals (three to six months) would be expected to be equally insensitive to performance changes and differences among language and learning disabled children.

The most relevant language evaluation is one in which specific questions have been posed about a child's assets and deficits by both parents and teachers. This permits the examiner to select appropriate formal test procedures and to interpret findings to provide answers. When formal tests are not available, informal techniques may be developed. Other factors, such as age, attention-span and reading ability of the child, and time of day of the evaluation, will need to be considered when selecting a test battery.

The following sections will discuss formal tests which may assist in evaluating the language processing abilities of learning disabled children and adolescents.

Assessment of Auditory Sensitivity

The auditory sensitivity of language disabled children and adolescents must be established before higher level auditory processing abilities can be meaningfully evaluated. Testing of auditory acuity requires accurate control of the acoustic stimuli, monitoring of the listener, and detailed measurement of the responses to the auditory input. This type of evaluation is best performed by an audiologist trained in the administration and interpretation of a wide range of auditory tests of sensation and perception. A detailed discussion of audiological evaluations (instrumentation, techniques, and interpretation) will not be presented here. The interested reader can obtain this information from reference works by Davis and Silverman (1970), Jerger (1963, 1973), Katz (1972), Newby (1972), and O'Neill and Oyer (1966), among others.

The Committee on Rehabilitative Audiology of the American Speech and Hearing Association has recently emphasized the scope of the competencies and responsibilities of the certified audiologist by stating that audiological evaluation should include:

(1) assessment of auditory sensitivity and dynamic range; (2) assessment of listening behavior, including descriptions of auditory attention, auditory awareness, speech perception in quiet and in the presence of competing messages, perception of connected speech, determination of the temporal capacities for speech comprehension, auditory closure, sequencing, memory span and retrieval, and definition of effective distance for auditory reception, (3) evaluation of phonologic, morphologic, syntactic, and semantic language abilities, and (4) gathering of functional evidence related to the anatomic site of pathology. [ASHA, 1974, p. 69]

While some of the areas of functioning listed above may be equally well assessed by a number of trained professionals, the evaluation of the sensitivity of auditory stimuli by the language disabled youngster is the responsibility of the audiologist. Among the several measures available to the audiologist for establishing the sensory and perceptual capacities of the auditory system are (1) thresholds for the awareness of sounds, (2) standard pure-tone thresholds, (3) sound localization, (4) identification of sound sources, (5) speech reception thresholds, and (6) speech discrimination scores. The advantage of obtaining these measures from an audiological assessment relate to the audiologist's control of stimulus characteristics and contexts such as frequency, intensity, duration, masking, and so forth.

Thresholds for the Awareness of Sound

Awareness of sound is the lowest level of response to auditory stimuli. The audiologist can employ a variety of auditory stimuli with measurable characteristics such as frequency and intensity to establish the threshold, that is, the intensity level required for sound detection. Among the possible familiar auditory stimuli are environmental and animal sounds, noisemakers, speech, and music. Among possible relatively unfamiliar acoustic stimuli are pure tones, "white" noise, and narrow-band noise.

Standard Pure-Tone Thresholds

The standard evaluation of auditory acuity uses pure tones presented through earphones at octave points in the frequency range from 250 to 8,000 Hz (cycles per second). The thresholds obtained by air conduction, using earphones, are compared against normative data and reported in the form of an audiogram, a chart in which the intensity levels required for the identification of the presence of pure tones are plotted against their frequencies.

The air-conduction thresholds are generally corroborated by bone—conduction thresholds obtained by placing a bone-conduction vibrator on the forehead or behind the ear. Comparison between air- and bone-conduction thresholds permits diagnosis of the type of loss as a *conduction loss* with middle-ear involvement or as a *sensory loss* with involvement of the sensory mechanisms and auditory pathways. This differential diagnosis is especially important for children in the elementary grades. Many learning disabled children have been reported to be afflicted with upper-respiratory and middle-ear problems, often resulting in fluctuating hearing losses (Katz & Illmer, 1972; Wunderlich, 1970). Evidence of a conduction loss associated with learning disabilities warrants medical attention to alleviate the situation and prevent future occurrences. Without medical attention, efforts at remedial intervention for auditory perception and language comprehension deficits may be futile.

Sound Localization

Sound localization measures reflect one aspect of the auditory-perceptual processing skills. The audiologist generally has an ideal environment at his disposal for the assessment of aspects of auditory perception. The testing environment is controlled for noise, and auditory stimuli may be presented to the subject either via earphones or in free-field with speakers located at different angles in relation to the listener. This latter plan allows the audiologist to evaluate sound localization abilities. The acoustic stimuli selected for localization may be familiar or unfamiliar. Sound localization ability may be assessed by noting subtle responses such as body movements, head turning, or eye movement towards the sound source or by requiring the listener to point towards the source.

Sound localization depends upon sensory integrity and central integration. The problems learning disabled children may encounter in localizing sounds are suggestive of deficient central integration and binaural summation. This relationship has been discussed by Bannatyne (1971) and Flowers, Costello, and Small, (1970). Bocca and others (1955) reported asymmetric articulation (speech discrimination) scores for distorted speech in some patients with brain tumors. Bocca (1955) and Calearo (1957) also observed that binaural summation did not occur when there was impairment of the cortical auditory area (temporal lobe). Jerger (1960) further observed that in order to balance loudness in the ipsilateral (side of lesion) ear in cases with temporal lobe lesions, more intensity was needed in the contralateral (opposite side of lesion) ear.

Matzker (1959) has suggested a method for assessing central integration and binaural summation. A succession of pure tones is transmitted to the ears, but they are introduced with a difference in the arrival time at each ear. Central lesions resulted in lateralization difficulties.

Clinical procedures for evaluating sound localization ability in free-field have been described by, among others, Bergman (1957), Bienvenue and Siegenthaler (1974), Link and Lenhart (1966), Nordlund (1964), Sanchez-Longo, Forster, and Auth (1957), and Zabrewski (1962). Dichotic listening procedures may be used as a means to infer which of the two cerebral hemispheres is dominant in processing symbolic and nonsymbolic auditory material. Procedures have been described by Broadbent (1954), Kimura (1963), Shankweiler and Studdert-Kennedy (1967), and Studdert-Kennedy and Shankweiler (1970), among others.

Identification of Sound Sources

The ability to associate environmental sounds with their sources may be evaluated in free-field or using headphones. The subject may be asked to associate familiar sounds with objects, animals, or pictures or to name the sound source. There are no standardized audiological tests for sound source identification. The test procedures and results and their interpretation will therefore depend upon the ingenuity and experience of the audiologist.

Speech Reception and Discrimination

Speech reception thresholds (the intensity levels at which 50% of selected verbal stimuli are perceived correctly) are generally established separately for each ear. A threshold may be established in free-field as a means of comparison. The speech stimuli may be presented against controlled, competing backgrounds of noise to assess the effects of masking on speech reception. The auditory stimuli generally used to establish speech reception thresholds are a recorded word list of spondees (combinations of two monosyllables such as *blackboard*). The subject is usually required to repeat the stimuli.

Speech discrimination measures are generally obtained using phonetically balanced, monosyllabic words (the distribution of speech sounds approximates the distribution in conversational American English). These words are presented well above threshold with or without masking (competing noise). The subject is required to repeat each word, and the percentage of words repeated correctly reflects speech discrimination ability. The speech discrimination scores reported by the audiologist in quiet and with noise may be used to corroborate other measures of speech discrimination obtained by the educator to assess auditory-perceptual abilities in language disabled youngsters. Among other relevant diagnostic procedures are the dichotic listening tasks that assess central auditory abilities (central integration and binaural summation).

Hennebert (1964) has reported findings indicating that dyslexic children differ from deaf and normal children in the speed with which they recognize undistorted words in the two ears. Witelson (1962) observed that children with learning problems experienced great difficulty in keeping two different auditory stimuli separate in a dichotic listening task. In a similar vein, Flowers (1964) and Flowers and Costello (1965) established significant relationships between central auditory abilities, phonic skills, and reading achievement in third graders.

Conners, Kramer, and Guerra (1969) observed significant differences between learning disabled children and their controls when they used a competing message task in dichotic listening. They concluded that "auditory tasks place the heaviest demand on attention, for they are temporally ordered, so that the subject does not have the option of reviewing the input, as he does with visual materials."

Katz and Illmer (1972), using the *Staggered Spondaic Word Test* (SSW) (Katz, 1962, 1968), have reported three patterns obtained in children with learning disabilities. The first pattern is indicative of a unilateral problem, suggesting "a severe dysfunction in auditory reception." The second pattern suggests problems in auditory attention. Children exhibiting this pattern may improve as a result of time (maturation), use of medication, or "added motivation." The third pattern, termed the A pattern, is generally associated with severe reading and spelling problems. In this pattern, the performance is normal for items presented first to the left ear while a large number of errors occur on items presented first to the right ear, the ear that is contralateral to the dominant left hemisphere. Katz and Illmer (1972) report that electroencephalogram (EEG) results suggest involvement of the left cerebral hemisphere with dysfunction in the area posterior to the primary auditory reception center, the tempero-occipital area. Morrill (1969) reported similar findings, suggesting that the SSW may be useful in the differential diagnosis of children and adolescents with language disabilities.

Assessment of Auditory-Perceptual Processing

The methods employed to assess auditory-perceptual abilities vary depending upon the age level of the person or population to be evaluated. There are three critical age groups for which assessment procedures are needed: (1) the preschool and early grades, (2) the middle grades, and (3) the junior-high and high-school ages. Current tests of auditory perception appear to have focused primarily on the two younger age groups, disregarding the difficulties that may be encountered by the older group.

Tests of auditory perception designed for the preschool and early and middle grades seem to reflect one of three orientations for their design: speech sound discrimination, segmentation and syllabication, and blending of sounds in words. The stimulus-response characteristics of these tests reflect a heavy emphasis on a combined auditory-visual (pictorial) input followed by a visual-motor or a same-different response.

Evaluation procedures for the middle grades, on the other hand, contain items assessing auditory skills related to the decoding skills for reading. The stimuli may be spoken words with or without pictorial choices, or words with associated printed-word choices. The responses required may be same-different judgments or identification of pictorial or printed-word units. The tests appear to reflect the background and orientation of their designers rather than comprehensive models of the nature and scope of the difficulties that may be observed in language disabled children.

At the high-school level, tests that tap aspects of auditory perception focus primarily on the auditory memory for semantic units (words) and on the ability to perceive and formulate implications and give evaluative responses to verbal materials on the basis of semantic evaluation. The last two skills reflect primarily cognitive-semantic abilities. The responses are generally of a multiple-choice, printed-word, visual-symbolic format. Basic auditory perceptual skills such as attention, figure-ground selection, and speech-sound discrimination are rarely assessed.

Tests for auditory perception may be classified as assessing primarily (a) auditory attention, (b) auditory figure-ground, (c) discrimination of nonverbal auditory stimuli, (d) discrimination of speech sounds (phonemes), (e) auditory synthesis, and (f) segmentation and syllabication. This classification does not presume that these auditory-perceptual abilities can be clearly delineated and separated. Witkin (1971) has stressed this point in the following statement:

> there is considerable intercorrelation among auditory perceptual abilities, such as discrimination, synthesis and memory span. Because speech production is rapid, the auditory perceptual task of attention, focusing, tracking, discrimination, sorting, scanning, and sequencing need to be accomplished in such a brief time span that for all practical purposes they occur simultaneously. It should, therefore, be kept in mind that tasks used in studies which attempt to isolate one or another aspect of auditory perception may really be testing two or more abilities. [p. 46]

Sabatino (1969) stresses the importance of assessing auditory-perceptual abilities in learning disabled children. When assessing thirty children with "known minimal brain damage," only eight of these were identified by performances on the *Bender Visual-Motor Test* (Bender, 1938). In contrast, twenty-three of the group were identified by auditory perceptual tests. When these tests were administered with background noise, twenty-nine of the thirty children were identified. Among the auditory measures, nonsense syllables, digits, and tapped patterns proved ineffective as identifiers. Sabatino concluded "auditory perception is a complex function with specific behavioral components that must be assessed independently if classroom management . . . is to be provided" (p. 736).

Hammill and Larsen (1974) reviewed thirty-three studies of the relationships between reading and measures of auditory perception. Among standardized measures of auditory perception used in the studies were the *Roswell-Chall Auditory Blending Test* (Roswell & Chall, 1963), the *WISC Digit Span* subtest (Wechsler, 1949), *ITPA Auditory Sequential Memory, Auditory Closure,* and *Sound Blending* subtests (Kirk, McCarthy, & Kirk, 1968), and the *Wepman Auditory Discrimination Test* (Wepman, 1958), tests commonly used in language assessment and selected for review in this section. Critical evaluation of the reported correlations indicated that, although significant, they were generally not of the magnitude (.35 or above) for use as predictions of reading achievement, one exception occurring for the *Roswell-Chall Auditory Blending Test.*

The results of correlational studies were observed to be in conflict with investigations comparing the mean performance differences on tests of auditory perception by, among others, Goetzinger, Dirks, and Baer (1960). The authors concluded that investigations evaluated "fail to validate the assumptions . . . that particular auditory skills, *as measured,* are essential to the reading process, and that *many* children actually fail to read proficiently because of auditory-perceptual deficits" (Hammill & Larsen, 1974, p. 45).

The current practice of assessing auditory perceptual abilities as part of the differential diagnosis of language disabilities is supported by several studies by, among others, Aram and Nation (1975), Marslen-Wilson (1975), and Stitt and Huntington (1969). Aram and Nation (1975) performed a factor analysis of the test scores of forty-seven children with developmental language disorders on selected measures of language comprehension, formulation, and repetition. The results suggested that language deficits at the phonological, syntactic, and semantic levels may be hierarchical. They concluded "if the semantic level is deficient, so will be the two lower levels, the syntactic and phonological. . . . Likewise, syntactic deficits subsume phonological problems. . . . Only the phonological level may be singly deficient" (p. 239).

Stitt and Huntington (1969) assessed the relationships between selected measures of auditory perception, articulation, and language abilities in forty-seven college students. They observed that phoneme discrimination ability correlated significantly and at levels well above .35 with articulation (.74, .69), college aptitude (.64, .59), and language abilities (.45, .64). Finally, Marslen-Wilson (1975) has presented evidence that sentences are processed simultaneously at all available levels (phonetic, lexical, syntactic, semantic) and that "information at each level can constrain and guide simultaneous processing at other levels" (p. 227). This evidence provides possibly the strongest argument for in-depth assessment of auditory perception in youngsters with language and learning disabilities.

Auditory Attention

In order to function adequately on a learning task, the child must select the relevant stimuli and resist other competing stimuli. Broadbent (1958) has stressed the necessity of focusing and maintaining attention on one stimulus source in a learning situation. Clements (1969) has described the learning disabled child as being "drawn to irrelevant stimuli in his environment. . . ." This description has been supported by evidence that LD children demonstrate problems in sustaining visual attention and resisting competing spoken messages (Lasky & Tobin, 1973; Ricks, 1974).

The assessment of learning disabled children's auditory attention should consider the ability to (1) sustain attention over time with or without distractors and (2) focus attention on relevant auditory stimuli and inhibit responses to irrelevant stimuli. The ability to sustain auditory and visual attention over a period of time has been measured in experimental studies using versions of the *Continuous Performance Test* (Kornetsky & Eliasson, 1969; Rosvold et al., 1956). Cognitive control, that is, the ability to focus attention on relevant stimuli while inhibiting responses to irrelevant ones, has been measured for the visual modality using the *Fruit Distraction Test* (Santostefano, 1964). Signal detection methods, used in audiological evaluations, may also provide measures of sustained auditory attention (Green & Swets, 1966; Mackworth, 1970). Unfortunately, these measures generally yield results that cannot be compared with normative data. The clinical interpretation is therefore tentative.

Continuous Performance Test

This test (Rosvold et al., 1956) employs a format in which a visual target stimulus, the letter *X*, is presented randomly among other letters either alone or in a stimulus sequence, such as *AX*. The observer is required to respond only to the target stimulus *X* or to the target stimulus sequence *AX*. The test is administered over a period of time, and auditory or visual distractors may be used. The original visual test format has been adapted by Kornetsky and Eliasson (1969) to employ auditory stimuli. The *Continuous Performance Test* or adaptions of it have been used in investigations of sustained visual attention in epileptic, aphasic, brain-damaged, and learning disabled children (Anderson, Halcomb, & Doyle, 1973; Campannelli, 1970; Crosby, 1969; Fedio & Mirsky, 1969; Ricks, 1974; Wiig & Austin, 1972).

Signal Detection Methods

These methods (Green & Swets, 1966) employ stimulus presentation sequences that are similar to those described for the *Continuous Performance Test*. The measures obtained differ in essential ways. The *Continuous Performance Test* yields scores reflecting errors of omission (failures to identify a target stimulus) and errors of commission (erroneous responses to irrelevant stimuli). Signal detection theory yields two measures, one reflecting auditory sensitivity, the other reflecting an internalized criterion for responding. The criterion for responding may be relatively lax, resulting in a high proportion of positive responses, some of which are correct and some of which are made to stimuli other than the target stimulus (so-called false alarms). Or the response criterion may be relatively strict, resulting in failure to identify some of the target stimuli (so-called false negatives). The responses to a signal detection task need not be compared to normative data since the statistics presume an "ideal listener" against which all individual responses are measured. Signal detection theory, therefore, promises a clinical method that may be used to assess auditory attention abilities of language disabled adolescents.

Fruit Distraction Test

The *Fruit Distraction Test* (Santostefano, 1964) measures the degree to which the child can continue to focus on a central task in the presence of intruding stimuli, that is, flexibility in cognitive control. It is appropriate for children in the age range from six to thirteen years. The test contains two ten-by-fifteen-inch cards with fifty drawings of various colored fruits on each. Card I presents only drawings of fruits while Card II introduces line drawings as distractors. A pretest is administered to assure that the child can name each fruit. The child is then asked to (1) name the fruits as rapidly as possible and (2) recall the distractors presented on Card II.

The test yields three measures: (1) reading time distractibility score (time to read Card II minus Card I), (2) reading errors distractibility score (total errors on Card II minus total errors on Card I), (3) number of distractors recalled. These measures have been found to differentiate between brain-damaged and normal children (Santostefano, 1964) and between under-achieving and achieving readers (Ricks, 1974). Evidence that a mechanism of inhibition becomes operative in the age range between five and seven (Kagan, 1967; White, 1965), and that children who lack inhibition in response selection are characterized by impulsivity (Kagan, 1965, 1967; Kagan et al., 1964) suggests that the *Fruit Distraction Test* may assist in identifying language and learning disabled children having deficits in cognitive control.

Auditory Figure-Ground

The ease with which relevant auditory information is differentiated from competing background noises or messages reflects auditory figure-ground abilities. In everyday life, the demands for adequate auditory figure-ground abilities are staggering, both in educational and social settings. Learning disabled children have demonstrated auditory figure-ground problems on a variety of auditory tests utilizing competing messages (Conners, Kramer, & Guerra, 1969; Katz, 1968; Katz & Illmer, 1972; Lasky & Tobin, 1973; Witelson, 1962). It is therefore important to assess auditory figure-ground abilities as part of a comprehensive evaluation of the learning disabled child. Among formal tests available to the educational specialist are (1) the *Goldman-Fristoe-Woodcock Test of Auditory Discrimination* (1970) and (2) the *Flowers—Costello Tests of Central Auditory Abilities* (Flowers, Costello, & Small, 1970).

Goldman-Fristoe-Woodcock Test of Auditory Discrimination

This picture-type discrimination test (Goldman, Fristoe, & Woodcock, 1970) was designed to assess speech-sound discrimination in one-syllable words under controlled listening conditions. The test may be administered to children four years old and above. Normative data are presented in percentiles per age level from three years eight months to seventy and older.

The test is composed of three parts: (1) training procedures, (2) *Auditory Discrimination-Quiet* subtest, and (3) *Auditory Discrimination-Noise* subtest. The training procedure, administered by the examiner, assures that the subject knows the vocabulary used. The *Auditory Discrimination-Quiet* subtest presents audio-taped items in isolation; in the *Auditory Discrimination-Noise* subtest, the items are presented with a background of tape-recorded school cafeteria noise. Comparison of the performances on these subtests provides a measure of the auditory figure-ground abilities of the listener.

The stimulus words are consonant-vowel and consonant-vowel-consonant combinations selected to provide a broad representation of the distinctive features of consonant sounds. Line drawings depict the stimulus words among three pictorial foils. The stimulus and sample words differ by one phoneme. When hearing a stimulus word, the subject must indicate his choice by pointing to the appropriate picture. The test contains a total of seventy-nine test items, and the different phonemes are in the same word position in each item to allow for sound-error analysis.

The results of the standardization procedures indicated that the performances on the *Quiet* subtest improved until age ten and that a gradual decrease in discrimination ability occurred after age thirty-four. On the *Noise* subtest, performances improved for a longer period, until age thirteen, and declined beginning at an earlier age of twenty-five. These findings suggest that auditory figure-ground abilities develop slowly and decline early. Test-retest reliability coefficients of .87 on the *Quiet* subtest and .81 on the *Noise* subtest were obtained, indicating stability of the test results.

Flowers-Costello Tests of Central Auditory Abilities

These tests (Flowers, Costello, & Small, 1970) present a theoretical rationale for assessing discrimination of (1) low pass filtered speech and (2) competing messages. The formats of the two subtests are similar in that each contains twenty-four sentences in which the target words are either distorted or deleted at the end of each sentence. The responses require identification of the distorted or deleted target words from among pictorial choices. In the *Low Pass Filtered Speech* subtest only the target words are subjected to increasing low-pass filtering and distortion. In the *Competing Messages* subtest all of the sentences are presented against a semantically competing background of an interesting story.

Normative data are available for kindergarten through the sixth grade. The norms indicate, however, that the sensitivity of the test diminishes after the third grade and that a ceiling is reached at the fifth. The internal reliability decreases from .87 for kindergarten to .60 and .37 for grades three and four, respectively, supporting the impression that the test may not be appropriate past grade three.

Performances on the Flower-Costello test have been found to correlate significantly with reading achievement scores on the *Gates Primary Reading Tests* and with achievement scores on the *Stanford Achievement Tests*. The value of the test for differential diagnosis is suggested by research indicating that resistance to distortion and to competing auditory stimuli differentiated normal and underachieving readers (Flowers, 1964; Flowers & Costello, 1965). It should be noted, however, that the test may tap semantic-cognitive and convergent production abilities (Guilford, 1967). Thus, the target words may be identified on the basis of the semantic and linguistic constraints provided by the context and structure of the carrier phrases immediately preceding the target word. Other aspects of the test design appear to facilitate selective responses. The syllable length, that is, duration, of the target words frequently differs considerably from the length of the foils, providing additional cues for accurate selection. As a result, test performances should be interpreted with caution.

Auditory Discrimination

Zigmond (1969) has stressed that auditory discrimination skills must be developed to facilitate auditory-visual integration and word attack skills in reading. Learning disabled children have been reported to exhibit significant reductions in phoneme (speech-sound) discrimination and sequencing (Aten & Davis, 1968; Birch & Belmont, 1964; Blank, 1968; Goetzinger, Dirks, & Baer, 1960). Speech discrimination ability has also been observed to relate directly to spelling and to measures of psycholinguistic ability (ITPA) (Cole, 1964; Rechner & Wilson, 1967). Blank (1968) further observed that retarded readers made significantly more discrimination errors involving the final rather than the initial parts of words.

Birch and Belmont (1964) also observed significant reductions in auditory-visual integration in retarded readers. They used an auditory-visual test in which the auditory stimuli consisted of a series of taps. The children were required to identify one of three visual patterns corresponding to the auditory signals. Their findings suggest a need for assessing the discrimination of both nonverbal and verbal auditory stimuli in learning disabilities.

Discrimination of Nonverbal Auditory Stimuli

Test of Non-Verbal Auditory Discrimination

The ability to discriminate nonverbal characteristics of auditory stimuli may be assessed by the *Test of Non-Verbal Auditory Discrimination* (TENVAD) (Buktenica, 1968). The test contains fifty tonal pairs, ten each assessing discrimination of pitch, loudness, rhythm, duration, and timbre. The TENVAD is patterned after the *Seashore Test of Musical Ability* (Seashore, 1960). It may be administered to groups or individuals and has been standardized for ages six through eight. The children are asked to tell whether the elements in a tonal pair are alike. The test may identify the kind of difficulty the child is having through careful examination of the error responses in each category.

The reliability of the test has been found to be significant, and it is maintained over the three-year span tested. The TENVAD correlates with the *Wepman Auditory Discrimination Test* (Wepman, 1958), the *Primary Abilities Test K—1*, and with a measure of first grade achievement, the *Metropolitan Achievement Test, Primary Battery I, Form A*. The TENVAD can be helpful in preschool screening and in identifying potential auditory perceptual deficits and language problems. Although informal procedures have been suggested to assess discrimination of nonverbal auditory stimuli (Bannatyne, 1971; Birch & Belmont, 1964; Luria, 1966; Zigmond, 1969), this test represents one of the few standardized measures for preschool and early grade children. Remediation strategies that may be appropriate for children identified by the TENVAD have been presented in the *Sound-Order-Sense: developmental program for auditory perception* (Semel, 1970).

Examining for Aphasia: Recognition of Sounds

Recognition of sounds in the environment constitutes a basis for the finer discriminations between the nonverbal stimuli of the TENVAD. Inability to recognize environmental sounds and noises has been recognized to constitute a sublinguistic disturbance (Eisenson, 1954). This inability, termed auditory agnosia, can be assessed by the *Recognition of Sounds* subtest of *Examining for Aphasia* (Eisenson, 1954).

In this test, the subject is required to name or imitate six activites performed by the examiner while the subject's eyes are closed. Among the sounds produced by the examiner are coughing, humming, and finger snapping. The test has not been standardized, but normally developing preschoolers are well able to recognize and imitate all six sounds. Language disabled children with subtle clinical signs of auditory agnosia may be able to recognize all of the sounds tested. They may, however, demonstrate difficulties in recognizing the subtle differences distinguishing the front door bell from the back door buzzer, the ringing of the telephone from that of an alarm clock, and the fire alarm from the dismissal gong. The ability to recognize these environmental sounds may provide an informal indicator of the child's nonverbal auditory discrimination abilities.

Discrimination of Verbal Auditory Stimuli

Speech-sound discrimination abilities may be assessed by a variety of formal tests. Among them are (1) the *Travis-Rasmus Speech Sound Discrimination Test* (Travis & Rasmus, 1931); (2) the *Short Test of Sound Discrimination* (Templin, 1943); (3) the *Wepman Auditory Discrimination Test* (Wepman, 1958); (4) the *Stanford Diagnostic Reading Test: Auditory Discrimination, Beginning and Ending Sounds*, and *Sound Discrimination* (Karlsen, Madden, & Gardner, 1966); (5) the *Durrell Analysis of Reading Difficulty: Hearing Sounds in Words* (Durrell, 1955); (6) the *Speech-Sound Discrimination Test* (Robbins & Robbins, 1948); (7) the *Boston University Speech-Sound Discrimination Picture Test* (Pronovost & Dumbleton, 1953; Pronovost, 1974); (8) the *Clymer-Barrett Prereading Battery: Discrimination of*

Beginning Sounds in Words and *Discrimination of Ending Sounds in Words* (Clymer & Barrett, 1967); and (9) the *Goldman-Fristoe-Woodcock Test of Auditory Discrimination*(Goldman, Fristoe, & Woodcock, 1970).

Travis-Rasmus Speech Sound Discrimination Test

This test (Travis-Rasmus, 1931) was among the first designed to consider the relationship between articulatory ability and speech-sound discrimination. It contains 366 nonsense-syllable pairs arranged in random sequence. Each consonant is compared with itself and with all other consonants. The syllable pairs are presented orally by an examiner, and the subject is required to indicate whether the syllable pairs are the same or different. The test was administered to 548 subjects from five years of age through childhood. A reliability coefficient of .72 was reported for the test, indicating adequate consistency of test performances.

Short Test of Sound Discrimination

Templin (1943) used a similar format in the *Short Test of Sound Discrimination*. This test contains seventy-two nonsense-syllable pairs. Approximately half of the items feature the target sounds in initial position, and the other half feature the target sounds in the medial and final positions. The test requires same-different judgments. Of the nonsense-syllable pairs, about 65% are different, 35% identical. The reported split-half reliability coefficient is .71, indicating adequate internal consistency. The *Short Test of Sound Discrimination* has been standardized for elementary school children in grades two through six.

Among the tests of speech-sound discrimination, the *Travis-Rasmus Speech Sound Discrimination Test* and the *Short Test of Sound Discrimination* (Templin) are unique in featuring nonsense rather than real word stimuli. The discrimination tasks involved in differentiating between minimally paired nonsense syllables and real words differ in an important aspect. The discrimination between two phonemes in minimally paired nonsense syllables depends upon efficient and adequate analysis-synthesis of the distinctive feature differences. The discrimination between two phonemes in a minimal word pair such as *fun-sun* is facilitated by the semantic interpretation of the units.

Templin later revised the *Short Test of Sound Discrimination* (Templin, 1957). The revised format contains fifty nonsense-syllable pairs such as *le-le* and *esh-ech*. Each pair is judged as either same or different. This revised form is appropriate for six- to eight-year-old children.

Because time constraints are imposed on the diagnostician, it is not always feasible to assess speech-sound discrimination for nonsense syllables as well as for meaningful words. A phoneme discrimination test employing nonsense syllables should, however, be considered for inclusion in a comprehensive test battery for children who have failed discrimination tests using real words or for children who persist in demonstrating auditory processing deficits and yet pass speech discrimination tests using real words.

Wepman Auditory Discrimination Test

The ability to make accurate discriminations between phonemes in initial, final, or medial positions may be assessed by the *Wepman Auditory Discrimination Test* (Wepman, 1958). Normative data on the development of phoneme discrimination are available for ages five to eight years. Research has indicated that the Wepman test has construct validity and that poor test performances are prevalent among children in the early grades who have articulation disorders or specific reading disabilities. The test contains forty word pairs that differ in only one phoneme. The responses require same-different judgments; of the forty items, ten require *same,* and thirty require *different* responses. Thirteen each assess discriminations between initial and final consonants, and only four assess discriminations between vowels. The test has two equivalent forms that can be used for test-retest evaluation within a short period of time. A test-retest reliability coefficient of .91 is reported, indicating a high degree of performance stability.

Several factors may limit the diagnostic value of the test. Children in preschool and first grade may not comprehend the concept *same-different,* as suggested by research on the development of language concepts (Carrow, 1968). Several of the word pairs contain words that may be well above the comprehension level of early grade children. The scoring of the test is very narrow, with each age level (five, six, seven, and eight) separated by a single point. From a clincial point of view, language disabled children with confusions between vowels and consonant blends are frequently missed by this test because these phonemes are not adequately represented.

Stanford Diagnostic Reading Test: Auditory Discrimination, Beginning and Ending Sounds, Sound Discrimination

The *Stanford Diagnostic Reading Test* (Karlsen, Madden, & Gardner, 1966) assesses several aspects of auditory perception at the phonological level. It is standardized for the second through the middle of the fourth grade and can be group administered. Auditory identification of identical sounds in initial, medial, and final position is appraised in the *Auditory Discrimination* subtest.

This subtest contains forty-five word pairs such as si*t*-ha*t* and provides word pairs of increasing length and complexity. The child is required to indicate the position in the words (beginning, middle, or end) of the two identical sounds. The error patterns permit identification of the location, type, consistency, and severity of the phoneme identification problem; however, the directions and the task required may surpass the abilities of some learning disabled children. Assets of the test include the attention given to vowels, blends, and medial consonants, aspects not generally emphasized in speech-sound discrimination tests.

The deficits identified by the *Auditory Discrimination* subtest can be further corroborated by performances on the *Beginning and Ending Sounds* subtest of the *Stanford Diagnostic Reading Test.* This subtest requires auditory-visual integration, association, and reauditorization to identify the beginning or ending sounds associated with words presented in pictorial stimuli. The child is required to mark the letter or letters associated with the beginning or ending sounds of the pictured stimuli; for example, the child must match a picture of an envelope with the appropriate beginning letters from among four choices, *ev, un, in,* and *en.* Unfortunately, the standard procedure requires that the scores for beginning and ending sounds be combined to obtain a grade equivalent. This procedure obscures some of the diagnostic potential, suggesting that error patterns should be identified for diagnostic purposes.

The *Sound Discrimination* subtest of the *Stanford Diagnostic Reading Test* further corroborates problems identified by the two other subtests. It assesses reauditorization and identification of identical phonemic elements based on visual-symbolic input. An illustrative test item follows: tell (sample), *hear, head, she* (multiple choices). The subtest contains thirty-six items, ten of which require consonant matches. All vowels and diphthongs are included. As a result, this subtest introduces a very extensive assessment procedure for vowel reauditorization and subsequent discrimination.

Durrell Analysis of Reading Difficulty: Hearing Sounds in Words

Auditory discrimination and identification of phonemes may also be evaluated by the *Hearing Sounds in Words* subtest of the *Durrell Analysis of Reading Difficulty* (Durrell, 1955). Words are presented orally by the examiner, and three written, nonidentical sample words are presented for matching initial, final, and a combination of initial and final phonemes. Seven of the items require identification of initial consonants, nine of either initial consonant blends or digraphs, and five of combined initial and final consonants. No vowels or final blends are included. The fact that the child must read and reauditorize the sample words limits the use of the test. It offers the unique facet of simultaneous identification of initial and final phonemes, a complex and rarely tested task. As a tool for differential diagnosis, comparison of the relative percentages of the misperception of initial consonants, initial blends and digraphs, final consonants, and combined initial and final consonants provides a guideline for the area of remediation. The subtest is optional, and it is therefore often not administered as a part of the assessment of reading ability.

Speech-Sound Discrimination Test

One of the first picture speech-sound discrimination tests was designed by Robbins and Robbins (1948). The test contains 108 paired speech sounds presented by naming 216 pictures. The speech sounds are arranged into nine groups, each containing twenty-four pictures: (1) vowels, (2) semivowels, (3) nasals, (4) unvoiced plosives versus unvoiced fricatives and sibilants, (5) voiced plosives, (6) cognate plosives, (7) cognate fricatives and sibilants, (8) unvoiced fricatives and sibilants, and (9) voiced fricatives and sibilants. Prior to test administration, the child is taught the name of each of the pictures. Discrimination is assessed by the examiner, who names a picture. The child points to the appropriate picture from among a set of foils.

The Robbins and Robbins *Speech-Sound Discrimination Test* also includes a section for older children in which the same stimulus words are presented in word contexts. Three words are presented orally by the examiner, two that are the same and one that differs by only one distinctive feature. The child is asked whether the words were alike or which word was different. The test may be administered using two words in minimal word pairs. The child is then asked whether the words were the same or different.

Boston University Speech-Sound Discrimination Picture Test

Pronovost and Dumbleton (1953) developed the *Boston University Speech-Sound Discrimination Picture Test* using a similar design. The test was based upon preliminary work by Mansur (1950). The test contains twenty word pairs and evaluates the discrimination of vowels, semivowels, plosives, fricatives, and blends. The examiner orally presents a word pair that the child identifies from among three pictorial choices, each consisting of two pictured objects. The test was administered to 434 first grade children for standardization. A split-half reliability coefficient of .88 is reported for the test, indicating high internal consistency. The authors recommend using a tape recording of the auditory stimuli to insure consistency of the test results. The test has recently been revised by Pronovost (1974), improving the pictorial choices.

Clymer-Barrett Prereading Battery: Discrimination of Beginning and Ending Sounds in Words

These two subtests of the *Clymer-Barrett Prereading Battery* (Clymer & Barrett, 1967) assess auditory discrimination of beginning and ending sounds in words in a picture-type test. The formats are the same for both subtests; each item consists of four pictorial stimuli, one stimulus item and three choices. All names of the pictures are read by the examiner. The first word read is the stimulus. The child is to choose the word among the remaining three words that begins or ends like the stimulus word.

The subtests can be administered to individuals or groups. Each subtest contains twenty items emphasizing consonant discrimination. The *Beginning Sound* subtest contains only one item with an initial vowel, two digraphs (ch and wh), and two blends (sk and fl). The *Ending Sound* subtest presents a more limited number of phonemes, presenting only one vowel and omitting $p, f, v, \theta, \eth, s$ among others. In order to design remediation strategies based on the test results, the nature of the errors must be phonetically analyzed.

The *Clymer-Barrett Prereading Battery* has been used extensively for predicting reading failure. It has not been used as extensively for differential diagnostic purposes. The age levels for which it is appropriate range from kindergarten through the first grade.

Goldman-Fristoe-Woodstock Test of Auditory Discrimination

Please refer to earlier discussion on page 89.

Auditory Synthesis

Auditory synthesis (resistance to distortion) depends on the ability to reconstruct distorted words. Auditory synthesis abilities have been found to
relate to oral reading and spelling (Bannatyne & Wichiarajote, 1969; Mulder
& Curtin, 1955). Learning disabled children may experience difficulties in
phonemic synthesis (sound blending) (Conners, Kramer, & Guerra, 1969;
Katz & Illmer, 1972). The assessment of auditory synthesis abilities may
employ audiological procedures such as dichotic listening or spoken words
in which phonemes are spoken at intervals, requiring blending, or words
with deleted phonemes, requiring closure. Auditory blending may be
assessed by using one of the following tests: (1) the *Roswell-Chall Auditory Blending Test* (Roswell & Chall, 1963); (2) the *Oliphant Auditory
Synthesizing Test* (Oliphant, 1971); (3) the *Sound Blending subtest of the
ITPA* (Kirk, McCarthy, & Kirk, 1968); and (4) the *Blending subtest of
the Stanford Diagnostic Reading Test* (Karlsen, Madden, & Gardner, 1966).

The *Auditory Closure Subtest of the ITPA* (Kirk, McCarthy, & Kirk, 1968)
may be used to evaluate the ability to synthesize words with deleted phonemes.

Roswell-Chall Auditory Blending Test

This test (Roswell & Chall, 1963) assesses auditory blending of sounds into
words. The test contains thirty items, ten each presenting two isolated phonemes, the initial phoneme or consonant blend in isolation with the remain-
der of the word synthesized, and three phonemes in isolation. Norms are
available for the first four grades. Significant correlations were established
between total scores on the *Auditory Blending, Gray Oral Reading*, and *Metropolitan Silent Reading Tests*, and measures of achievement in word analysis skills obtained by using the *Roswell-Chall Diagnostic Test*, for the first
three grades. This test may provide valuable diagnostic information to the
speech and language pathologist.

Oliphant Auditory Synthesizing Test

The ability to synthesize phonemes into words may also be assessed by the
Oliphant Auditory Synthesizing Test (Oliphant, 1971). It contains three subtests, ten items each requiring synthesis of two, three, and four phonemes.
Normative data are only available for first graders. A cut-off point of twenty
correct responses is arbitrarily considered indicative of significant weaknesses
in the areas tested. The task requires synthesis of isolated phonemes
presented by the examiner at one-half-second intervals. The child must identify the intended word from three spoken choices. The author suggests that
error patterns may reflect auditory reversals, auditory memory deficits,
and perseveration of sounds from word to word.

The test design reflects weaknesses at various levels in the choice of target
and foil words. Two of the three practice words, *out* and *toy*, contain diphthongs (combinations of two vowels). and may therefore confuse the child.
The third contains the vowel [ɝ] which is sensitive to regional variations and,
for that reason, may cause difficulties and result in inaccurate synthesis.

Among the four-phoneme items, five words (school, green, sleep, grade, black) begin with consonant blends, presenting an artificial phoneme segmentation. The ten three-phoneme items appear most relevant in design.

Sound Blending Subtest of the ITPA

This subtest of the *Illinois Test of Psycholinguistic Abilities* (Kirk, McCarthy, & Kirk, 1968) was developed to assess the ability to analyze and synthesize phoneme sequences into meaningful or nonmeaningful units. Phonemes are presented at half-second intervals. The task requires ability to segment and resynthesize a phoneme sequence, a task that may be more easily related to the reading process than to the auditory-verbal process. Pictures are presented with demonstration items. All items require verbal production of the intended, synthesized phoneme sequence. Normative data are available from two years four months to eight years seven months. The reliability coefficients reported for five month stability are generally low, ranging from .30 to .69, suggesting less than adequate consistency of the results for differential diagnostic purposes.

Stanford Diagnostic Reading Test: Blending Subtest

The *Blending* subtest of the *Stanford Diagnostic Reading Test* (Karlsen, Madden, & Gardner, 1966) presents an unusual design for the assessment of sound blending and subsequent auditory-visual integration. It is a test that can provide the language pathologist with data for in-depth analysis of the interfacing between auditory-perceptual and auditory-visual integration deficits. The sample item below illustrates the format of the items:

a. Stimulus: Bird
b. Response format: O r   O ir   O d
                                 O b   O a   O n

The task is to mark the appropriate circles to form the test word. As can be seen, the item above contains two potential words *bird* and *ran*, both of which could have been identified before hearing the stimulus word *bird*. The majority of the items contain only one acceptable printed word while the foils provide opportunities for phoneme substitutions. Diagnostically, the error patterns may reflect problems in the initial synthesis (blending) of the heard units or impaired auditory-visual integration, frequently resulting in random or positional markings. The errors may indicate that initial or final segments are consistently omitted or confused or that various phoneme clusters are consistently confused.

Auditory Closure Subtest of the ITPA

This test (Kirk, McCarthy, & Kirk, 1968) was designed to assess the ability to reconstruct spoken words with deleted phonemes, for example, *cho late*. Its use is suggested for evaluation of the resistance to noise in language processing. Twelve different consonants and one vowel are deleted; most of the deletions involve phonemes with high-frequency acoustic emphasis. There appears to be little rationale for the selection of the type and frequency of the specific phoneme deletions. Normative data are presented for the ages of two to ten. The five month stability coefficients range from low to adequate (.36 to .71). The internal consistency coefficients decrease with age, from .84 at three years seven months to .45 at eight years, suggesting that this subtest should be used with discretion. There is little discussion in the test manual regarding the differential effects of the selected deletions in the test items upon speech intelligibility to assist in the interpretation of the significance of specific errors.

Segmentation and Syllabication

Segmentation refers to the ability to analyze and divide perceived words into their smallest grammatical units. It can be considered a perceptual-linguistic processing ability. This ability seems currently overlooked in formal testing. Syllabication, that is, the ability to identify syllables, reconstruct words from separate syllables, and detect the number of syllables in words, is often assessed as part of a comprehensive evaluation of reading abilities. This ability reflects auditory-perceptual processing and overlaps with segmentation ability, which requires both auditory-perceptual and linguistic processing. The detection of syllable boundaries and the identification of other quantitative and qualitative word aspects, such as the location of stress within syllable sequences, may facilitate word and sentence recall. Syllabication skills may be assessed by, among others, the *Syllabication* subtest of the *Stanford Diagnostic Reading Test* (Karlsen, Madden, & Gardner, 1966) and the *Syllabication* subtest of the *Gates-McKillop Reading Diagnostic Test* (Gates & McKillop, 1962).

Stanford Diagnostic Reading Test: Syllabication Subtest

This subtest of the *Stanford Diagnostic Reading Test* (Karlsen, Madden, & Gardner, 1966) evaluates the ability to identify the first syllables in printed one-, two, or three-syllable words. The task requires reauditorization and indirectly assesses the ability to detect syllable boundaries in perceived words.

Gates-McKillop: Syllabication Subtest

The *Syllabication* subtest of the *Gates-McKillop Reading Diagnostic Test* (Gates & McKillop, 1962) evaluates the ability to combine and blend syllables presented in a syllable list into spoken, nonsense words. The demonstration items introduce syllables spoken by the examiner. Examples of nonsense words that have to be combined and pronounced are *immo, foter, nilow,* and *elling.* Normative data are available for the first through the middle of the sixth grade. The performances should be compared with performances on the subtests for *Oral Reading, Spelling,* and *Recognizing and Blending Common Word Parts.* In the clinical setting, problems in syllabication are often found in association with retrieval deficits. Since syllabic cueing provides one means of facilitating word identification and recall, deficits will influence the design of remedial strategies.

References

Anderson, R. P., Halcomb, C. G., & Doyle, R. B. The measurement of attentional deficits. *Exceptional Children*, 1973, **39**, 534-39.

Aram, D. M., & Nation, J. E. Patterns of language behavior in children with developmental language disorders. *Journal of Speech and Hearing Research*, 1975, **18**, 229-41.

American Speech & Hearing Association, Committee on Rehabilitative Audiology. The audiologist: responsibilities in the habilitation of the auditorily handicapped. *ASHA*, 1974, **16**, 68-70.

Aten, J., & Davis, J. Disturbances in the perception of auditory sequence in children with minimal cerebral dysfunction. *Journal of Speech and Hearing Research*, 1968, **11**, 236-45.

Bannatyne, A. *Language, reading and learning disabilities*. Springfield, Ill.: Charles C Thomas, 1971.

Bannatyne, A. D., & Wichiarajote, P. Relationships between written, spelling, motor functioning and sequencing skills. *Journal of Learning Disabilities*, 1969, **2**, 6-18.

Bender, L. A visual-motor Gestalt test and its clinical use. *American Orthopsychiatric Association Research Monograph*, 1938, No. 3.

Bergman, M. Binaural hearing. *Archives of Otolaryngology*, 1957, **66**, 572-78.

Bienvenue, G. R., & Siegenthaler, B. M. A clinical procedure for evaluating auditory localization. *Journal of Speech and Hearing Disorders*, 1974, **39**, 469-77.

Birch, H. G., & Belmont, L. Auditory-visual integration in normal and retarded readers. *American Journal of Orthopsychiatry*, 1964, **34**, 852-61.

Blank, M. Cognitive processes in auditory discrimination in normal and retarded readers. *Child Development*, 1968, **39**, 1091-101.

Bocca, E. Binaural hearing: another approach. *Laryngoscope*, 1955, **65**, 1164-75.

Bocca, E., Calearo, C., Cassinari, V., & Migliavacca, F. Testing cortical hearing in temporal lobe tumors. *Acta Oto-Laryngologica*, 1955, **45**, 289-303.

Broadbent, D. E. The role of auditory localization in attention and memory span. *Journal of Experimental Psychology*, 1954, **47**, 191-96.

Broadbent, D. E. *Perception and communication*. Elmsford, N. Y.: Pergamon Press, 1958.

Buktenica, N. A. *Test of non-verbal auditory discrimination*. Nashville, Tenn.: Author, 1968.

Calearo, C. Binaural summation in lesions of the temporal lobe. *Acta Oto-Laryngologica*, 1957, **47**, 392-95.

Campanelli, P. A. Sustained attention in brain-damaged children. *Exceptional Children*, 1970, **36**, 317-24.

Carrow, M. A. The development of auditory comprehension of language structure in children. *Journal of Speech and Hearing Disorders*, 1968, **33**, 99-111.

Clements, S. D. A new look at learning disabilities. In L. Tarnopol (Ed.), *Learning disabilities: introduction to educational and medical management*. Springfield, Ill.: Charles C Thomas, 1969. Pp. 31-40.

Clymer, T., & Barrett, T. C. *Prereading battery*. Princeton, N. J.: Personnel Press, 1967.

Cole, M. Specific educational disability involving spelling. *Neurology*, 1964, **14**, 968-70.

Conners, C. K., Kramer, K., & Guerra, F. Auditory synthesis and dichotic listening in children with learning disabilities. *Journal of Special Education*, 1969, **3**, 163-69.

Crosby, K. K. Attention and distractibility in mentally retarded children. Unpublished doctoral dissertation, Boston University, 1969.

Davis, H., & Silverman, S. R. (Eds.) *Hearing and deafness*. (3rd ed.) New York: Holt, Rinehart & Winston, 1970.

Durrell, D. D. *Durrell analysis of reading difficulty*. New York: Harcourt Brace Jovanovich, 1955.

Eisenson, J. *Examining for aphasia*. (Rev. ed.) New York: Psychological Corp., 1954.

Fedio, P., & Mirsky, A. F. Selective intellectual deficits in children with temporal lobe or centrencephalic epilepsy. *Neuropsychologia*, 1969, **7**, 287-300.

Flowers, A. Central auditory abilities of normal and lower group readers. Cooperative Research Project No. S—076. Albany: State University of New York, 1964.

Flowers, A., & Costello, M. R. The resistance to distortion factor in auditory perception and its relationship to specific phonic abilities. Technical Research Report, No. K001, Office of Research and Evaluation. Oak Park School, Oak Park, Mich., 1965.

Flowers, A., Costello, M. R., & Small, V. *Flowers-Costello tests of central auditory abilities*. Dearborn, Mich.: Perceptual Learning Systems, 1970.

Foster, C. R., Giddan, J. J., & Stark, J. *ACLC: assessment of children's language comprehension*. Palo Alto, Calif.: Consulting Psychologists Press, 1972.

Gates, A. I., & McKillop, A. S. *Gates-McKillop reading diagnostic tests*. New York: Teachers College Press, Columbia University, 1962.

Goetzinger, C., Dirks, D., & Baer, C. J. Auditory discrimination and visual perception in good and poor readers. *Annals of Otology*, 1960, **69**, 121-36.

Goldman, R., Fristoe, M., & Woodcock, R. W. *Goldman-Fristoe-Woodcock test of auditory discrimination*. Circle Pines, Minn.: American Guidance Service, 1970.

Green, D. M., & Swets, J. A. *Signal detection theory and psychophysics*. New York: John Wiley & Sons, 1966.

Guilford, J. P. *The nature of human intelligence*. New York: McGraw-Hill, 1967.

Hammill, D. D., & Larsen, S. C. The relationship of selected auditory perceptual skills and reading ability. *Journal of Learning Disabilities*, 1974, **7**, 40-46.

Hennebert, P. E. Troubles de l'audition et dyslexie. *Bulletin of the Orton Society*, 1964, **45**, No. 104.

Jerger, J. Observations of auditory behavior in lesions of the central auditory pathways. *Archives of Otolaryngology*, 1960, **71**, 797-806.

Jerger, J. (Ed.) *Modern developments in audiology*. (2nd ed.) New York: Academic Press, 1973.

Kagan, J. Reflection-impulsivity and reading ability in primary grade children. *Child Development*, 1965, **36**, 609-28.

Kagan, J. Biological aspects of inhibition systems. *American Journal of Diseases of Children*, 1967, **114**, 507-12.

Kagan, J., Rosman, B. L., Kay, D., Albert, J., & Phillips, W. Information processing in the child: significance of analytic and reflective attitudes. *Psychological Monographs: General and Applied*, 1964, **78**, 1-37.

Karlsen, B., Madden, R., & Gardner, E. F. *Stanford diagnostic reading test*. New York: Harcourt Brace Jovanovich, 1966.

Katz, J. The use of staggered spondaic words for assessing the integrity of the central auditory nervous system. *Journal of Auditory Research*, 1962, **2**, 327-37.

Katz, J. The SSW test—an interim report. *Journal of Speech and Hearing Disorders*, 1968, **33**, 132-36. (a)

Katz, J. The use of methyl-phenidate with children having learning disabilities: speech, hearing, language and auditory perception. Paper presented at the Annual Convention of the American Speech and Hearing Association, Denver, 1968. (b)

Katz, J. (Ed.) *Handbook of clinical audiology*. Baltimore: Williams & Wilkins, 1972.

Katz, J., & Illmer, R. Auditory perception in children with learning disabilities. In J. Katz (Ed), *Handbook of clinical audiology*. Baltimore: Williams & Wilkins, 1972. Pp. 540-63.

Kimura, D. Speech lateralization in young children as determined by an auditory test. *Journal of Comparative Physiology Psychology*, 1963, **56**, 899-902.

Kirk, S. A., McCarthy, J. J., & Kirk, W. D. *Illinois test of psycholinguistic ability* (Rev. ed.) Urbana: University of Illinois Press, 1968.

Kornetsky, C., & Eliasson, M. Reticular stimulation and chlorpromazine: an animal model for schizophrenic over-arousal. *Science*, 1969, **165**, 1273-74.

Lasky, E. Z., & Tobin, H. Linguistic and nonlinguistic competing message effects. *Journal of Learning Disabilities*, 1973, **6**, 243-50.

Lee, L. *Northwestern syntax screening test*. Evanston, Ill.: Northwestern University Press, 1969.

Link, R., & Lenhart, E. The examination of directional hearing, a simple clinical method. *International Audiology*, 1966, **5**, 67-70.

Luria, A. R. *Higher cortical functions in man*. New York: Basic Books, 1966.

Mackworth, J. F. *Vigilance and attention*. Middlesex: Penguin Books, 1970.

Mansur, R. The construction of a picture test for speech sound discrimination. Unpublished master's thesis, Boston University, 1950.

Marslen-Wilson, W. D. Sentence perception as an interactive parallel process. *Science*, 1975, **189**, 226-28.

Matzker, J. Two new methods for the assessment of central auditory functions in cases of brain disease. *Annals of Otolaryngology*, 1959, **68**, 1185-97.

Morrill, J. C. A staggered spondaic word test as an indicator of minimal brain dysfunction in children. Unpublished master's thesis, Texas Technological College, 1969.

Mulder, R. L. & Curtin, J. Vocal phonic ability and silent-reading achievement: a first report, *Elementary School Journal*, 1955, **56**, 121-23.

Newby, H. *Audiology*. New York: Appleton-Century Crofts, 1972.

Nordlund, B. Directional audiometry. *Acta Oto Laryngologica*, 1964, **57**, 1-8.

Oliphant, G. *Oliphant auditory synthesizing test*. Cambridge, Mass.: Educators Publishing Service, 1971.

O'Neill, J., & Oyer, H. *Applied audiometry*. New York: Dodd, Mead & Co., 1966.

Pronovost, W. *The Boston University speech sound discrimination picture test*. Cedar Falls, Iowa: Go-Mo-Products, 1974.

Pronovost, W., & Dumbleton, C. A picture-type speech sound discrimination test. *Journal of Speech and Hearing Disorders*, 1953, **18**, 258-66.

Rechner, J. & Wilson, B. A. Relation of speech sound discrimination and selected language skills. *Journal of Communication Disorders*, 1967, **1**, 26-30.

Ricks, N. Sustained attention and the effects of distraction in under-achieving second grade children. Unpublished doctoral dissertation, Boston University, 1974.

Robbins, S. D., & Robbins, R. S. *Speech sound discrimination tests*. Boston: Expression Co., 1948.

Rosvold, H. E., Mirsky, A. F., Sarason, I., Bransome, E., & Beck, L. A continuous performance test of brain damage. *Journal of Consulting Psychology*, 1956, **20**, 343-50.

Roswell, F. G., & Chall, J. S. *Roswell-Chall auditory blending test*. New York: Essay Press, 1963.

Sabatino, D. The construction and assessment of an experimental test of auditory comprehension. *Exceptional Children*, 1969, **35**, 729-37.

Sanchez-Longo, L., Forster, F. M., & Auth, T. L. A clinical test for sound localization and its applications. *Neurology*, 1957, **7**, 655-63.

Santostefano, S. Cognitive controls and exceptional states in children. *Journal of Clinical Psychology*, 1964, **20**, 213-18.

Seashore, C. E. *Seashore measures of muscial talent*. New York: Psychological Corp., 1960.

Semel, E. M. *Sound-Order-Sense: a developmental program in auditory perception*. Chicago: Follett Educational Corp., 1970.

Semel, E. M., & Wiig, E. H. Comprehension of syntactic structures and critical verbal elements by children with learning disabilities. *Journal of Learning Disabilities*, 1975, **8**, 53-58.

Shankweiler, D., & Studdert-Kennedy, M. Identification of vowels and consonants presented to left and right ears. *Quarterly Journal of Experimental Psychology*, 1967, **19**, 59-63.

Stitt, C. L., & Huntington, D. A. Some relationships among articulation, auditory abilities, and certain other variables. *Journal of Speech and Hearing Research*, 1969, **12**, 576-93.

Studdert-Kennedy, M., & Shankweiler, D. Hemispheric specialization for speech perception. *Journal of the Acoustical Society of America*, 1970, **48**, 479-94.

Templin, M. A study of sound discrimination ability of elementary school pupils. *Journal of Speech and Hearing Disorders*, 1943, **8**, 127-32.

Templin, M. *Certain language skills in children*. Minneapolis: University of Minnesota Press, 1957.

Travis, L. E., & Rasmus, B. The speech sound discrimination abilities of cases with functional disorders of articulation. *Quarterly Journal of Speech*, 1931, **17**, 217-26.

Wechsler, D. *Wechsler intelligence scale for children*. New York: Psychological Corp., 1949.

Wepman, J. *Auditory discrimination test*. Chicago: University of Chicago, 1958.

White, S. Evidence for a hierarchical arrangement of learning processes. In L. P. Lipsett & C. C. Spiker (Eds.), *Advances in child development and behavior*, Vol. 2. New York: Academic Press, 1965. Pp. 187-220.

Wiig, E. H., & Austin, P. W. Visual attention and distraction in aphasic and non-aphasic children. *Perceptual and Motor Skills*, 1972, **35**, 863-66.

Wiig, E. H., & Semel, E. M. Development of comprehension of logico-grammatical sentences by grade school children. *Perceptual and Motor Skills*, 1974, **38**, 171-76. (a)

Wiig, E. H., & Semel, E. M. Logico-grammatical sentence comprehension by learning disabled adolescents. *Perceptual and Motor Skills*, 1974, **38**, 1331-34. (b)

Witelson, S. Perception of auditory stimuli in children with learning problems. Unpublished master's thesis, McGill University, Montreal, 1962.

Witkin, B. R. Auditory perception—implications for language development. *Language Speech and Hearing Service*, 1971, **4**, 31-52.

Wunderlich, R. C. *Kids, brains, and learning*. St. Petersburg, Fl.: Johnny Reads, 1970.

Zabrewski, A. Clinical tests for the acuity of directional hearing. Bull. Soc. Amis. Sci. Pozan, 1960, **10**, 7-14. *Exerpta Medica*, 1962, **15**, 134.

Zigmond, N. K. Auditory processes in children with learning disabilities. In L. Tarnopol (Ed.), *Learning disabilities: introduction to educational and medical management*. Springfield, Ill.: Charles C Thomas, 1969. Pp. 196-216.

5 Assessing Cognitive and Linguistic Processing Abilities

Overview

This assessment chapter introduces selected tests and subtests which may assist in diagnosing deficits in the cognitive-semantic and linguistic processing abilities of children and adolescents. The desirable characteristics as well as the limitations of the selected tests are presented. The discussions of the interpretation of test results focus on the analysis of error patterns and on the sensitivity of the tests in identifying cognitive-semantic and linguistic processing deficits that may be associated with learning disabilities.

The selection of tests is not to be interpreted as exhaustive. The discussions are meant to assist the diagnostician in selecting a test battery that will sample language abilities at various levels of cognitive-semantic and linguistic processing. For additional tests, the interested reader may consult references and test reviews by Berry (1969), Buros (1965), Darley (1964), Irwin and Marge (1972), Johnson and Bommarito (1971), Johnson, Darley and Spriestersbach (1963). The authors recognize that the diagnostician must exhibit judgment and caution when using selected subtests of comprehensive test batteries to assess specific cognitive-semantic or linguistic processing abilities.

Cognitive-Semantic Processing

There is increasing evidence that some of the language deficits of children and adolescents with learning disabilities may reflect reductions in cognition and logical growth (Wiig & Semel, 1973, 1974b; Wiig, Lapointe, & Semel, 1975). As a result, the diagnostician responsible for the identification or differential diagnosis of language disabilities in school-age children and adolescents must sample language abilities reflecting cognitive-semantic processing. Furthermore, the cognitive-semantic processing abilities must be evaluated at various levels. Guilford (1967) has reported independent cognitive abilities for:

1. semantic units (words and concepts)
2. semantic classes (associations between related words and concepts)
3. semantic relations (logical relationships between words and concepts)
4. semantic systems (verbal problems)
5. semantic transformations (redefinitions of words and concepts)
6. semantic implications (cause-effect relationships, etc.)

The psychologist has generally been responsible for evaluating cognitive abilities and interpreting deficits or reductions in cognition based on his specialized training and experience. There is, however, an increasing desire among educators and language pathologists to know the nature as well as the degree of specific cognitive-semantic deficits to better design and implement educational or remedial programs. This need has resulted in the availability of tests of cognitive-semantic processing that are not restricted in use to any one profession. It is the responsibility of each diagnostician to select a test battery that reflects his or her training, experimental background, and professional competencies and qualifications.

Cognition of Semantic Units

The cognition of semantic units requires specific as well as broad, general knowledge of the meaning of words and concepts. Receptive vocabulary tests such as (1) the *Peabody Picture Vocabulary Test* (Dunn, 1965), (2) the *Full-Range Picture Vocabulary Test* (Ammons & Ammons, 1958), and (3) the *Preschool Preposition Test* (Aaronson & Schaefer, 1971) assess the knowledge of the specific referential meaning of words, for example, nouns, verbs, adjectives, and prepositions.

Broad, general knowledge of the meaning of words and concepts requires abstraction and generalization of a variety of attributes and relationships, including knowledge of the temporal, spatial, quantitative, and negative aspects denoted by words. Among tests for the cognition of semantic units, which may be used to assess the development of concept formation for a wide range of basic concepts, attributes, and relationships, are (1) the *Irwin-Hammill Abstraction Test* (Irwin & Hammill, 1964; Hammill & Irwin, 1966); (2) the *Boehm Test of Basic Concepts* (Boehm, 1970); (3) the *Basic Concept Inventory* (Engelman, 1967); (4) the *Meaning of Opposition* test (Kreezer & Dallenbach, 1929); (5) the *Word Opposites: Reading-Listening* subtest of the *Botel Reading Inventory* (Botel, 1970); (6) the *Oral Vocabulary* subtest of the *Gates-McKillop Reading Diagnostic Tests* (Gates & McKillop, 1962); and (7) the *Social Adjustment B* subtest of the *Detroit Tests of Learning Aptitude* (Baker & Leland, 1959).

Guilford (1967) has indicated that cognition of semantic units implies specific knowledge of the meaning of words and concepts as well as knowledge of their broad general meanings. In reference to Guilford's view of the abilities comprising the cognition of semantic units, the picture vocabulary tests reviewed below satisfy the criteria for knowledge of the specific, referential meaning of words.

Peabody Picture Vocabulary Test

This test (Dunn, 1965) was designed to evaluate single word, receptive vocabulary comprehension in the age range from two years three months to eighteen years five months. The test materials consist of 3 demonstration plates and 150 test plates. Each plate contains four black-and-white line drawings, three foils, and one target item. The stimulus words are presented in order of increasing difficulty. The predominant proportion of the stimulus words are nouns, followed by verbs in the progressive tense and adjectives. The examiner reads the stimulus words aloud, and the child is required to point to the picture best representing the meaning of the stimulus word. The test has two forms with normative data for each, and the test scores can be converted to mental age, IQ, and standard score and percentile equivalents.

The reliability of the test has been established in several studies. Test-retest reliability coefficients for both forms are high (.97), indicating good consistency of the results. Performances on the *Peabody Picture Vocabulary Test* correlate with performances on the *Stanford-Binet* (.71) and with WISC full-scale IQ (.61).

Although learning disabled children may show a scatter of errors below ceiling on the *Peabody Picture Vocabulary Test,* the performances are generally within normal limits (within -6 months of chronological age). The pattern of errors on the PPVT will at times provide information regarding the nature of specific vocabulary problems. As an example, LD children may fail Item 27 of Form A, *building.* The target picture associated with the stimulus word is of a small boy repairing a wagon. Learning disabled children often say there is no picture of *a building,* suggesting problems with words having multiple meanings. Other LD children have difficulty comprehending the meaning of action verbs, and others fail on items requiring knowledge of adjectives.

Full-Range Picture Vocabulary Test

This test (Ammons & Ammons, 1958) assesses the receptive vocabulary in the age range from two years through adulthood. The test consists of sixteen test plates, each containing four cartoonlike, black-and-white line drawings. Each of the two forms of the test contains a total of eighty-five stimulus words of increasing difficulty. The examiner says the stimulus word, and the subject is required to point to the corresponding drawing on the appropriate test plate. Each test plate contains drawings of from one to eleven test words.

The reported test-retest reliability coefficient is high (.93), suggesting a high level of consistency of the results. Performances on the *Full-Range Picture Vocabulary Test* correlate positively with *Stanford-Binet Vocabulary* subtest scores. The raw scores can be converted into mental age or into adult percentile ratings for age levels above 16½ years. There are separate norms for Spanish-American children, black children and adults, and white rural children. Some of the pictorial items are, unfortunately, dated.

Preschool Preposition Test

Standardized picture vocabulary tests tend to assess the comprehension of a rather limited category of words. Word categories such as prepositions are generally not tested. *The Preschool Preposition Test* (Aaronson & Schaefer, 1971) may be used to identify problems in the comprehension of prepositions such as *up, into, inside,* and *under,* in preschool and early grade LD children. The test contains twenty-three items. Normally developing children show increasing ability to comprehend the test items as a function of age with a ceiling effect occurring at ages 5½ or 6. Performances on the test correlate positively with scores on the *Stanford-Binet* and *Peabody Vocabulary Test* (.57). The relatively low ages at which normal children show a ceiling effect limits the use of the test, suggesting a need to consider informal procedures to evaluate the comprehension of prepositions by learning disabled youngsters in the middle and upper grades.

Irwin-Hammill Abstraction Test

This test (Irwin & Hammill, 1964; Hammill & Irwin, 1966) assesses sequential, coordinate, and mixed categorization and abstraction. In the sequential category, the child is required to identify the missing item in a sequence such as identifying the numeral between three and five. In the coordinate category, the child is required to identify words that do not belong to the class, in sequences such as *cat, dog, horse, tree;* this identification requires cognition of semantic classes. In the mixed category, the child is required to match attributes and their descriptions with nouns, reflecting the cognition of semantic units. An example of an item is: A baseball is: round, sour, hot, mushy. The test consists of two forms, each containing twenty-five items.

The test has been administered to 122 cerebral palsied children (Irwin & Hammill, 1964) and 109 mentally retarded children (Hammill & Irwin, 1966), ranging in age from six to seventeen. Split-half and alternate form reliability coefficients have been reported of .95, indicating excellent internal consistency. Performances on the test correlate positively with scores on the WISC *Similarities* subtest and the *Peabody Picture Vocabularly Test* at .72 and .74, respectively. Normative data are not available. The test may assist in clinical differentiation between difficulties in the cognition of semantic units, that is, mixed categorization and abstraction, and semantic classes, that is, coordinate categorization and abstraction. Analysis of error patterns may also suggest areas for remedial emphasis and strategies for remedial intervention for children with learning disabilities and related language disorders.

Boehm Test of Basic Concepts

The *Boehm Test of Basic Concepts* (Boehm, 1970) evaluates comprehension of the labels for concepts of quantity and number, space (dimension, direction, location, orientation), and time, among others. The test has two forms, each containing twenty-five test items consisting of a stimulus word spoken by the examiner and three pictorial samples from which the child is required to select the most appropriate. Among the basic concepts evaluated, twenty-eight have a spatial reference (thirteen prepositions, three superlatives, and twelve others), thirteen reflect quantity, and nine reflect time. Of these fifty items, eight relate to combinations of space, quantity, or time. It may be administered individually or to small groups, and normative data are available for children in kindergarten through the second grade.

Basic Concept Inventory

This test (a research edition) (Engelman, 1967) assesses the comprehension of labels for basic concepts in ten items. Each of the items contain one or more subitems, and nine items are associated with a stimulus picture. Among the concepts evaluated are conjunction (and), dimension, direction, function, location, negation (not), time, and quantity. The inventory contains no normative data. It is considered a criterion-referenced measure as defined by Glaser (1963). Measures of reliability and validity are not available. The test is recommended for preschool children through the third grade.

The administration manual discusses in detail how responses may be elicited using alternate strategies for questioning. As a result, both quantitative and qualitative aspects of a child's abilities can be analyzed to provide a basis for intervention. Educational strategies are presented for specific difficulties in comprehending the labels associated with the concepts.

Meaning of Opposition

This test (Kreezer & Dallenbach, 1929) contains twenty-five word items representative of common kindergarten and first grade vocabulary. Before the test items are presented, the examiner gives examples of opposites and limited instruction about opposition. The child can respond to the test items by naming antonyms or by demonstrating knowledge of opposition by using *not* or other forms; for example, *not smooth* and *unsmooth* are as acceptable as the antonym *rough* in response to the stimulus word *smooth*. Norms are available at six-month intervals for the age range from 5 to 7½ years. The test provides an alternative format to verbal opposite tests requiring exact naming of antonyms.

Botel Reading Inventory: Word Opposites

Word Opposites: Reading-Listening subtest of the *Botel Reading Inventory* (Botel, 1970) provides a multiple-choice format for assessing knowledge of verbal opposites. It contains 100 test items, 10 each for the first grade through high school. The test is easy to administer and score, is applicable to a wide age range, and permits identification of the grade level of the vocabulary at which problems occur. The multiple-choice format reduces the demands upon memory, recall, and retrieval since the correct answer can be identified by recognition.

Gates-McKillop: Oral Vocabulary

The *Oral Vocabulary* subtest of the *Gates-McKillop Reading Diagnostic Test* (Gates & McKillop, 1962) assesses the knowledge of vocabulary meaning using a multiple-choice, sentence-completion format. The examiner says an incomplete sentence to the youngster and provides four choices for the selection of the appropriate response; for example, "A turbine is part of a _____," is followed by the choices *flower, machine, building, stomach*. The test has two forms, each containing thirty items, permitting reevaluation at intervals or following a period of intervention. The authors indicate that this subtest need not be used if results of the *Stanford-Binet* vocabulary test are available. They also stress that the subtest is most appropriate for youngsters in the fourth grade or above.

The subtest is considered to be supplementary and may not be administered as part of the assessment of reading abilities. The raw scores may be translated into grade scores. Grade norms are available for the second grade third month through the twelfth grade third month. Above the seventh grade, a difference of one raw score may result in grade scores that differ by five months, suggesting inadequate sensitivity to changes occurring in the higher grades.

DTLA: Social Adjustment

The *Social Adjustment* subtest of the *Detroit Tests of Learning Aptitude* (Baker & Leland, 1959) may be used to assess broad knowledge of the meaning of words related to the social environment. It contains twenty stimulus words such as *jail, money, board of health,* and *committee* spoken by the examiner. The child is required to define the words. Responses are scored according to whether they are (1) beside the point or incorrect, (2) vague, apply too generally, or are very limited, (3) specific, brief, and correct but limited in expression, or (4) generalized, showing use of explanations, or use of superior vocabulary. Examples of responses within each category are presented in the test manual. Norms are available for the age range from 3½ years to 17 years 9 months. The responses permit analysis of the knowledge of word meaning along a simple-concrete to complex-abstract continuum.

Cognition of Semantic Classes

The cognition of semantic classes reflects ability to categorize and classify semantically related words and concepts. As an example, the words *apples, lion, tiger, bananas, elephant,* and *pears* may be categorized into two semantically related classes, wild animals and fruits. Words and concepts may also be used to label dimensions, attributes, or aspects which may form the basis for the categorization of objects, events, or ideas, a related cognitive ability.

McCarthy Scales: Conceptual Grouping

The *Conceptual Grouping* subtest of the *McCarthy Scales of Children's Abilities* (McCarthy, 1970) evaluates the child's ability to categorize blocks according to a single dimension, such as size, and according to a combination of dimensions such as size, form, and color. The materials used in administering the subtest are six square and six circular blocks. Each shape is provided in three colors (blue, red, yellow) and in two sizes for each color (big, little). The subtest contains nine items, the initial three of which require identifcation of each one of the dimensions (little-big, red-blue-yellow, square-round) in response to oral directions given by the examiner. An example of an item is: Find the square one . . . Show me the round one. The next three items require identification of all of the blocks containing a specified dimension or combination of dimensions (square, big yellow, big red round); for example, "Now see how many big red round ones you can find. Remember, you're looking for big red round ones." The last three items require addition of appropriate blocks to a category specified by a visual display. An example of an item presents five scrambled blocks (big blue circle, big red circle, big yellow circle, big red square, big yellow square) in combination with the verbal instruction "Which one here (point to the scrambled blocks) goes best with the ones on the card? Find it and put it on the card."

The subtest performances are described to reflect perceptual performance and general cognitive functioning. Verbal ability is included to the degree that the child must understand the spoken instructions. The child's ability to "deal logically with objects, to classify, and to generalize" (p. 12) is evaluated. The McCarthy scales were standardized using a total sample of 1,000 children, equally distributed at half-year intervals between the ages of 2½ to 5½ when rapid developmental growth occurs, and at one-year intervals between the ages of 5½ to 8½. Normative data are available for each of five subscales: (1) verbal, (2) perceptual performance, (3) quantitative, (4) memory, and (5) motor, as well as for the general cognitive scale. No norms are provided for individual subtests. As a result, the *Conceptual Grouping* subtest performances must be pooled with performances on other subtests of the perceptual-performance scale (Block Building, Puzzle Solving, Tapping Sequence, Right-Left Orientation, Draw-A-Design, Draw-A-Child), a fact which limits the clinical-educational interpretation of the performances. Adequate reliability coefficients have been reported for the perceptual–performance scale, ranging from .75 to .90 for the various age levels tested. This scale may be useful in assessing whether language disabled children with deficits in forming verbal-semantic classes (categorizing words and concepts) have acquired the basic perceptual-cognitive grouping strategies.

Cognition of Semantic Relations

The ability to comprehend logical relationships between words and concepts, as in the verbal analogy "Grass is green. Sugar is _____" and in the sentence "Cats are bigger than kittens," expressing a comparative relationship, reflects cognition of semantic relations. This ability may be assessed by tests such as: (1) the *Opposite Analogies* subtest of the *Stanford-Binet Intelligence Scale* (Terman & Merrill, 1960); (2) the *Auditory Association* subtest of the ITPA (Kirk, McCarthy, & Kirk, 1968); (3) the *Wiig-Semel Test of Linguistic Concepts* (Wiig & Semel, 1973, 1974a, 1974b); and (4) the *Otis Alpha Short Form* (Otis, 1954).

Stanford-Binet: Opposite Analogies

The *Stanford-Binet Intelligence Scale* (Terman & Merrill, 1960) features *Opposite Analogies* subtests at years IV (five items), VI (four items), and VII (four items) and for Superior Adult III (three items and three alternates). Examples of items at year IV and Superior Adult III are "The sun shines during the day; the moon at _____," and "A debt is a liability; an income is _____." The opposite analogy items are said by the examiner and the child or adult is required to perceive and formulate the specific verbal opposite needed to complete the analogy. Scoring standards are presented for each subtest. Performances reflect knowledge of verbal opposites, ability to perceive the semantic relations (logical relationships) involved in the analogy, and convergent production of semantic relations. The subtests may be administered in isolation to evaluate whether these abilities are developed or delayed according to expectations for chronological age.

ITPA: Auditory Association

The *Auditory Association* subtest of the ITPA (Kirk, McCarthy, & Kirk, 1968) also assesses the ability to perceive and formulate verbal analogies. The subtest contains forty-two items of progressive difficulty. The following example illustrates the format of the test items: "A rabbit is fast; a turtle is

_____." In order to respond correctly to the items, the child must possess an adequate repertory of verbal associations, including verbal opposites. In addition, he must be able to perceive the logical relationship that exists among the three critical words in the analogy and to identify, retrieve, and formulate the target element. Failure to perform adequately may therefore reflect deficits in the available repertory of verbal associations, difficulties in performing the logical operations involved in discerning the semantic relationships, or problems in the recall and retrieval of the target words. The differential diagnosis of the problem area will depend on corroborative data from other tests.

The *Auditory Association* subtest has been standardized for the age range from two years four months to ten years eleven months, when a ceiling effect may be expected in the normal child. Five-month stability coefficients have been reported which range from .83—.90, suggesting good consistency. The internal consistency is adequate with split-half correlations ranging from .74 to .85. Wiig and Semel (1975) have reported findings which suggest that deficits of LD children in perceiving and formulating verbal analogies may persist into adolescence. Performances on the *Auditory Association* subtest have also been observed to correlate positively with measures of receptive vocabulary (PPVT), comprehension of syntactic structures (NSST), and controlled verbal associations, suggesting that the test has predictive value (Wiig, Lapointe, & Semel, 1975).

Wiig-Semel Test of Linguistic Concepts

This test (Wiig & Semel, 1973, 1974a, 1974b) evaluates the comprehension of fifty linguistic concepts requiring logical operations. Of the fifty sentence items, ten each represent (1) comparative, (2) passive, (3) temporal—sequential, (4) spatial, and (5) familial relationships. The test was designed to (1) control the sentence length to five to seven words, (2) limit the relationships to involve only two critical elements, (3) provide a large ethnic variety of proper names, and (4) permit yes/no responses for the majority of the items. The following questions illustrate representative items: (1) comparative relationships: "Are watermelons bigger than apples?" (2) passive relationships: "Jerry was pushed by Bob. Was Bob pushed?" (3) temporal relationships: "Does Thursday come after Tuesday?" (4) spatial relationships: "Hal stood in back of Beth. Was Beth in front?" (5) familial relationships: "Give another name for your mother's father." The total test is presented in Table 11.

TABLE 11

Wiig-Semel Test of Linguistic Concepts

Comparative relationships

1. Are watermelons bigger than apples?
2. Are jets slower than turtles?
3. Are trees smaller than flowers?
4. Are trains faster than airplanes?
5. Are parents older than their children?
6. Are lemons sweeter than candy?
7. Is ice cream colder than coffee?
8. Is night darker than day?
9. Are feathers heavier than books?
10. Is water wetter than snow?

Passive relationships

1. John was hit by Eric. Was John hit?
2. Bill was caught by Tom. Was Tom caught?
3. Jerry was pushed by Bob. Was Bob pushed?
4. Judy was pulled by Sue. Was Judy pulled?
5. Betty was brought by Ruth. Was Betty brought?
6. Mary was driven by Alice. Was Alice driven?
7. Pearl was phoned by Fran. Was Fran phoned?
8. Don was upset by Jane. Was Jane upset?
9. Paul was chosen by Steve. Was Paul chosen?
10. Ann was left by Kate. Was Ann left?

Temporal relationships

1. Does lunch come before breakfast?
2. Does evening come before afternoon?
3. Does dinner come before lunch?
4. Does noon come after morning?
5. Does Saturday come before Sunday?
6. Does Thursday come after Tuesday?
7. Does summer come after spring?
8. Does Thanksgiving come before Halloween?
9. Does May come after June?
10. Does December come before November?

Spatial relationships

1. Pat came after James. Was James first?
2. The elephant sat on the mouse. Was the mouse on top?
3. Sally ran in front of Brian. Was Sally first?
4. The chair fell on the toy. Was the chair on the bottom?
5. Philip rode behind Charles. Was Philip last?
6. Leslie swam between Burt and Angel. Was Angel in the middle?
7. Sharon finished before Henry. Was Henry last?
8. The ball rolled to the left of the fence. Was the ball on the left side?
9. Hal stood in back of Beth. Was Beth in front?
10. Mike walked to the right of Joe. Was Joe on the right side?

TABLE 11 (Continued)

Familial relationships

(Demonstration: What do you call your mother's mother?)

1. Give another name for your mother's father.
2. Give another name for your father's father.
3. Give another name for your father's mother.
4. Give another name for your mother's brother.
5. Give another name for your mother's sister.
6. Give another name for your father's brother.
7. Give another name for your aunt's daughter.
8. Give another name for your uncle's son.
9. Give another name for your aunt's son.
10. Give another name for your uncle's daughter.

TABLE 12

Correct responses to logico-grammatical sentences by 210 grade
school children by grade (nS = 30)

Relationship				Grade				
		1	2	3	4	5	6	7−8
Total test	M	26.30	34.90	37.13	41.06	45.40	46.97	46.27
	SD	4.99	4.76	6.14	3.99	3.86	2.06	2.00
Comparative	M	7.70	8.10	8.50	8.67	9.47	9.60	9.40
	SD	1.55	1.33	1.28	1.38	0.72	0.61	0.55
Passive	M	6.60	7.80	7.83	8.37	8.67	9.17	9.00
	SD	1.43	1.64	2.03	1.28	1.47	0.90	1.03
Temporal	M	6.50	6.53	6.77	7.60	8.73	9.07	8.73
	SD	1.50	1.83	1.75	1.33	1.41	0.82	0.99
Spatial	M	4.73	7.23	8.13	8.60	9.17	9.43	9.27
	SD	2.06	1.52	1.43	0.99	1.10	0.92	0.7?
Familial	M	1.43	5.23	5.97	7.83	9.07	9.70	9.87
	SD	1.50	2.92	2.98	2.68	2.21	0.74	0.43

SOURCE: Reprinted with permission of publishers from: Wiig, E. H., & Semel, E. M.
Development of comprehension of logico-grammatical sentences by grade school
children. *Perceptual and Motor Skills*, 1974, **38**, 171-76.

NOTE: M = mean; SD = standard deviation.

Construct validity was determined by evaluating age differentiation (Wiig
& Semel, 1974a). As language comprehension skills are reported to be developmental, test scores were expected to show an increase with age. Two hun-
dred and ten grade school children were randomly selected, thirty each from
the first through eighth grades. Analysis of variance indicated significant differences between grades. Norms for all grades are presented in Table 12.

The test was administered to thirty-two learning disabled children and their academically achieving controls and to thirty LD adolescents (Wiig & Semel, 1973, 1974b). In both instances, LD youngsters were differentiated from their age peers at statistically significant levels. Concurrent validity has been established with a widely used test of psycholinguistic ability (ITPA) (Wiig & Semel, 1974b). Correlations ranged from r = .43 for auditory association to r = .59 for psycholinguistic age.

The internal consistency of the test was determined by the split-half method and corrected by the Spearman-Brown formula. The correlation for thirty children from the second and third grades was adequate (r_2 = .82).

Otis Alpha Short Form

This test (Otis, 1954) assesses the comprehension of a wide range of linguistic concepts in forty-five sentences. Among the linguistic concepts presented are spatial relationships (eighteen items), comparative relationships (nine items), temporal-sequential relationships (four items), familial relationships (one item), and other linguistic concepts such as *if, not,* and *but* (thirteen items). Each sentence is said by the examiner, and the child indicates comprehension by pointing to one of a set of four pictures.

Age norms are available from five years to twelve years eleven months, at one-month intervals. The age scores suggest that the test becomes less sensitive at ages eleven and twelve. Split-half reliability coefficients of .87 and .88 are reported for two samples of third grade pupils. Performances on this test correlated significantly with *Metropolitan Achievement Test* scores at .63. The *Otis Alpha Short Form* is a group test generally used to estimate intelligence. The nature of the test suggests that it may be of value in identifying children with difficulties in processing and interpreting linguistic concepts. Analysis of the error patterns may indicate the types of relationships that are particularly difficult and suggest areas for intervention.

Cognition of Semantic Systems

The ability to comprehend the structure of a verbal problem and to arrive at its correct solution reflects the cognition of semantic systems. This ability is indicated to be an inherent part of solving many verbal math problems (Guilford, 1967). Among tests which evaluate verbal problem-solving ability, the *Metropolitan Achievement Tests: Mathematics Problem Solving* (Durost et al., 1970) illustrates the design of verbal math problems requiring cognition of semantic systems.

MAT: Mathematics Problem Solving

This subtest of the *Metropolitan Achievement Tests: Primary II* (Durost et al., 1970) assesses the ability to perceive and analyze the structure of verbal math problems and formulate a correct solution. This subtest contains thirty-five items, the last eighteen of which are verbal math problems. These must be analyzed structurally to be able to compute the calculations and arrive at an appropriate numerical response. An example of an item is: "Kathy has 50 cents in her bank. If she puts 30 cents more in, how many cents will she have in her bank?" Although failure to give the correct mathematical response may reflect difficulties at several levels, that is, analysis of the structure (semantic system) or mathematical computation, the test may be adapted to reflect problems in the structural analysis of the verbal problems.

In the adaptation, the problems would be said by the examiner. First, the child would be asked to give the answer to the problem. Next, he would be asked to explain how he arrived at this answer, reflecting analysis of the structure of the verbal statements. The math problems of this test contain vocabulary and syntactic structures that may pose problems to LD children. Among these are verbs and verb forms such as *need, earn,* and *should,* multiple—meaning words such as *cross, rate,* and *change,* comparative constructions such as *taller than, if—then,* and noun determiners such as *some* and *every.* Errors in analyzing the structural aspects of the problems may reflect difficulties in interpreting any of these words, and the error patterns may suggest areas for intervention.

Among other achievement tests containing mathematical problem-solving subtests are the *Metropolitan Achievement Tests: Advanced Battery* (Durost et al., 1958), the *Peabody Individual Achievement Test* (Dunn & Markwardt, 1970), the *SRA Achievement Series* (Thorpe et al., 1963), the *Stanford Achievement Test* (Kelley et al., 1964), the *Stanford Diagnostic Arithmetic Tests* (Beatty, Madden, & Gardner, 1966), and the *Wide Range Achievement Test* (Jastak, 1965).

Cognition of Semantic Transformations

The ability to recognize redefinitions of words and concepts when different attributes and aspects are stressed reflects the cognition of semantic transformations (Guilford, 1967). Tests which may be used to assess this ability are (1) the *WISC Similarities* subtest (Wechsler, 1949); (2) the *Stanford-Binet: Differences, Similarities,* and *Similarities* and *Differences* subtests (Terman & Merrill, 1960); and (3) the *Detroit Tests of Learning Aptitude: Likenesses and Differences* subtest (Baker & Leland, 1959).

WISC: Similarities

The *Similarities* subtest of the WISC (Wechsler, 1949) contains twelve word pairs requiring verbal identification of likenesses between objects, substances, facts, or ideas, a task that reflects ability to perform semantic transformations. For example, one word pair requires abstraction of similarities between *piano—violin.* The responses to each of the twelve items can be scored to indicate the level of abstraction reflected by the response. Thus, lower order abstraction on the item described above would be reflected by a response that they both are "for playing." Higher level abstraction would be indicated by the response that they are both "musical instruments."

Cohen (1959) has reported factor analysis results which suggest that the *Similarities* subtest measures "verbally retained knowledge impressed by formal education" at 7½ and 10½ years. At 13½ years the test is considered to assess "application of judgment to situations following some implicit verbal manipulation."

Stanford-Binet: Differences, Similarities, Similarities and Differences

The *Stanford-Binet Intelligence Scale* (Terman & Merrill, 1960) presents a series of *Differences, Similarities,* and *Similarities and Differences* subtests, requiring that the child or adult perceive, abstract, and describe either (1) similarities and/or differences between two things or abstract words, or (2) similarities between three things. At year VII, the child is required to describe similarities between four word pairs (concepts) such as *ship— automobile*. At year VIII, the task requirements are increased and the child must describe both similarities and differences between four item pairs such as *ocean—river*. At year XI, the complexity of the task is further increased to require description of similarities between three concepts such as *wool— cotton—leather*. At the Average Adult level, the requirement is to describe differences between three abstract word pairs such as *character—reputation*. At this level, a second subtest containing three items requires description of essential differences between such pairs as *optimist—pessimist*. At the Superior Adult I level, descriptions of essential similarities are required for three pairs of items such as *melting—burning*. Performances are scored according to the scoring standards provided in the manual and reflect the ability to abstract essential shared or different attributes and to redefine the concepts, that is, cognition of semantic transformations (Guilford, 1967).

DTLA: Likenesses and Differences

The *Likenesses and Differences* subtest of the *Detroit Tests of Learning Aptitude* (Baker & Leland, 1959) evaluates the ability to abstract and describe ways in which concepts denoting objects, qualities, or ideas share essential characteristics or are essentially different. One of the items requires comparison of the terms *morning* and *afternoon*. The scoring key specifies the most essential shared characteristic, *part of a day*, and the differences, *early—before noon* and *late—after midday*. Responses are scored for correctness using a four-point scale; the highest point score is given for responses with essential (determining, limiting) similarities and differences. Norms are available for the age range between six years nine months and nineteen years.

Cognition of Semantic Implications

The ability to comprehend inferred cause-and-effect relationships, predict outcomes, note inconsistencies, recognize absurdities, and understand puns, proverbs, and idioms reflects the cognition of semantic implications. Among tests assessing this level of cognitive processing are (1) the *Boston Diagnostic Aphasia Examination: Complex Ideational Material* (Goodglass & Kaplan, 1972); (2) the *Proverbs Test* (Gorham, 1956a, 1956b); and (3) the *Stanford-Binet: Verbal Absurdities, Finding Reasons, Problems of Fact, and Proverbs* (Terman & Merrill, 1960).

Boston Diagnostic Aphasia Examination: Complex Ideational Materials

This subtest (Goodglass & Kaplan, 1972) of the *Boston Diagnostic Aphasia Examination* contains four short stories with associated questions which tap the inferred or implied cause-effect relationships. An example of a story reads as follows:

A soldier tried to cash a check in a bank near his camp. The teller, firm but sympathetic, said, "You will have to have identification from some of your friends from the camp." The discouraged soldier answered, "But I don't have any friends in camp—I'm the bugler."
Was the soldier's check cashed at once?
Did the teller object to cashing the check?
Did the soldier have a friend with him?
Did the soldier have trouble finding friends? [p. 10]

The test has not been standardized for children and adolescents. It is sensitive to the auditory processing deficits incurred by adults with aphasia. It may provide information of similar deficit areas in adolescents with language and learning disabilities.

Proverbs Test

A method for evaluating verbal abstraction ability is presented in the *Proverbs Test* (Gorham, 1956a, 1956b). Interpretation of proverbs requires ability to translate concrete symbols into generalized, abstract concepts. The process of abstraction has been described by Goldstein (1948).

In the abstract attitude, we transgress the immediately given specific aspects or sense impression; we abstract from particular properties. We detach ourselves from the given impression, and the individual thing represents to us an accidental sample or representative of a category. [pp. 18-19]

There are two formats of the *Proverbs Test,* one requiring free responses and the other a multiple-choice format. Each format contains thirty-six items with twelve items each in three parallel forms. Examples of the proverbs are "Strike while the iron is hot," "All is not gold that glitters," and "It never rains but it pours." The free responses to the proverbs are scored using a three-point system designed according to the following principles:

a. If a proverb contains two symbols, both must be converted into their "meanings" to achieve an adequate response.
b. Excellence of expression is not scored, only the ability to abstract the concrete symbols into general concepts.
c. Bizarre responses are given the same value as popular responses as long as the concrete symbols are converted into abstract, general concepts.

Norms are available for the fifth through the twelfth grades and above. Inter—correlations between the three forms of the free response subtest have been reported at .92. A correlation of .90 has been reported for the consistency between the free response and the multiple-choice forms. Inter-tester reliability has been found to be high with a correlation of .95.

The authors consider proverbs to be of value in assessing verbal comprehension and abstraction because (1) they are interesting to the subject, (2) they reflect, in familiar sayings, the distilled wisdom of various cultures, (3) the individual words and concepts in proverbs are relatively easy to understand since they describe familiar objects and events, (4) subjects seem to easily understand the task of telling the meaning of a proverb, and (5) the test has a wide range of applicability. The *Proverbs Test* has been found to differentiate schizophrenic adults from normals (Gorham, 1956c); the test manual describes qualitative differences between responses (Gorham, 1956a). An adaptation of the *Proverbs Test* may be used in diagnostic evaluations of learning disabled adolescents. In this adaptation the stimuli are presented orally. Free responses given verbally by the subjects are tape recorded. Multiple choices are also presented orally by the examiner. This adaptation has been observed to be of clinical value in identifying problems of verbal abstraction in adolescents with reading retardation.

Stanford-Binet: Verbal Absurdities

The *Stanford-Binet Intelligence Scale* (Terman & Merrill, 1960) introduces several *Verbal Absurdities* subtests that require perception and identification of illogical or erroneous cause-effect relationships, that is, cognition of semantic implications (Guilford, 1967). At year VIII, four statements containing verbal absurdities are said by the examiner. The youngster must perceive and describe the stated absurdity. An example of a test item at this level is "Walter now has to write with his left hand because two years ago he lost both his arms in an accident." Verbal absurdities are also introduced at years IX (five items), X (three alternate items), and XI (three items).

Stanford-Binet: Finding Reasons, Problems of Fact

The *Finding Reasons* subtests and the *Problems of Fact* subtest also require cognition of semantic implications but utilize different formats. *Finding Reasons* subtests are introduced at years X (two items) and XI (two alternate items). An example of an item is "Give two reasons why children should not be too noisy in school." In order to provide appropriate answers to the questions, the youngster must perceive and identify alternate, implied cause−effect relationships. The *Problems of Fact* subtest featured at Year XIII (three items) utilizes a sentence completion and paragraph format such as "An Indian who had come to town for the first time in his life saw a boy riding along the street. As the boy rode by, the Indian said, 'The white boy is lazy; he walks sitting down.' What was the boy riding on that caused the Indian to say, 'He walks sitting down'?" In order to respond to these items, the youngster must perceive and describe the implied causes for the stated effects.

The *Verbal Absurdities*, *Finding Reasons* and *Problems of Fact* subtests may be administered in isolation to evaluate whether the ability to perceive and identify the implications of verbal statements are developed according to age expectations.

Stanford-Binet: Proverbs

The *Stanford-Binet Intelligence Scale* also features subtests that evaluate the comprehension of proverbs. These subtests are introduced at the Average Adult (three items), the Superior Adult II (two items), and the Superior Adult III levels (three items). The adults are required to describe the abstract, generalized meaning of proverbs such as "Don't judge a book by its cover" and "It's an ill wind that blows nobody good." Detailed procedures for standard scoring are introduced in the test manual.

Linguistic Processing

Efficient linguistic processing depends upon ability to perform analysis-by-synthesis in which the input is processed at several levels simultaneously. Concurrent processing requires ability to utilize linguistic structure for sentence comprehension. The assessment of linguistic processing abilities should consider (1) the knowledge of morphological rules, (2) the comprehension of words (concepts) in sequence and knowledge of syntax, and (3) semantic aspects. Learning disabled children have demonstrated significant delays in both the acquisition of English morphology and syntax (Semel & Wiig, 1975; Vogel, 1974; Wiig, Semel, & Crouse, 1973). They have also been reported to experience significant reductions in the ability to comprehend sequences of four critical words (Semel & Wiig, 1975).

Morphology

Knowledge of English morphology reflects knowledge of word-formation rules and the ability to interpret changes in word meaning when morphemes (minimal units of meaning) are combined. Tests of morphology must cover a wide range of inflectional and derivational rules to provide information of problem areas. Among tests that may be used to assess the child's knowledge of English morphology are (1) the *Berko Experimental Test of Morphology* (Berko, 1958); (2) the *Grammatic Closure* subtest of the ITPA (Kirk, McCarthy, & Kirk, 1968); and (3) the *Michigan Picture Language Inventory* (Lerea, 1958; Wolski, 1962).

Berko Experimental Test of Morphology

This test (Berko, 1958) utilizes an ingenious format in which nonsense words and pictures are used to evaluate the child's knowledge of morphology. It contains thirty-three items, ten assessing the rules for the formation of noun plurals, eight assessing past tense, three each assessing singular possessives, plural possessives, and derivation, two each assessing third singular of verbs and adjectival inflection, and one each assessing progressive tense and compounding. An example of a test item presents a black line drawing of a bird-like figure with the accompanying text "This is a wug. "Now there is another one. There are two of them. There are two _____." The child is required to provide the missing word applying the appropriate morphological rules for each item (see chapter 8, figure 7).

Berko's test has been shown to differentiate between the acquisition of morphology by mentally retarded and normal children (Newfield & Schlanger, 1968) and by high-risk, learning disabled, and normal children (Wiig, Semel, & Crouse, 1973). Unfortunately, the test is not commercially available. It must be reproduced according to Berko's descriptions of test items, thus limiting the use of the test for clinical purposes.

ITPA: Grammatic Closure

The Grammatic Closure subtest of the ITPA (Kirk, McCarthy, & Kirk, 1968) evaluates the child's knowledge of morphology and syntactic structures using real words. It contains thirty-three items which tap the knowledge of the formation and use of regular and irregular noun plurals (ten items), noun possessive singular (one item), noun derivation (one item), progressive tense (one item), regular and irregular past tense (five items), past participle (one item), adjectives *any* and comparative and superlative (seven items), adverbs (two items), prepositions (two items), and pronouns (three items). The *Grammatic Closure* subtest has been reported to correlate closely with tests of reading and writing ability (Newcomer et al., 1975).

Normative data are available for the age range from two years two months to ten years four months. The reported five-month stability coefficients range from .46 to .87 and the internal reliability coefficients from .60 to .74.

Michigan Picture Language Inventory

This test (Lerea, 1958) assesses the comprehension and expression of vocabulary and language structure. The *Language Structure* subtest contains nine sections that evaluate four main word classes and three function word groups (Fries, 1952). The word classes and parts of speech represented are (1) singular and plural nouns, (2) personal pronouns, (3) possessives, (4) adjectives, (5) demonstratives, (6) articles, (7) adverbs, (8) prepositions, and (9) verbs and auxiliaries. Items are presented first to elicit oral responses, using a sentence completion procedure with previously presented contextual cues. Comprehension of the grammatical structures is assessed only when the oral response to an item is incorrect.

Reliability coefficients for language structure comprehension range from .72 to .99. Content validity is suggested by significant performance increases with age. Normative data have been presented for four-, five-, and six-year-olds (Wolski, 1962). These data suggest that a ceiling effect was not established in six-year-olds and that the test may be used with children in the early grades.

The test follows a clearly discernible psycholinguistic classification scheme. Noun plurals are tested for a few regular and several irregular forms, arranged to reflect increasing difficulty. Pronouns are divided into personal and possessive, and all personal pronouns are assessed. In the two adjective sections, comparative and superlative forms are elicited for six highly common—size adjectives. These sections assess transfer of the rules for adjectival inflection in examples contrasting adjectives with their opposites, for example, "The block is the largest and the triangle is the (smallest)." The comparative and superlative of two adverbs, *fast* and *slow,* are tested in a similar design. The comprehension of demonstratives (this, that, these, those) is tested with considerable detail. Two indefinite articles, *a* and *an*, are tested in combination with eleven frequent nouns.

The preposition section introduces nine prepositions, of which six are definite and static in location and three are dynamic, reflecting a change in location, an aspect not generally tapped. The verbs and auxiliaries reflect a relatively wide variety of tenses (present, present progressive, past, past progressive, future, and future progressive) for three regular and five irregular verbs.

The test is relatively easy to administer, the suggested total test time ranging from about twenty-five to forty-five minutes depending upon age. The pictorial representations are particularly clear with relatively few ambiguous drawings. Guidelines for interpretation and implications for clinical management have not been presented. The structure of the test, however, lends itself to easy identification of problem areas, and the patterns used may be extended to clinical-educational management.

Syntax, Sentence, and Paragraph Comprehension

The comprehension of words in sequence, syntactic structures, and paragraphs may be assessed by one of the following tests: (1) the *Assessment of Children's Language Comprehension* (Foster, Giddon, & Stark, 1972); (2) the *Test for Auditory Comprehension of Language* (Carrow, 1973); (3) the *Northwestern Syntax Screening Test* (Lee, 1969, 1971); (4) the *Meeting Street School Screening Test: Follow Directions I and II* (Hainsworth & Siqueland, 1969); (5) the *Token Test* (DeRenzi & Vignolo, 1962); and (6) the *Durrell Analysis of Reading Difficulty: Listening Comprehension* (Durrell, 1955).

Assessment of Children's Language Comprehension

The ability to process and interpret sequence of critical verbal elements may be assessed by the *Assessment of Children's Language Comprehension* (ACLC) (Foster, Giddan & Stark, 1972). The test contains four sections which evaluate: (1) vocabulary comprehension, (2) comprehension of two critical elements in sequence such as *dog eating*, (3) comprehension of three critical elements such as *ball under the table*, and (4) comprehension of four critical elements such as *monkey sitting on the fence*. The vocabulary section assesses comprehension of the verbal elements subsequently introduced and contains thirty nouns, ten verbs, five adjectives, and five prepositions. The items containing verbal elements in sequence require comprehension of the vocabulary, analysis-and-synthesis, and memory of the various elements. The test has been standardized for ages three years through six years five months. The critical elements' items are presented verbally, and the child is required to point to the appropriate pictorial presentation from among four or five pictorial choices.

Although the majority of the pictorial representations are clear, some items such as for *broken cup* and *dirty box* and for *animals sleeping* (two items) are unclear. The test contains two items requiring perception and interpretation of facial expressions of emotions, a task that often presents problems for learning disabled children. Accordingly, errors on these items may reflect problems other than auditory comprehension of the critical elements. The test is simple to administer, easy to score, and requires limited administration time. The ACLC has been reported to identify receptive language deficits in research with LD children (Semel & Wiig, 1975). Performances correlated with achievement measures on the *Peabody Individual Achievement Test* (PIAT) for *Math, Reading Comprehension,* and *Spelling* (Dunn & Markwardt, 1970) and with performances on the *Receptive* subtest of the *Northwestern*

Syntax Screening Test (NSST) (Lee, 1971). The error patterns may provide guidelines for remediation by suggesting the parts of speech and sequences causing difficulty and the number of critical verbal elements that can be easily processed in sentences.

Test for Auditory Comprehension of Language

This test (Carrow, 1973) was designed to assess auditory comprehension for a variety of language categories. It contains 101 items grouped by grammatical category rather than by difficulty level. The test contains four sections:

1. Form classes and function words. These are nouns, adjectives, verbs, and adverbs. The adjective category assesses comprehension of common attributes such as color, size, and quantity and taps knowledge of the concepts of *same-different*. In the verb category, all but one item are in the progressive tense, and we are unsure why *jump* requires deviation from the format. Only three adverbs and two demonstratives are assessed. The classification of several items in the form-class section may be questioned. As examples, vocabulary items such as *left*, *up*, and *middle* are introduced in uncommon contexts. A total of six prepositions are evaluated, five referring to definite locations in space and one, *at the side of*, to an indefinite location.
2. Morphology. Only eight items are contained in this section, all of which assess noun derivation or adjectival inflection. To some children, it may be confusing to be presented with three derived nouns with the suffix *er*, followed by two comparative forms of adjectives with the same suffix, a fact that may provide diagnostic insight.
3. Grammar. This section evaluates comprehension of pronouns (gender and number), noun plurals, and verb number, tense, voice, and status.
4. Syntax. Comprehension of imperatives, noun-verb agreement, complementation, modification, and coordination are included in this section. The classification of several items within both the grammar and syntax sections seems arbitrary.

The test items are presented verbally by the examiner; in responding, the child must identify one of three pictorial choices. Normative data are available for the range from three years to six years eleven months. Concurrent validity has been established with several clinical groups, ranging from deaf children to children with clinical language disorders. Test-retest reliability has been established with correlation coefficients ranging from .77 to .94.

From a diagnostic point of view, it is an asset that age expectations are presented for each item in the form of percentiles. The scope of the test makes it a valuable clinical tool for the identification of auditory comprehension deficits in the early grades. The organization of the test items and the very limited guidance provided for the interpretation of errors and the implications for clinical-educational management are seen as drawbacks.

Northwestern Syntax Screening Test

The *Northwestern Syntax Screening Test* (NSST) (Lee, 1969, 1971) assesses the ability to process, interpret, and recall syntactic structures of increasing complexity. Performances reflect knowledge of linguistic rules, simultaneous analysis and synthesis, and auditory memory. The test consists of two subtests, *Receptive* and *Expressive*, each containing twenty items with two semantically and syntactically minimally-paired sentences. (Mother says, "Look *who* is here," and Mother says, "Look *what* is here.") The test was standardized on children between the ages of three years and seven years eleven months from middle- and upper-income communities. It is considered a screening test only and is not considered to provide a detailed analysis of syntactical skills. The *Receptive* subtest items are presented verbally and the child must identify the appropriate pictorial representation from among four choices. A Spanish version of the test is available (Toronto, 1973).

Among the syntactic structures included in the *Receptive* subtest are prepositional phrases, pronominalization, negation, subject-verb agreement, noun singular versus plural, reflexive pronouns, past versus present tense, subject-object reversals, possessive, present versus future tense, wh- questions, declarative versus interrogative, demonstratives, active versus passive, and direct-indirect object sequences. The NSST has been found to differentiate learning disabled and achieving children (Semel & Wiig, 1975). Performances on the NSST *Receptive* and *Expressive* subtests correlated positively and significantly, and performances on both correlated with measures of achievement on the *Peabody Individual Achievement Test* (PIAT) (Dunn & Markwardt, 1970).

For clinical use, certain aspects of the test design should be taken into account in interpreting results. One of the sentence pairs and the associated pictorial representations, "The boy sees himself" versus "The boy sees the shelf," may be confused based upon either auditory or visual perceptual difficulties. Similarly, one item that contrasts *who* versus *what* is represented by a visually ambiguous choice in which a package outside a door may be perceived as the bottom step of a staircase. Guidelines for error interpretation and implications are not presented, leaving the examiner to analyze and interpret them. Critical cut-off points (tenth percentile) are presented at one-year intervals for the range from three to eight years. Recent research has supported that selected items on the NSST can be valuable in differentiating children with language impairments from normally developing and mentally retarded children (Ratusnik & Koenigsknect, 1975).

Meeting Street School Screening Test: Follow Directions I and II

These tests (Hainsworth & Siqueland, 1969) assess the child's ability to comprehend and retain verbal directions of spatial concepts and execute them by actions (Follow Directions I) and by drawing (Follow Directions II). *Follow Directions I* contains six items including commands for action with one, two, and three directions. The directions contain the prepositions *right, left, above, behind, between, forward, backward, to* (turn to, nearer to), and *from* (away from). *Follow Directions II* contains five items including commands for drawing with one, two, and three directions. The items contain the following prepositions: *behind, from — to, in, right, left, inside,* and *around.*

Normative data are not presented for each subtest of the test battery. Total test scores are converted to scaled scores, and five normative percentile tables are available for the ages from five years to seven years five months. Total test performances have been found to differentiate children with learning disabilities and to correlate positively with performances on the ITPA ($r = .77$). Test-retest reliability is adequate for all subtests with coefficients ranging from .75 to .85.

The test manual describes the diagnostic uses of the *Meeting Street School Test,* designed to be a screening device. Analysis of error patterns on the *Follow Directions* subtests may suggest deficits in memory and recall and difficulties in comprehending specific prepositions and prepositional phrases. The three-level commands contain differences in structure. In one command the three components are connected with *and* as in "Take three steps toward me and then turn and face away from me." In two others a connecting *and* is deleted as in "Turn right, take two steps backwards, and then turn left." The sequence in which the three components of the command are connected by *and* are easier to retain and recall for some LD children. Others retain better the interrupted sequence with deletion of *and,* a difference which is of importance in determining the structural aspects that may facilitate responses to oral directions.

Token Test

The ability to process verbal directions of increasing length and complexity is evaluated in the *Token Test* (DeRenzi & Vignolo, 1962). This test has been used extensively in investigations of adult aphasics (Boller & Vignolo, 1966; Orgass & Poeck, 1966; Swisher & Sarno, 1969; Wertz, Keith, & Custer, 1971; Wertz & Perkins, 1972). It has been revised and normative data have been established by Noll (1970).

The *Token Test* was designed to assess the comprehension of linguistic materials with minimal redundancy, requiring that the semantic value of each word be grasped. The test contains five parts. The items in the first four parts contain commands of a verb-subject format. Although all items are of the same basic format, the length increases from four to ten words. Conjunctions are contained in parts two, three, and four. The versions of the *Token Test* that have been adapted for children use only one verb, *touch,* in the commands, limiting the motor complexity of the responses. Parts two and four introduce one and two modifier strings, respectively. The modifier strings contain at most two adjectives in sequence, denoting combinations of color, shape, and size.

Part five of the test introduces particles, complex syntactic structures, and compound oral commands. Processing of linguistic concepts requiring logical operations is tapped for the concepts *If-then, All-except, When I-you, Except for,* among others. A variety of spatial prepositions are included in the items, among them *beside, between,* and *in front of.* Two adverbs, *slowly* and *quickly,* are also included, and subordinate clauses are introduced. From a diagnostic viewpoint this section assesses, among others, logical-cognitive processing and simultaneous analysis and synthesis. It appears most sensitive to subtle, higher level linguistic and cognitive-semantic processing deficits, generally not assessed by other tests.

Procedures facilitating administration and scoring of the test for children between the ages of five to eleven years have been presented by Hahn and Weiss (1973). These authors have also presented guidelines for remediation.

The *Token Test* has been found to identify subtle receptive language deficits in learning disabled adolescents (Lapointe, 1975). Performances by these adolescents on the *Token Test* (Part VI) correlate positively with performances on the Wiig-Semel Test of Linguistic Concepts (Wiig & Semel, 1974a, 1974b) and on the *NSST Expressive* subtest (Lee, 1971) (Wiig, Lapointe, & Semel, 1975). The test is versatile, has great scope and depth, may be used with a wide age range, and assesses subtle deficits in higher level language processing relevant to processing linguistic data in academic tasks.

Durrell: Listening Comprehension

Auditory listening comprehension of graded paragraphs may be assessed by the *Listening Comprehension* subtest of the *Durrell Analysis of Reading Difficulty* (Durrell, 1955). Very few tests designed to evaluate the language abilities of children include standardized, graded paragraphs for the assessment of auditory comprehension. The paragraphs have been standardized for the first six grades. At each grade level, the subtest contains one paragraph of increasing length and complexity. The increase in length is reflected in the number of words rather than in the number of sentences, the number of sentences ranging from six to eight. The increased complexity is reflected in the vocabulary and at the syntactic level.

Comprehension is evaluated based on the oral responses to a series of *wh*-questions from the examiner. The predominant question format uses *what*. *Where, why,* and *how* are used sparingly at the lower grade levels, *who* is used only once, and *which* and *why* are never used. This choice of *wh*- interrogatives provides an excellent model. The complexity of the questions increases according to the hierarchy of difficulty observed and suggested in chapter 3. The results provide a measure of the developmental level of the child's ability to grasp information from verbally presented material.

The introduction of several numerically presented informational items at the fourth-grade reading level provides the possibility for premature failure by LD youngsters. Testing should be continued if this is suspected. Inability to retain numerically presented information should be considered clinically significant since this pattern is common among learning disabled children and deserves special attention in remediation. Performances on the test reflect auditory memory, linguistic and semantic processing abilities, and recall.

Auditory comprehension of paragraphs may also be evaluated using tests designed for the differential diagnosis of aphasia. Among these are (1) *Examining for Aphasia* (Eisenson, 1954), (2) the *Boston Diagnostic Aphasia Examination* (Goodglass & Kaplan, 1972), and (3) the *Minnesota Test for Differential Diagnosis of Aphasia* (Schuell, 1965).

Semantics

At the semantic level, linguistic processing relates to the connotative meanings of words to a person and to the affective and attitudinal reactions to signs (Osgood & Miron, 1963). These reactions have been evaluated exten-

sively using the *Semantic Differential*, a method combining controlled association and scaling procedures (Osgood, Suci, & Tannenbaum, 1957). The
subject is provided a concept (stimulus word) that must be evaluated against
a set of bipolar scales such as *hard-soft, good-bad, strong-weak*. A seven-step
scale is provided for the evaluation so that the subject can indicate the direction of his association as well as the intensity of the judgment. Research has
substantiated that concepts (words) as well as other aspects of reality tend to
be structured around three semantic categories: evaluation (represented by
scales such as good-bad, optimistic-pessimistic, and timely-untimely); po-
tency (toughness, represented by scales such as hard-soft, heavy-light, and
severe-lenient); and activity (oriented activity, represented by scales such
as active-passive, excitable-calm, and hot-cold) (Snider & Osgood, 1969).

Semantic Habits Inventory

Tests and techniques that evaluate semantic habits, for example, the *Semantic Differential* (Osgood, Suci, & Tannenbaum, 1957), are generally
cumbersome to administer and score. The *Semantic Habits Inventory* (Nunnally, Flaugher, & Hodges, 1963, 1971) provides an exception. It measures
verbal response tendencies or semantic habits, using either forced binary or
multiple choices, or free-associative responses. The inventory contains 143
stimulus items for which the response alternatives contrast various combinations of scales (words) implying positive evaluation (e.g., *sweet* and
good) negative evaluation (e.g., *sour* and *bad*), observable denotative qualities (e.g., *round* and *long*), and classificatory evaluation of some denotative
attributes (e.g., *fruit* and *reptile*).

The inventory has been used with preschool, elementary, and high school
children and college students. Normative data are available only for adults
(Nunnally, Flaugher, & Hodges, 1963), suggesting that the test can be used
with learning disabled college students. Although the relationships between
semantic habits and other verbal skills are hypothetical, stereotyped, or
widely atypical, evaluations may reflect sensory, perceptual, associative, or
cognitive limitations. In a similar vein, differences in semantic habits may influence the quality of verbal interactions and of reading comprehension.

References

Aaronson, M., & Schaefer, E. Preschool preposition test. In O. G. Johnson & J. W. Bommarito (Eds.), *Tests and measurements in child development: a handbook.* San Francisco: Jossey-Bass, 1971. P. 75.

Ammons, R., & Ammons, H. *Full-range picture vocabulary test.* Missoula, Mont.: Psychological Test Specialists, 1958.

Baker, H. J., & Leland, B. *Detroit tests of learning aptitude.* Indianapolis: Test Division of Bobbs-Merrill, 1959.

Beatty, L., Madden, R., & Gardner, E. *Stanford diagnostic arithmetic test.* New York: Harcourt Brace Jovanovich, 1966.

Berko, J. The child's learning of English morphology. *Word,* 1958, **14,** 150-77.

Boehm, A. E. *Boehm test of basic concepts.* New York: Psychological Corp., 1970.

Boller, F., & Vignolo, L. A. Latent sensory aphasia in hemisphere damaged patients: an experimental study with the token test. *Brain,* 1966, **89,** 815-30.

Botel, M. *Botel reading inventory.* Chicago: Follett Educational Corp., 1970.

Buros, O. K. (Ed.) *The sixth mental measurements yearbook.* Highland Park, N.J.: Gryphon Press, 1965.

Carrow, E. *Test for auditory comprehension of language.* Austin, Tex.: Urban Research Group, 1973.

Cohen, J. The factorial structure of the WISC at ages 7½, 10½, and 13½. *Journal of Consulting Psychology,* 1959, **23,** 285-99.

Darley, F. L. *Diagnosis and appraisal of communication disorders.* Englewood Cliffs, N.J.: Prentice-Hall, 1964.

DeRenzi, E., & Vignolo, L. A. The token test: a sensitive test to detect receptive disturbances in aphasics. *Brain,* 1962, **85,** 665-78.

Dunn, L. *Peabody picture vocabulary test.* Circle Pines, Minn.: American Guidance Service, 1965.

Dunn, L. M., & Markwardt, F. C. *Peabody individual achievement test.* Circle Pines, Minn.: American Guidance Service, 1970.

Durost, W. N., Bixler, H. H., Hildreth, G. H., Lund, K. W., & Wrightstone, J. W. *Metropolitan achievement tests: advanced battery.* New York: World Book, 1958.

Durost, W. N., Bixler, H. H., Wrightstone, J. W., Prescott, G. A. & Balow, I. H. *Metropolitan achievement tests: primary II. form F.* New York: Harcourt Brace Jovanovich, 1970.

Durrell, D. D. *Durrell analysis of reading difficulty.* New York: Harcourt Brace Jovanovich, 1955.

Eisenson, J. *Examining for aphasia.* (Rev. ed.) New York: Psychological Corp., 1954.

Engelmann, S. *The basic concept inventory.* Chicago: Follett Publishing Co., 1967.

Foster, C. R., Giddan, J. J., & Stark, J. *ACLC: assessment of children's language comprehension.* Palo Alto, Calif.: Consulting Psychologists Press, 1972.

Fries, C. C. *The structure of English.* New York: Harcourt Brace Jovanovich, 1952.

Gates, A. I., & McKillop, A. S. *Gates-McKillop reading diagnostic tests.* New York: Teachers College Press, Columbia University, 1962.

Glaser, R. Instructional technology and the measurement of learning outcomes: some questions. *American Psychologist,* 1963, **18,** 519-21.

Goldstein, K. *Language and language disturbances.* New York: Grune & Stratton, 1948.

Goodglass, H., & Kaplan, E. *Boston diagnostic aphasia examination.* Philadelphia: Lea & Febiger, 1972.

Gorham, D. R. *Proverbs test.* Missoula, Mont.: Psychological Test Specialists, 1956. (a)

Gorham, D. R. A proverbs test for clinical and experimental use. *Psychological Reports,* 1956, **2,** 1-12. (b)

Gorham, D. R. Use of the proverbs test for differentiating schizophrenics from normals. *Journal of Counseling Psychology,* 1956, **20,** 435-40. (c)

Guilford, J. P. *The nature of human intelligence.* New York: McGraw-Hill, 1967.

Hahn, W. J., & Weiss, M. New scoring criteria for use of the token test in identifying language disabilities in children of low socioeconomic status. Paper presented at the Annual Convention of the American Speech and Hearing Association, Detroit, 1973.

Hainsworth, P. K., & Siqueland, M. L. *Early identification of children with learning disabilities: the Meeting Street School screening test.* Providence, R. I.: Crippled Children and Adults of Rhode Island, 1969.

Hammill, D. D., & Irwin, O. C. An abstraction test adapted for use with mentally retarded children. *American Journal of Mental Deficiency,* 1966, **70,** 866-72.

Irwin, J. V., & Marge, M. (Eds.) *Principles of childhood language disabilities.* New York: Appleton-Century Crofts, 1972.

Irwin, O. C., & Hammill, D. D. An abstraction test for use with cerebral palsied children. *Cerebral Palsy Review,* 1964, **25,** 3-9.

Jastak, J. F. *Wide range achievement test.* Wilmington, Del.: Guidance Associates, 1965.

Johnson, O. G., & Bommarito, J. W. (Eds.) *Tests and measurements in child development: a handbook.* San Francisco: Jossey-Bass, 1971.

Johnson, W., Darley, F. L., & Spriestersbach, D. C. *Diagnostic methods in speech pathology.* New York: Harper & Row, 1963.

Kelley, T. L., Madden, R., Gardner, E. F., & Rudman, H. C. *Stanford achievement test: intermediate battery.* New York: Harcourt Brace Jovanovich, 1964.

Kirk, S. A., McCarthy, J. J., & Kirk, W. D. *Illinois test of psycholinguistic ability.* (Rev. ed.) Urbana: University of Illinois Press, 1968.

Kreezer, G., & Dallenbach, K. M. Learning the relation of opposition. *American Journal of Psychology,* 1929, **41,** 432-41.

Lapointe, C. Token test performances by learning disabled and academically achieving adolescents. Master's thesis, Boston University, 1975.

Lee, L. *Northwestern syntax screening test.* Evanston, Ill.: Northwestern University Press, 1969, 1971.

Lerea, L. Assessing language development. *Journal of Speech and Hearing Research*, 1958, **1**, 75-85.

McCarthy, D. *McCarthy scales of children's abilities.* New York: Psychological Corp., 1970.

Newcomer, P., Hare, B., Hammill, D., & McGettigan, J. Construct validity of the Illinois test of psycholinguistic abilities. *Journal of Learning Disabilities*, 1975, **8**, 32-43.

Newfield, M. U., & Schlanger, B. B. The acquisition of morphology by normal and educable mentally retarded children. *Journal of Speech and Hearing Research*, *1968*, **4**, 693-706.

Noll, J. D. The use of the token test with children. Paper presented at the Annual Convention of the American Speech and Hearing Association, New York, 1970.

Nunnally, J. C., Flaugher, R. L., & Hodges, W. F. Measurement of semantic habits. *Educational and Psychological Measurement*, 1963, **23**, 419-34.

Nunnally, J. C., Flaugher, R. L., & Hodges, W. F. Semantic habits inventory. In O. G. Johnson & J. W. Bommarito (Eds.), *Tests and measurements in child development: a handbook.* San Francisco: Jossey-Bass, 1971, Pp. 80-81.

Orgass, B., & Poeck, K. Clinical validation of a new test for aphasia: an experimental study on the token test. *Cortex*, 1966, **2**, 222-43.

Osgood, C. E., & Miron, M. S. *Approaches to the study of asphasia.* Urbana: University of Illinois Press, 1963.

Osgood, C. E., Suci, G. J., & Tannenbaum, P. H. *The measurement of meaning.* Urbana: University of Illinois Press, 1957.

Otis, A. S. *Otis quick scoring mental abilities tests: alpha short form.* New York: Harcourt Brace Jovanovich, 1954.

Ratusnik, D. L., & Koenigsknecht, R. A. Internal consistency of the Northwestern syntax screening test. *Journal of Speech and Hearing Disorders*, 1975, **40**, 59-68.

Schuell, H. *Minnesota test for differential diagnosis of aphasia.* Minneapolis: University of Minnesota Press, 1965.

Semel, E. M., & Wiig, E. H. Comprehension of syntactic structures and critical verbal elements by children with learning disabilities, *Journal of Learning Disabilities*, 1975, 8, 53-58.

Snider, J. G., & Osgood, C. E. *Semantic differential technique: a sourcebook.* Chicago: Aldine-Atherton, 1969.

Swisher, L. P., & Sarno, M. T. Token test scores on three matched patient groups: left brain damaged with aphasia; right brain damaged without aphasia; non-brain damaged. *Cortex*, 1969, **5**, 264-73.

Terman, L. M., & Merrill, M. A. *Stanford-Binet intelligence scale.* Boston: Houghton Mifflin Co., 1960.

Thorpe, L. P., Lefever, D. W., & Naslund, R. A. *Science Research Associates achievement series.* Chicago: Science Research Associates, 1963.

Toronto, A. A. *Spanish syntax screening test.* Evanston, Ill.: Northwestern University Press, 1973.

Vogel, S. A. Syntactic abilities in normal and dyslexic children. *Journal of Learning Disabilities*, 1974, **7**, 47-53.

Wechsler, D. *Wechsler intelligence scale for children.* New York: Psychological Corp., 1949.

Wertz, R. T., Keith, R. L., & Custer, D. D. Normal and aphasic behavior on a measure of auditory input and a measure of verbal output. Paper presented at the Annual Convention of the American Speech and Hearing Association, Chicago, 1971.

Wertz, R. T., & Perkins, M. P. Measures of auditory input and verbal output in children. *Journal of the Colorado Speech and Hearing Association*, 1972, **5**, 11-18.

Wiig, E. H., Lapointe, C., & Semel, E. M. Relationships among language processing and production abilities of learning disabled adolescents. Paper presented at the Annual Convention of the American Speech and Hearing Association, Washington, D.C., 1975.

Wiig, E. H., & Semel, E. M. Comprehension of linguistic concepts requiring logical operations. *Journal of Speech and Hearing Research*, 1973, **16**, 627-36.

Wiig, E. H., & Semel, E. M. Development of comprehension of logico-grammatical sentences by grade school children. *Perceptual and Motor Skills*, 1974, **38**, 171-76.

Wiig, E. H., & Semel, E. M. Logico-grammatical sentence comprehension by learning disabled adolescents. *Perceptual and Motor Skills*, 1974, **38**, 1331-34. (b)

Wiig, E. H., Semel, E. M., & Crouse, M.A. The use of morphology by high-risk and learning disabled children. *Journal of Learning Disabilities*, 1973, **6**, 457-65.

Wolski, W. Language development of normal children four, five, and six years of age as measured by the Michigan picture language inventory. Unpublished doctoral dissertation, University of Michigan, 1962.

6 Remediation of Perceptual and Linguistic Processing Deficits

Overview

The present chapter advocates that remediation of language processing deficits should precede intervention for language production deficits since language processing and comprehension involve recognition while language production requires recall and retrieval. This view is based on supportive evidence presented by, among others, Asher (1972), Brown, Cazden, and Bellugi (1968), Fraser, Bellugi, and Brown (1963), and Winitz (1973). It also advocates that remedial procedures and materials should be presented to reflect developmental sequences or order of difficulty as indicated by clinical observations and/or research. In addition, it is proposed that problem solving, made easier by providing minimal differences in linguistic structures and by interfacing cognitive and linguistic features, facilitates improvement of language processing (Winitz, 1973).

Procedures and methods that lend themselves to improving auditory attention, identification and localization of sound sources and auditory figure-ground judgments are suggested, and the potential role of the clinical audiologist in remedial intervention is emphasized. In the area of auditory discrimination, the discussions focus on assisting the educator-clinician in the development, evaluation, and/or selection of appropriate programs and activities for improving speech-sound discrimination. Aspects emphasized for designing or evaluating materials, methods, or programs are (1) the scope of the sound elements included or presented, (2) the sequencing of phoneme contrasts based on distinctive feature analysis, (3) the level of difficulty of the task or tasks, and (4) the response characteristics. Selected phonics and auditory perception programs which are commercially available are compared against these criteria.

Methods and procedures are also suggested for the improvement of auditory—visual integration. The procedures combine nonsymbolic and symbolic auditory stimuli with representative nonsymbolic or pictorial visual displays.

Finally, methods and procedures are suggested and illustrated that lend themselves to improving knowledge of morphology and syntax. Evidence of

131

linguistic processing deficits observed in language and learning disabilities is introduced as a background for the discussions of areas which may need emphasis in remediation. Observations of normal developmental sequences and order of difficulty in processing syntactic structures are presented as a basis for suggesting sequencing of remedial materials.

General Considerations in Planning Intervention

Designing procedures for remedial intervention requires awareness of the assets and deficits of the individual in need of the intervention as well as knowledge of remedial methods and strategies. Ideally, the diagnostic evaluation should result in identification of specific deficit areas, knowledge of the degree and extent of specific deficits and of the relationships between them, and recognition of areas of strength. It is the responsibility of the educator or clinician to select those intervention methods, strategies, and materials which best match the youngster's profile of assets and defits. In this fashion, areas of strength may be used for compensation of specific deficits. The following sections suggest and discuss methods and strategies for the improvement of auditory-perceptual and linguistic processing.

The methods, strategies, and specific procedures suggested reflect the views that (1) language processing and comprehension precede oral language production and involve recognition rather than recall and retrieval. These views are supported by observations by Asher (1972), Brown, Cazden, and Bellugi (1968), Fraser, Bellugi, and Brown (1963), and Winitz (1973), among others. The discussions also reflect the view that the remedial materials and procedures can be sequenced to reflect increases in the level of difficulty on the basis of either clinical observations, research findings, cognitive or linguistic theories, or psycholinguistic principles. Furthermore, they reflect the view that problem solving (Winitz, 1973), facilitated by providing minimal differences in linguistic structures and by interfacing cognitive and linguistic aspects, may accelerate the improvement of language processing. This view is supported by observations by, among others, Asher (1972), Bever (1970), and Winitz (1973), and by research of the effects of remedial language intervention with learning disabled children (Wiig & Semel, 1973).

Principles and Methods for Improving
Auditory-Perceptual Processing

Based on a critical review of research of the relationship between selected auditory-perceptual skills and reading ability, Hammill and Larsen (1974) recently concluded:

> Apparently a large percentage of children who perform adequately on tests of auditory perception experience difficulty in learning to read; and an equally sizable percentage who do poorly on these same tests have *no* problem in reading. As a consequence the time and expense currently devoted to auditory training in the schools should be re-evaluated, if the purpose of such training is to improve reading proficiency. [p. 434]

Although this conclusion is well supported, there is support for training auditory-perceptual skills if significant deficits are observed and if the purpose is to facilitate auditory-perceptual processing. This support originates from a variety of sources and reflects clinical observations and the findings of basic and applied research.

Johnson and Myklebust (1967) have expressed the view that if a child is diagnosed to exhibit auditory-perceptual deficits, remediation should be provided for the specific deficits. De Hirsh, Jansky, and Langford (1966) concur with this view and advocate that areas of strength and weakness should be assessed and specific intervention provided for deficits. In a similar vein, Chalfant and Scheffelin (1969) stress that "there is a need to identify and distinguish the different auditory activities and develop specific remedial approaches for these activities" (p. 19). These views are opposed by several educators, among them Mann (1970) and Mann and Phillips (1967). Their views are summarized in the statement by Mann (1970) that "These 'learning disabilities' are hypothesized as being basic to academic and other types of achievement or malachievement and are presumed to be finitely separable, diagnosable and (by many) trainable" (p. 88).

Investigations of the efficacy of training in auditory perception on specific auditory abilities have yielded positive results. Durrell and Murphy (1958) reported that children with auditory discrimination deficits demonstrated gains in the auditory analysis of words as a function of training. Children with proficient auditory discrimination, on the other hand, showed minimal gains from extra training. Silvaroli and Wheelock (1966) provided speech-sound discrimination training to kindergarteners with lower socioeconomic backgrounds. The experimental group made significantly larger gains on the *Wepman Auditory Discrimination Test* than the controls who did not receive training.

Semel (1972) investigated the effects of listening intervention, using the *Sound-Order-Sense Developmental Program in Auditory Perception* (Semel, 1970), on the performance on nine selected tests of auditory perception by second graders. The experimental training program was administered to sixty-eight randomly selected children with thirty-four children serving as controls. Analysis of covariance of the pre- and post-training performances indicated significantly larger performance gains by the experimental group on (1) the *Competing Messages* subtest of the *Flowers-Costello Tests of Central Auditory Abilities*, (2) the *Stanford Diagnostic Auditory Discrimination* subtest, and (3) the *Durrell-Hayes Listening Test for Sentences*. It was concluded that the training program was effective in improving performances on task-related standardized tests of auditory perception.

In a different vein, Winitz and Preisler (1967) reported that pretraining in auditory discrimination of successively closer distinctive features resulted in significantly improved sound discrimination ability. Similar training procedures were employed effectively with forty-one second graders by Ritterman (1970). He further reported retroactive facilitation effects in an observation group, suggesting that vicarious experience may facilitate speech-sound discrimination. These findings, in combination with evidence that sentence processing occurs simultaneously at all available levels of analysis (phonetic, lexical, syntactic, semantic) (Marslen-Wilson, 1975), are considered to support the current practice among language pathologists of providing intervention for deficits observed at any level of language processing.

Auditory Attention and Identification of Nonsymbolic Stimuli

Procedures designed to improve auditory attention and identification of nonsymbolic stimuli may utilize a wide range of auditory stimuli with varying stimulus characteristics. Auditory stimuli lending themselves to improving the awareness of the presence of specific sounds in the environment and to establishing associations between sounds and sound sources may include the following:

1. Sounds made by familiar objects such as cars, doorbells, and telephones.
2. Sounds made by moving body parts such as shuffling feet, clapping hands, and snapping fingers.
3. Sounds generated in particular environments such as on a playground; for example, balls bouncing, children playing games, screeching of an unoiled swing, the thump of a seesaw, etc., or in a cafeteria; for example, dishes being stacked, water boiling, cash register ringing, etc.
4. Sounds with controlled differences in pitch (frequency), intensity, duration, and quality.

Materials for implementing activities that incorporate the various sounds described may be obtained from several educational and commercial sources. A variety of sounds and sound sources is also available on commercial recordings of sound effects.

Activities designed to improve sustained auditory attention may use recordings or audiotapes of familiar environmental sounds. One of the sounds may be identified as the target sound. This sound should occur at irregular intervals. The child or children may be asked to identify the presence of the target sound by either (1) raising a hand, (2) imitating the sound, (3) naming the sound source, or (4) identifying a picture of the sound source. As sustained auditory attention improves, the intervals between the target stimuli may be increased. Auditory stimuli of different pitch (frequency), intensity, duration, and rate may be used as alternatives, depending upon the child's auditory acuity and auditory discrimination skills.

An alternate activity has been suggested by Kirshner (1972) in which a series of tape-recorder taps are presented. The listener must count the series of taps, generally twenty-five or more, and report the number heard in the series. The rate of presentation of the stimuli may be varied to accommodate those having difficulties in rapid processing of auditory input. The activity is discontinued when the reported number of taps corresponds to the number of auditory stimuli presented. The progress may be charted to provide feedback and reinforcement.

A sequence for the remedial intervention of auditory attention and sound-source association deficits has recently been described by Chappell (1972).

Remedial procedures have also been suggested by Bangs (1954, 1968), Berry and Eisenson (1956), and Johnson and Myklebust (1967), among others.

Localization of Sounds

Activities designed to improve the ability to localize sounds in the environment may use the following sources and procedures:

1. The sound sources may utilize familiar or unfamiliar environmental sounds differing in frequency, intensity, and duration; connected speech; or music.
2. The position of sound sources may vary in distance and/or direction.

The environments in which the activities may be conducted range from a sound-treated audiological suite to a hallway or a classroom. The location of the activity will determine the nature of the stimuli and the procedures used. The rehabilitation audiologist may design activities to improve sound localization for pure tones, noise, music, and speech. In the audiological setting, the location of the sound sources and the stimulus parameters may be controlled by instrumentation. The duration of the auditory stimuli may also be shortened, and the sound intensity may be varied as the child's ability to localize sounds improves.

Activities applicable to the educational setting have been described by Semel (1970):

1. The teacher is instructed to take a group of children to the gym. The children are blindfolded and instructed to go to the teacher when he blows a whistle from various locations, reflecting coordinates of space (front-back, right-left, up-down).
2. A child is sitting with eyes covered in the center of the room. Other children call out the child's name from different directions and at different distances. The child in the center must indicate the location of the caller by pointing.

Auditory Figure-Ground

Auditory figure-ground ability is reflected by skill in recognizing a relevant (target) stimulus against a competing background of sounds. It is a necessary skill, since auditory-perceptual processing must be accomplished daily in situations in which both target and background stimuli vary continuously. Activities designed for improving auditory figure-ground skills may use: (1) target stimuli (nonverbal or verbal), and (2) background stimuli (nonverbal or verbal, continuous or interrupted, repetitive or changing, and predictable or random).

In audiological settings, the controlled environment and the instrumentation permit the design of activities in which the parameters of the target stimuli (pure tones, environmental sounds, music, or speech) can be controlled against backgrounds of competing stimuli and presented through the same, or different, earphones or loudspeakers.

In the initial activities conducted in the audiological setting, the signal-to-noise ratios may be controlled to facilitate identification of the target stimulus. The target stimuli and auditory backgrounds may also be introduced with separation in space to facilitate differentiation of figure and ground by selective use of the ears. Knowledge and control of masking (auditory background) characteristics and of signal-to-noise ratios may be utilized by the audiologist to design tasks of increasing difficulty.

Semel (1970) provides a set of activities for educational settings, with the stimuli being a set of sequential oral directions performed against a variety of recorded auditory backgrounds. The program of sequential oral directions requires ability to focus on the relevant verbal stimuli and to inhibit responses to competing auditory inputs ranging from environmental sounds to speech.

Among the activities suggested is one in which the class pretends to take a bus ride. The children provide the auditory background by imitating engine and traffic sounds. Each child is given a target stimulus, the name of the street where he lives. The teacher calls out street names for the children to identify. One variation of this activity is identification of beginning sounds of street names.

The records accompanying the program may provide auditory backgrounds for activities designed by the teacher. Other sounds that can be used as backgrounds are noises of a vacuum cleaner or of other electrical appliances, the playing of a musical instrument, hand clapping, and sounds of a metronome, buzzer, or timer.

Auditory Discrimination of Phonemes

In designing or evaluating commercially available programs and activities for improving speech-sound discrimination, the following aspects should be considered: (1) scope, (2) sequencing of sounds, (3) response characteristics, and (4) procedures.

1. The *scope* of the sound elements included or presented must be considered. Programs and activities may be designed to improve discrimination of a limited set of phonemes by focusing on initial consonants and short and long vowels or by emphasizing graphemes rather than phonemes. They may also emphasize phoneme-grapheme correspondences in the discrimination activities. Educational programs for improving speech-sound discrimination rarely cover a wide selection of speech sounds (vowels, consonants in initial and final word positions, and blends).

    The scope of the sound elements included in available programs for auditory discrimination varies considerably. Traditional phonics programs tend to limit the selection of speech sounds to short and long vowels and consonants (Hay & Wingo, 1967; Stern & Gould, 1965). Programs based on phonetic models seem to include a wider range of sounds and include consonants, consonant blends, and vowels. They emphasize a one-to-one relationship between phonemes and their corresponding graphemes (Gattegno, 1963; Lindamood & Lindamood, 1969; Semel, 1970, in press). The selection of speech sounds suggested for auditory discrimination in the speech pathology literature is generally determined by relationships between articulation and speech-sound dicrimination errors (Berry & Eisenson, 1956; Van Riper, 1963).

2. The *sequencing* of sounds in the discrimination activities must be considered. Evidence suggests that phonemes and phoneme sequences (blends) which differ maximally in terms of distinctive features should be contrasted before phonemes which differ minimally (Winitz, 1969; Winitz & Preisler, 1967).

The approaches to sequencing auditory stimuli for improving discrimination vary widely in available programs. Few programs utilize distinctive feature analysis to determine the relative ease with which phonemes may be discriminated (Semel, 1970, in press). Reading programs generally do not consider one-to-one correspondences between phonemes and graphemes. Among the exceptions are the following reading programs: *Words in Colour* (Gattegno, 1963), *Psycholinguistic Color System* (Bannatyne, 1968), *Open Court Kindergarten Program* (Bereiter & Hughes, 1970), and *Initial Teaching Alphabet* (Pitman, 1969; Warburton & Southgate, 1969).

Discrimination training activities suggested by speech pathologists sometimes suggest hierarchies of sounds to be included for auditory discrimination. Thus, Winitz (1969) has emphasized distinctive feature analysis in selecting minimal pairs for auditory discrimination and has stressed that phoneme discrimination is basic to the improvement of phoneme production.

The number of distinctive feature differences separating English consonants has been analyzed by Jakobson, Fant, and Halle (1952). A chart of the units of distinctive feature differences presented by Saporta (1955) is included in Table 13. This chart may be used to program the sequence of consonant presentation in minimal word pairs to reflect a gradual decrease in the number of distinctive features that separate target phonemes.

3. *The response characteristics and differences* should be considered and sequenced in order of difficulty. Observations suggest that:

(a) Initially, the responses may identify the presence of sounds in single words, minimally paired words, word triplets, and sentences. The presence of a target sound may be signaled in a variety of ways: by raising a hand, saying yes-no, or by repeating the word.

(b) Same-different responses to minimal word and sentence pairs require knowledge of the concepts involved in the response and adequate memory and are therefore more complex.

(c) Later response modes may include identification of the position (initial, medial, final) of sounds in single words, selection of target sounds by repetition and reauditorization, and production of words with omitted target sounds.

(d) Responses requiring auditory-visual integration and association between speech-sounds and letters and between speech-sound and letter sequences should be required last.

4. The *procedures* suggested should reflect a progression in the order of task difficulty required. Thus, recognition of words containing a specific target sound should precede discrimination of target sounds in minimally paired words or word triplets and discrimination of target sounds in minimally paired sentences.

TABLE 13

English Phonemes: Units of Difference

	m	p	b	f	v	θ	ð	n	t	d	s	z	š	ž	ě	ǰ	ŋ	k	g
m	—																		
p	4	—																	
b	4	2	—																
f	4	2	4	—															
v	4	4	2	2	—														
θ	7	5	7	3	5	—													
ð	7	7	5	5	3	2	—												
n	2	6	6	6	6	5	5	—											
t	7	3	5	5	7	2	4	5	—										
d	7	5	3	7	5	4	2	5	2	—									
s	7	5	7	3	5	2	4	5	4	6	—								
z	7	7	5	5	3	4	2	5	6	4	2	—							
š	8	6	8	4	6	5	7	8	7	9	3	5	—						
ž	8	8	6	6	4	7	5	8	9	7	5	3	2	—					
ě	8	4	6	6	8	7	9	8	5	7	5	7	2	4	—				
ǰ	8	6	4	8	6	9	7	8	7	5	7	5	4	2	2	—			
ŋ	3	7	7	7	7	8	8	3	8	8	8	8	5	5	5	5	—		
k	8	4	6	6	8	5	7	8	3	5	7	9	4	6	2	4	5	—	
g	8	6	4	8	6	7	5	8	5	3	9	7	6	4	4	2	5	2	—

SOURCE: Reprinted with permission of the *Linguistic Society of America* from: Saporta, S. Frequency of consonant clusters. *Language*, 1955, **31**, 25-30.

The procedures used in programs for improving the discrimination of speech sounds are generally limited in range. Van Riper (1963) has outlined the following basic procedural steps for auditory discriminiation training: (1) isolation of sounds from their contexts, (2) stimulation with sounds and sound sequences, (3) identification of correct-incorrect sounds, and (4) discrimination of correct-incorrect sounds. Berry and Eisenson (1956) outline a similar sequence of procedural steps: (1) analysis and auditory recognition of defective and correct speech sounds, (2) sound stimulation, (3) phonetic replacement, and (4) analysis of sound combinations.

Phonics programs often emphasize visual (pictures and written words) rather than auditory input. The children may be required to identify like sounds from a list of written words or a group of pictures, match sounds with pictures, select the letter that represents an initial sound, or to group word families.

The response modes utilized by phonics programs often require ability to read or at least ability to reauditorize the words associated with pictures. Johnson and Mykebust (1967) have reported that reauditorization may represent a problem area for children with learning disabilities, and many may not be able to read. As a result, the characteristics of the required responses should be carefully considered and preferably a choice of responses should be provided. The following examples illustrate the variety of possible procedures and suggest sequencing for the target sound *m:*

1. Identification of words with the target sound from among randomly selected words:
    a. fun - cat - *milk*
    b. cake - *man* - dog
    c. *mix* - ring - eat
2. Same or different judgment of word pairs containing the target sound:
    a. mix - fix
    b. marble - marble
    c. wake-up - make up
3. Identification of the target sound in minimal word pairs:
    a. *mean* - bean
    b. fight - *might*
    c. *mess* - less
4. Identification of the target sound in word triplets:
    a. *mink* - pink - sink
    b. wet - *met* - pet
    c. sail - pail - *mail*
5. Identification of the position (initial or final) of the target sound in word pairs:
    a. *mustard* - custard
    b. drug - dru*m*
6. Reauditorization and production of an omitted target sound:
    a. (m)agic
    b. (m)acaroni
    c. (m)ustache
7. Same or different judgment of minimally paired sentences:
    a. Can Mary *make* a cake?
       Can Mary bake a cake?
    b. Mike can't see the *mountain*.
       Mike can't see the fountain.
8. Identification of the target sound in minimally paired sentences:
    a. Mother is never sad.
       Mother is never *mad*.
    b. *Monkeys* have long tails.
       Donkeys have long tails.

Activities for Auditory Sequencing

Activities designed to improve auditory sequencing should consider the following:

1. Materials should be included that require judgments of phoneme, syllable, and word sequences.
2. Nonverbal as well as verbal responses, requiring identification of same-different and correct-incorrect sequences and rearrangement of incorrectly sequenced materials, should be included.

3. To facilitate retention of sequential aspects, the auditory stimuli should be introduced in a series so that the initial stimulus sequences are irreversible. Later stimuli may be reversible to demand retention of all aspects of the sequence (Goodglass & Kaplan, 1972).

Among the few programs designed to improve auditory sequential processing, the *Sound-Order-Sense* and the SAPP programs (Semel, 1970, in press) introduce programmed activities requiring judgments of phoneme, syllable, and word sequences. At the phonemic level, youngsters are asked to judge sequential aspects in a same-different example. At the syllable level, word segments (syllables and morphemes) are presented in incorrect order, and the youngsters are asked to rearrange the sequences to form words. Examples are board black, cream ice, and nic pic.

Words in Colour (Gattegno, 1963), another educational program stressing sequencing abilities, utilizes only phoneme sequences. The auditory stimuli are individual letters in different spatial arrangements. As an example, the letters *p, a, t* are written on a chalkboard in different sequences. The child is required to sound out the sequence of letters and say the corresponding word. The program also presents a substitution-sequencing pattern in which a phoneme sequence (p - a - t) is first reversed (t - a - p). Next, a substitution of the final phoneme is made (t - a - n), and this sequence is reversed (n - a - t). Finally, the initial phoneme is substituted (b - a - t), and this sequence is reversed (t - a - b). The teacher initiates the sequence and provides the associated written stimuli using a different color for each phoneme. After the rules has been established, the children may generate the stimuli.

Auditory Discrimination in Depth (Lindamood & Lindamood, 1969) presents activities focused on teaching basic auditory-perceptual skills. The areas stressed in the program include speech-sound discrimination, sound sequencing, and sound-symbol association.

Among other commercially available programs which may be of value in planning remedial procedures are the *Listening Skills Program* (Bracken, Hays, & Bridges, 1970), *Auditory Perception* (Saleh, 1970), and *Auditory Perception Training* (Willette, Jackson, & Peckins, 1970). Of these programs, the *Listening Skills* and the *Auditory Perception* programs were designed to cover the widest age range, from six to twelve years and five to twelve years, respectively. Both programs cover a wide range of skills.

The *Listening Skills Program* (Bracken, Hays, & Bridges, 1970) was designed to develop awareness of pitch, volume, and sentence patterns and to improve auditory discrimination, memory, and listening for directions, details, and main ideas, among others. The program developed by Saleh (1970) stresses the development of auditory discrimination, memory span and comprehension, and of differentiation of inflection and rhythm patterns.

The *Auditory Perception Training* program (Willette, Jackson, & Peckins, 1970) was designed for the age range from five to eight. It contains taped lessons for developing (1) auditory memory, (2) figure-ground, (3) auditory discrimination, (4) auditory imagery, and (5) auditory-motor integration.

Improving Auditory-Visual Integration

Learning disabled children have been reported to experience deficits in auditory–visual integration by Birch and Belmont (1964), Birch and Lefford (1963), and McGrady and Olson (1970). In a similar vein, Holloway (1971) has observed that schoolchildren with language delays of unknown origin exhibit significant reductions in auditory-visual integration but not in visual-motor integration. These observations suggest that learning disabled children with language deficits may need considerable assistance in transferring auditory processing skills to an auditory-visual task such as reading.

Understanding that a one-to-one relationship can exist between an auditory stimulus and a visual display constitutes a basic ability in auditory-visual integration. In order to establish this relationship, the educator may combine nonsymbolic auditory stimuli with representative nonsymbolic visual displays. These procedures may include:

1. Discriminating and matching tonal pairs to visual displays representing their durations:
   Auditory stimulus: *long* tone—*short* tone
   Visual displays: __ _____ / _____ __
2. Discriminating and matching tonal pairs with visual displays representing their intensities:
   Auditory stimulus: *loud* tone—*soft* tone

   Visual displays: ■ ☐ / ☐ ■

3. Discriminating and matching tonal pairs to visual displays representing their frequencies (pitch):
   Auditory stimulus: *upward* modulated tone—*downward* modulated tone

   Visual displays: ↗ ↘ / ↘ ↗

4. Discriminating and matching tonal pairs with visual displays representing changes in rate:
   Auditory stimulus: *fast* tone—*slow* tone.

   Visual displays: 〰 ～ / ～ 〰

The next step in the progression towards the integration of auditory-verbal and visual-symbolic stimuli requires matching between auditory-verbal stimuli and nonsymbolic visual displays. Among possible activities are

1. Discriminating and matching auditory-verbal sequences with visual displays representing the temporal patterns:
   Instruction: When you hear the word *gum* mark the place where you heard it. First, in the middle, or at the

Auditory stimulus: shoe—table—gum
Visual displays: _____ _____ ___X___

2. Discrimination and identification of the identities or differences (same-different) of the words in the minimal word pair with representative visual displays:
   *Auditory stimulus:*cat—bat
   Visual displays: O O / X O

3. Discrimination and matching of a series of digits, letters, or words of which the majority are identical while one differs with representative visual displays.
   Auditory stimulus: three-three-three-seven
   Visual displays: O O O X / O O O O

4. Discrimination and matching of an auditory-verbal sequence with visual displays representing similarities and differences in the composition of speech sounds (phonemes):
   Auditory stimulus: gate—rate—date—house
   Visual displays: O O O O / O O O X

5. Discrimination and matching of minimal word pairs with pictorial displays.
   a. *Auditory stimuli:*   mountain—fountain
                              Mark: fountain
      Pictorial displays: (two choices)
   b. *Auditory stimuli:*   face—race—lace
                              Mark: face
      Pictorial displays: (three choices)
   c. *Auditory stimuli:*   man—pan—fan—can
                              Mark: fan
      Pictorial displays: (four choices)

The procedures designed to establish integration between auditory-verbal and visual-symbolic stimuli may initially introduce additional nonsymbolic visual cues. These facilitating cues may be gradually faded, as in the following steps:

1. Discrimination and matching of minimal word pairs that differ in visual configuration with combined pictorial—written stimuli:
   Auditory stimuli: mountain—fountain
                         Mark: mountain
   Visual displays: pictures of both items

2. Discrimination and matching of minimal word pairs that differ in visual configuration with visual-symbolic stimuli emphasized for configurational differences:
   Auditory stimulus: coat—boat—goat
                         Mark: boat
   Visual displays: pictures of all items

3. Discrimination and matching of minimally paired words with visual-symbolic stimuli:
   Auditory stimuli: tail—mail—pail
                         Mark: mail
   Visual displays: pictures of all items

It is desirable that the inventory of speech sounds used in these activities be as large as possible and that consonants, vowels, and blends are incorporated. The design should focus on using sounds with phoneme-grapheme correspondence. Sources for additional materials and procedures include *Speech to Print* (Durrell & Murphy, 1964), *Words in Colour* (Gattegno, 1963), *Auditory Discrimination in Depth* (Lindamood & Lindamood, 1969), and the *Sound-Order-Sense* and *Semel Auditory Processing* programs (Semel, 1970, in press).

Improving Linguistic Processing

Improving Knowledge of Morphology

Learning disabled youngsters have been reported to experience significant delays in the acquisition and use of English morphology (Vogel, 1974; Wiig, Semel, & Crouse, 1973). They may exhibit delays in acquiring the word-formation (morphological) rules for:

1. Noun plurals (regular and irregular) and possessives (singular and plural).
2. Derivation of nouns and adverbs.
3. Third person singular of the present tense and past tense of regular verbs.
4. Irregular verb tenses.
5. Adjectival inflections (comparative and superlative).

Clinical observations further indicate that they may experience problems in interpreting the mood and aspect of verbs.

In remediation, the word-formation rules sharing common properties may be introduced together to facilitate transfer and generalization. On this basis the suggested sequence for remediation progresses as follows:

1. Noun plurals (regular and irregular) and noun-verb agreement.
2. Noun derivation.
3. Prefixes and suffixes
   a. derivational suffixes
   b. prefixes
   c. inflectional suffixes
4. Verb tenses and auxiliary verbs
5. Comparative and superlative of adjectives.

Noun Plurals and Noun-Verb Agreement

Knowledge of the word-formation rules for noun plurals may be established using a variety of activities and formats. Initially, the children may be required to identify which words, in a list of regular and irregular nouns said to them, mean *one* or *more than one*. This procedure permits identification of noun categories (regular or irregular) that present difficulties.

In the second step, a multiple-choice cloze procedure may be used. Regular nouns should be introduced initially, and nouns which share the same phonological conditioning rules (-s, -z, -iz) should be introduced together. Irregular noun plurals should be introduced last. It is also important that the noun (plural or singular) is introduced with a variety of markers such as *a, an, the, this, that, these, those, all, some,* and so forth. Examples:

1. Mary takes one (book/books) to school.
2. Is the (book/books) she takes very heavy?
3. Yes, it is a very big (book/books).
4. Why doesn't she take all her (book/books) to school?

A subsequent, but closely related step, is to establish noun-verb agreement for third person singular and plural of present tense verbs. The rules may be established in a cloze procedure with multiple choices, using sentences such as:

1. The boy (swims/swim) in the lake.
2. The dogs (barks/bark) at the mailman.

Finally, the children may be asked to change sentences containing singular nouns to ones containing plural nouns and vice versa. This step requires knowledge of the rules for forming noun plurals and of the rules for noun-verb agreement.

Noun Derivation

Establishing the rules for noun derivation seems a natural extension of the previous focus on the noun category. Compounding of nouns provides a transitional step between the previous focus on noun plurals and the subsequent focus on rules for deriving nouns from other word classes. Materials and activities for establishing compounding of nouns may use sentence completion procedures with or without multiple choices. Learning disabled youngsters generally di not experience difficulties in compounding nouns, and multiple-choice procedures may be unnecessary. The purpose of the transitional step is to develop awareness that new nouns can be formed that reflect the added meaning of a function, job, skill, and so forth. Examples:

1. A man who sells milk is a _____ (mailman/milkman).
2. A ship that sails through space is a _____ (flagship/spaceship).

Prefixes and Suffixes

Prefixes and suffixes are minimal grammatical units that carry meaning such as *un-. dis-, -ness, -ly.* These units do not occur in isolation, but must be bound to a root word (base) as in *un*(like), *dis*(like), (like)*ness.* Suffixes may be divided into two categories: (1) *inflectional suffixes* which are used for inflecting a base (root word) to indicate plurality (boy-boys), tense (walk-walk*ed*), comparative (great-great*er*) or superlative (great-great*est*) forms, and so forth, and (2) *derivational suffixes* which are used to derive new words such as forming a noun (teach)*er,* from a common verb base, *teach.*

Derivational suffixes

Among derivational suffixes which may pose problems for the learning disabled youngster are:

1. *-er* as in teach*er*. The problems seem related to confusion between derived nouns such as *singer, teacher,* etc., and comparatives such as *greater* in which the bound morpheme *-er* is used to inflect an adjective.
2. *-ly* as in happi*ly,* a derived adverb.
3. *-y* as in wind*y,* an adverb derived from the noun *wind*.

The LD child may consider each derived word to be a novel word with a new and unrelated meaning. He may fail to see the relationship in meaning between the derived word and the root word and may be unable to easily identify root words (bases) in derived words. Therefore, the focus of remediation is to improve (1) identification of root words (bases), (2) segmentation, that is, dividing words into their smallest meaningful units, and (3) analysis and synthesis of the meanings of base suffix combinations. Intervention strategies may proceed as in the following steps and may require:

1. *Identification* of root words in words such as *happiness, happily, happier*.
2. *Segmentation* of words used previously for identification of root words. The segmentation process should include a discussion of the meaning of the identified bases and the various suffixes. Subsequently, sentence completion procedures may be introduced in which the youngster is required to supply only a derivational suffix: "Ted bought his mother a birthday card because he is thought _____ (ful)."
3. *Analysis and synthesis* of the meaning of derived words and *knowledge of the rules for derivation* may be established by:
   a. multiple-choice cloze procedures: "A person who begins is a (starter/beginner/finisher)."
   b. cloze procedures in which the appropriate derived word must be provided spontaneously: "Someone who climbs mountains is a mountain climber."
   c. cloze procedures using sentences in which several appropriate derived forms of the same root word must be supplied: "Mother took her _____ list to go _____. She is a good _____."

Prefixes

For the learning disabled youngster, prefixes may present difficulties that seem to reflect:

1. Confusions between the meanings of the various prefixes or lack of differentiation between similar prefixes.
2. Confusion between phonologically similar prefixes such as *pre-,* and *re-* and *under-* and *un-*.

3. Problems in comprehending that the addition of a prefix changes the meaning of the word as in *cover, uncover, discover, recover.* The prefixed words may be more and more distantly related to the root word or may function as synonyms for entirely different words. In the example above, *uncover* is oppositionally related to *cover. Discover* is a synonym for *find,* a word which is quite unrelated to the base, *cover. Recover* may be used as a synonym for *find* in the sentence "I *recovered* my lost jewels," for *get well* in "I hope you *recover* quickly from your illness" or for *cover again* in "The upholstery on my couch was just *recovered.*"

4. Problems in perceiving or retaining the prefix and the base in the correct sequence. As a result, the word *recover* may be confused and interpreted as *recovery* or *covery.*

Remediation strategies designed to establish differentiation between the meaning of a root word and a prefixed form of the root word and between various prefixes may use sentences that are minimally paired. The responses may require same-different judgments, identification of the difference in meaning, or restatement of the initial sentence, "Lock the door," to reflect the opposite meaning, "Unlock the door." Examples:

1. Zip your jacket.
2. Unzip your jacket.
3. Mother planted the shrubs.
4. Mother replanted the shrubs.

A different format may be introduced using sentence pairs in which one makes sense and the other does not. The child is required to indicate which sentence makes sense and why. Examples:

1. I will *untie* my shoes before I take them off.
   I will *tie* my shoes before I take them off.
2. Al *buttoned* his coat before he took it off.
   Al *unbuttoned* his coat before he took it off.

Subsequently, the children may be asked to form as many varieties of root words as possible using prefixes and suffixes. Printed, color-coded cue cards may assist in establishing sequencing of prefix + base, base + suffix, and prefix + base + suffix. Among root words lending themselves to this activity are *cover, clean,* and *interest.*

Inflectional suffixes

Inflectional suffixes, such as -*ing* which is added to a root verb to form the progressive tense and -*er* which is added to a root adjective to form the comparative form, do not change the meaning of the base (root word) or change the grammatical category of the word. As an example, adding -*er* to the word *tall* does not change the basic meaning of the adjective. The inflectional suffix denotes that two persons or objects with similar qualities are being compared. Adding -*er* to *tall* also does not change the grammatical category of the base (root word). It remains an adjective. In this way, inflectional suffixes differ from derivational suffixes, the addition of which changes the grammatical category of the word, for example, *teach*- teach*er*. Unfortunately, the same root words (bases) may lend themselves to both derivation and inflection. Example: *teach:* teach*er* (derived noun); teach*ing* (derived noun: "His teaching was clear."); teach*ing* (inflected verb: "He was teaching his class.")

Inflectional suffixes are used to form (1) noun plurals and noun possessives, (2) verb tenses, and (3) comparative and superlative adjectives.

Learning disabled youngsters may experience problems in recognizing the differences in tense denoted by the inflectional suffixes. The verb tenses that denote inflectional suffixes are (1) progressive tense with the addition of *-ing* to the root verb (base), (2) third person singular of the present tense with the addition of /s/, /z/, or /iz/; for example, "He walks," "He runs," and "He dresses," and (3) past tense with the addition of /t/, /d/, or /id/ to regular verbs; for example, "He walked," "He climbed," "He ended the session," and internal changes in irregular verbs (run; ran; bring; brought).

Verb Tenses and Auxiliary Verbs

Learning disabled children may experience a variety of other problems in processing verbs and verb tenses. They may not:

1. Differentiate the durational distinctions denoted by the progressive and present tenses and may consider them to be synonymous. As a result, they may have difficulty differentiating the sentences "He is walking to school (now)" and "He walks to school (generally)."
2. Differentiate the temporal differences expressed by the past, present, and future tenses.
3. Perceive the phonological factors which condition the use of a specific inflectional suffix (/s/, /z/, /iz/ and /t/, /d/, /id/).
4. Perceive the rules that govern the changes in irregular verbs.
5. Perceive the rules that apply to forms of the copula (to be) and of auxiliary verbs (do, have, be, can, could, may, might, must, will, would, shall, and should).

Remediation strategies designed to improve verb tense comprehension should reflect a sequence that corresponds to the relative levels of difficulty of the various rules and forms. The description of difficulties provided above reflects clinical observations of the order of difficulty for LD youngsters.

Initially, the differentiation between the present and progressive tenses may be established using formats such as:

1. Cloze procedures with multiple choices: "The boy was *walk/walking* to the store."
2. Cloze or sentence completion procedures requiring spontaneous responses:
   a. Right now he is (sleeping).
   b. During the night he generally (sleeps).
   c. He often (sleeps) through class.

Differentiation between the temporal aspects denoted by verb tenses may be established by using sentences featuring either *yesterday,* or *today,* or *tomorrow* as cues to the appropriate tense. Initially, these cues can occur at the beginning of sentences; later, they may occur at the end of sentences or be deleted. Responses may require (a) same-different judgments, (b) identification of when an action occurred, (c) classification according to a time scale, (d) sentence completion from multiple choices, (e) spontaneous sentence completion, and (f) reforming of sentences into the past, future, or present tenses. Examples:

1. Same-different judgments of sentence pairs, such as "I went away," and "I have gone away."
2. Classification of verbs according to whether they denote *yesterday, today,* or *tomorrow* using verbs such as *ate, eats,* or *will eat.*
3. Classification of sentences according to whether they express a past, a current/present, or a future event, using sentences such as "Joe was reading his book," "Joe will read his book," "Joe is reading his book," and "Joe reads his book."

The rules for irregular verbs and auxiliary verbs may be established using similar procedures and formats. Methods for establishing the rules governing transformations of the verb phrase to express mood and aspect appear to follow in a natural extension of the procedures described above. The mood expressed by the forms *must, have to,* and *ought to* and the aspect indicated by the forms *have, will,* and *am* may combine with various tenses to express subtle differences. These differences have been discussed in Chapter 3. The procedures suggested for establishing differentiation of verb tenses and use of auxiliaries may be adapted and extended to establish comprehension of mood, aspect, and combinations of mood and aspect.

Comparative and Superlative of Adjectives

Comparative and superlative forms of adjectives may pose the following problems for LD children:

1. They may not easily discern the underlying seriation, an aspect discussed above in relationship to the comprehension of comparative relationships.
2. They may not comprehend the superlative form unless it is presented in a sequence progressing from the base to the comparative and finally to the superlative.
3. They may not perceive the rules governing the use of irregular forms of the comparative and superlative (good, better, best; courageous, more courageous, most courageous).

In order to establish the cognitive basis for the comparative form of adjectives, the child may need experiences in comparing differences in size, length, weight, or quality. In this activity, the educator may use a series of common objects, two each, which differ in some attribute. The child may be required to answer a series of questions such as:

a. Is this apple bigger than that one?
b. Is this book smaller than that one?

These questions may be varied to include the following:

a. Which apple is bigger?
b. Is this pencil longer than your book?
c. Is this apple big? Is it bigger than a watermelon?
d. Which is bigger, a tree or a twig?

The cloze procedure with or without multiple choices may be introduced next to establish identification of comparative and superlative adjective forms. The irregular comparative and superlative forms of adjectives may be introduced in sentences that contain the correct and an obviously incorrect form:

a. Is Sally the beautifulest or the most beautiful girl in town?
b. Is two littler or less than four?

Finally, the children may be required to correct sentences which feature only the root adjectives such as:

a. Which do you like (good), oranges or bananas?
b. Was that the (fast) race he ever ran?

Among sources for training procedures that may be used to establish seriation are (1) *Learning and the Development of Cognition* (Inhelder, Sinclair, & Bovet, 1974) and (2) the *Lavatelli Early Childhood Curriculum* (Lavatelli, 1970). Both the *Sound-Order-Sense* (Semel, 1970) and the SAPP (Semel, in press) provide materials and activities designed to improve the knowledge of English morphology and linguistic processing. These sources may be used to complement the procedures and methods discussed here.

Improving Syntactic Processing

The infinite variety of sentences encountered in the English language may be traced back to five basic sentence patterns from which they were developed. These basic patterns are illustrated in the following sentences:

1. Boys run.
2. Boys play games.
3. The boy is my brother.
4. The boy is tall.
5. The boy became ill.

According to transformational grammar (Chomsky, 1957), these sentences may be generated using phrase-structure rules (PS-rules). Each of the five sentences (Σ) may be divided into two units, a noun phrase (NP) and a verb phrase (VP), according to the rewrite rule: $\Sigma \rightarrow$ NP + VP. The noun phrase (NP) of the last three sentences may be divided into a determiner (T) and a noun (N) according to the rule: NP $\rightarrow$ T + N. The verb phrases (VP) of the last four sentences may also be further subdivided according to PS-rules. The sentences are all simple, active, declarative sentences, that is, *kernel* sentences.

Transformational grammar contains a set of supplementary rules (the transformational component) which may operate on the basic sentence patterns after the PS-rules have been applied. Among the transformational rules outlined by Chomsky (1957) are rules for forming passive, interrogative, conjoined (compound), and embedded (complex) sentences. All of the syntactic rules of English emphasize word order.

Learning disabled youngsters may experience problems in interpreting wh- sentences, and sentences with indirect object transformations as well as the types mentioned above. (Semel & Wiig, 1975; Wiig & Roach, 1975). Clinical observations also indicate that they may experience difficulties in interpreting (1) adjective sequences and may not discern the rules applying to modifier strings, (2) elements of conjoined sentences, and (3) syntactically ambiguous sentences. They may also have problems discerning whether or not a sentence is complete (Wiig & Semel, 1975).

Word Sequencing

Some learning disabled children may not recognize the word-sequencing rules that are implicit in the phrase-structure rules. Activities that may assist in establishing sequential patterns for simple, active, declarative (kernel) sentences may require:

1. Correct-incorrect judgments of sentence pairs:
   a. She in the yard played.
      She played in the yard.
   b. Karen wanted to play the game.
      Karen the game to play wanted.
2. Rearranging words and phrases into simple, active, declarative sentences using formats:
   a. Jumps Jack.
   b. Good bananas taste.
3. Rearranging words and phrases into as many simple, active, declarative, or interrogative sentences as possible:
   a. The soldiers - coming - town - are - to.
      The soldiers are coming to town.
      Are the soldiers coming to town?

The differentiation between simple, active, declarative sentences may be further developed by saying a series of sentences and requiring the youngster to identify which are statements and which are questions. The interrogative sentences presented should include a variety of transformations such as *Is* . . . , *Are* . . . , *Does* . . . , *Did* . . . , *Has* . . . , *Have* . . . , *Can* . . . , *Could* . . . , *Will* . . . , *Would* . . . , *May* . . . , *Might* . . . , *Must* . . . , and wh- question forms.

Differentiation between sentences and sentence fragments should also be established within the series of activities which form a buildup to establish comprehension of transformations. Imperatives should be included since they are often judged to be sentence fragments rather than sentences. Example:

a. The boys are.
b. The boys run.
c. What if the boys.
d. Come here!
e. Go!

Passive Sentences

The problems that LD youngsters may experience in processing passive sentences may reflect (1) delays in logical cognitive growth or (2) delays in the acquisition of syntactic, transformational rules (Wiig & Semel, 1973, 1974). Remedial strategies to expand the logical processing abilities will be discussed later. Based on word recall data (Savin & Perchonock, 1965), the order of difficulty in processing passive sentences progresses as follows:

1. Active-declarative: The girl drove the car.
2. Passive: The car was driven by the girl.
3. Passive question: Was the car driven by the girl?
4. Negative passive question: Wasn't the car driven by the girl?
5. Emphatic passive: The car *was* driven by the girl.
6. Negative passive: The car was not driven by the girl.

Savin and Perchonock conclude:

Various grammatical features of English sentences—negative and passive transformations, and others—are encoded in immediate memory apart from one another, and apart from the rest of the sentences. The evidence for this claim is that sentences having these features require a larger part of the capacity of immediate memory than do otherwise identical sentences lacking these features. [p. 348]

Clinical observations of learning disabled youngsters suggest a hierarchy of difficulty for the various passives which differs slightly from the foregoing sequence. It progresses as follows:

1. The packages were sorted by the mailman. (passive)
2. What was sorted by the mailman? (wh- passive question)
3. Were the packages sorted by the mailman? (passive interrogative)
4. The packages were not sorted by the mailman. (passive negative).
5. Weren't the packages sorted by the mailman? (passive negative interrogative)
6. The packages *were* sorted by the mailman. (emphatic passive)
7. The packages *were not* sorted by the mailman. (emphatic negative passive)

For designing remediation, the preceding list may be used as a guide in sequencing the materials according to difficulty.

Strategies and procedures which may be used to establish knowledge of the transformational rules may emphasize:

1. Rearranging words and phrases into an active declarative sentence and a contrasting passive sentence. As an example, the following scrambled words "The book-the girl-gave to the boy-was given-the book-the boy-by the girl" may be rearranged into:
   a. An active declarative sentence: The girl gave the boy the book.
   b. A passive sentence: The book was given to the boy by the girl. A model sentence pair, active-passive, may be provided in the initial stages of intervention. The following sentence pair may serve as models:
   a. The boy hit the ball
   b. The ball was hit by the boy.
2. Comparison, discrimination, and description of similarities and differences between sentences which include the active-declarative and variations of the passive sentence format. Examples:
   a. The girl gave the book to the boy.
   b. The girl gave the boy the book.
   c. The book was given to the girl by the boy.
   d. The book was given to the boy by the girl.
   e. The book was not given to the girl by the boy.
   f. Wasn't the book given to the girl by the boy?
   g. Didn't the girl give the book to the boy?
   h. The book *was* given to the boy by the girl.
   i. The book *was not* given to the girl by the boy.
3. Transformation of kernel sentences to various types of passive sentences. Example:
   a. The policeman directed the traffic. (active-declarative)
   b. The traffic was directed by the policeman. (passive)
   c. The traffic was not directed by the policeman. (negative passive)
   d. Was the traffic directed by the policeman? (passive question)
   e. Wasn't the traffic directed by the policeman? (negative passive question)
4. Abstraction of a kernel sentence from an elaborate passive transformation.
   a. The shot for distemper was given by the veterinarian to my dog, that is, my dog got a shot.

Interrogatives

Learning disabled children may demonstrate problems in processing interrogatives that require (1) *transposing*, that is, interchange of subject and an auxiliary; for example, "*Has* Daddy finished dinner," and (2) *preposing* as in wh- questions (Semel & Wiig, 1975). Observations of the problems they may experience suggest the following hierarchy of difficulty for *wh- questions:*

1. What . . .
2. Where . . . and When . . .
3. Who . . . and Which . . .
4. Why . . .
5. How . . . , How many . . . , How much . . . , Whose . . .

The order of difficulty is slightly different from the sequence of development observed in normal children (Brown, 1968; Brown, Cazden, & Bellugi, 1968). At age three, normally developing children used and were able to answer *who, what,* and *where* questions, but they were unable to answer *when* and *how* questions. Lee (1974) suggests that *what . . . do* questions may appear later than *who* or *what* questions followed by *where, when,* and *why* (p. 33).

The remedial procedures designed to improve the comprehension of wh- questions may stress:

1. Identification of wh- questions in sentence pairs that include a statement and a question:
   a. Who lives next door?
   b. The girl lives next door.
2. Matching wh- question forms to words and phrases.
   a. Does this tell *where* or *when?* . . . *at the movies,* . . . *on the table,* . . . *outside,* etc.
   b. Does this tell *who* or *why? George Washington, because we are moving, no one told her, Santa Claus,* etc.
3. Categorizing words and phrases according to the appropriate wh- question forms:
   a. Sample: Where did they go?
      Choices: They went to my house.
                    They went last week.
                    They went south.
   b. Sample: When did they leave?
      Choices: They left home.
                    They left quickly.
                    They left at noon.
4. Presentation of oral sentences followed by questions focusing on specific wh- question forms:
   a. Joe said: "I am going."
      Who was going?
      Who said so?
5. Presentation of an oral paragraph followed by a series of questions focusing on specific wh- questions (what . . . /who . . . /where . . , etc.):
   a. He is somebody you see at the circus.

He has on old clothes and big shoes.
He hops when he walks and has a red nose.
He does funny things.
He makes people laugh.
　　Who is he?
　　Who has a big red nose?
　　Who hops when he walks?
　　Who laughs at him?

6. Identification of wh- question words when presented in sentence pairs, one of which contains a relative clause:
   a. Who is the girl next door?
      I know who the girl next door is.
   b. What is the matter with Tom?
      I know what I am looking for.
7. Presentation of an oral sentence or paragraph followed by a variety of wh- questions. This step may provide a necessary transition for the learning disabled child to be able to respond to educational procedures that tap knowledge through wh- questions:
   a. The flowers mother planted in the garden in the spring are red and pink.
      　　What did mother plant?
      　　Who planted the flowers?
      　　When were they planted?
      　　Where were they planted?

Similar remediation procedures may be designed to focus on the identification and interpretation of other wh- question forms: (1) *Whom* . . ., and *Whose*, (2) *How* . . . , *How Many*, and *How much* . . . , and (3) *Why* . . . , and *Why do you think* . . . , and so forth.

Interrogatives requiring *yes-no* responses are generally easy to comprehend if the active-declarative sentence contains an auxiliary or a form of *be*. These interrogatives are formed by shifting the position of the auxiliary or the copula. Interrogatives transformed from active-declarative sentences that do not contain auxiliaries or a form of *be* may present problems in processing and interpretation. These interrogatives require insertion of an auxiliary, for example, "The girl baked these cookies" to "Did the girl bake these cookies" or "Has the girl baked these cookies."

Observations suggest that these interrogatives should be categorized and sequenced for remediation as follows:

1. Does . . .—Did . . .
2. Can . . .—Could . . .
3. Has . . .—Have . . .
4. Will . . .—Would . . .
5. May . . .—Might . . .

The remediation strategies may be designed according to many of the principles outlined above for wh- questions and may include:

1. Identification of questions in minimal sentence pairs:
   a. Jane can go to the movies.
   b. Can Jane go to the movies?
2. Presentation of oral sentences followed by questions which focus on specific auxiliaries:
   a. The teacher gives apples to all the children.
      Does the teacher give apples?
      Did the children get pears?
3. Presentation of oral paragraphs followed by questions focusing on specific auxiliaries:
   a. One day Jack took all his friends to the new bicycle shop. They each bought a shiny new bell and an odometer for their bikes. When they came home they had no money left.
      Did the boys buy a loaf of bread?
      Do all the boys have bicycles?
      Does Jack know how to get to the bicycle store?
      Did the boys use all their money?
4. Presentation of oral sentences and paragraphs followed by a variety of *yes-no* questions:
   a. The girl was in the barn looking for kittens.
      Has the girl found the kittens?
      Can the girl find the kittens?

Conjunctions

Learning disabled youngsters may experience difficulties in interpreting sentences with conjunctions. They seem to have problems in discerning that these sentences contain two ideas, and their problems may be further compounded by conjunction deletions as in "I went to the store and bought a pizza." Learning disabled children may fail to grasp the implied referents. As a result, they may comprehend the sentence "Eric shot the ball, and he scored the basket" but may show confusion when confronted with the sentence "Eric shot the ball and scored the basket."

Lee (1974) suggests a sequence of increasing semantic difficulty for various conjunctions. They progress in difficulty as follows: (1) *and*, (2) *but*, (3) *because*, (4) *so*, (5) *or*, (6) *if*, (7) *until*, (8) *after*, (9) *since*, (10) *although*, and (11) *as* (p. 40).

Observations by Clark (1973) suggest that the principles (1) order of mention, (2) derivational simplicity, and (3) choice of theme must be considered in designing materials for intervention. Clark postulated that sentences with conjunctions would be "simpler" if the *order of mention* of two events coincided with the chronological order, as in the sentence "Jane set the table before she called everyone to dinner." This hypothesis was based upon the results of a memory study (Clark & Clark, 1968) and on data indicating that both adults and schoolchildren preferred sentences with agreement between the order of mention and chronological sequence of occurrence.

The principle of *derivational simplicity* relates to the number of transformations that have been applied to the deep structure. Based on this principle, the sentence (1) "He got up from his chair when he saw the door open" is considered "simpler" than the sentence (2) "When he saw the door open, he got up from his chair" (Clark, 1973, p. 587). The third principle, *choice of theme*, suggests that sentences with "rhematic-thematic continuity" are simpler than sentences in which there is no continuity between the two successive utterances. As an example, the sentences, "She saw a boy. The boy was building a wagon," in which the theme (a boy) of the first sentence is the theme (subject) of the second are easier to understand than sentences without continuity such as "She saw a boy. The wagon was being built by the boy." Analysis of young children's speech supported the stated hypotheses. Clark (1973) concludes:

> of the three principles, choice of theme basically makes the speaker use one syntactic construction rather than the other. Developmentally, it directly affects the order in which a child will learn to use certain syntactic structures. The two other principles are equally important; psychologically, there is a strong preference for mentioning events in chronological order unless there is some (pragmatic) reason not to, and linguistically, there is a preference for using the subordinate clause in second position. . . . [p. 604]

Conjoined sentences with *and - or* in which the expressed ideas have equal status seem easier to interpret for learning disabled youngsters than sentences conjoined by *if, when,* and so forth, in which one clause (idea) is subordinated. Observations also suggest that the hierarchy of difficulty for conjunctions follows the sequence: *and, or, but, besides, also, so, if, when, before, until.* The remediation procedures may use the following formats:

1. Oral presentation of *and - or* conjunctions without deletions followed by identification of the two coordinated sentences (ideas):
   a. John is tall and Bill is short.
   John is tall.
   Bill is short.
2. Oral presentation of *and - or* conjunctions with deletions followed by identification of the two coordinated sentences:
   a. John drives a car or rides a motorcycle.
   John drives a car.
   John rides a motorcycle.
3. Oral presentation of sentences with deletion of *and - or* using a cloze procedure.
   a. We had a good dinner _____ then we washed the dishes.
4. Oral presentation of sentences with subordinate clauses followed by identification of the component sentences:
   a. I don't want a Coke, but I'd like an ice cream cone.
   I don't want a Coke.
   I'd like an ice cream cone.
5. Presentation of oral paragraphs with conjunction omissions using a cloze procedure:
   a. The waitress said: "You can have a salad, potato, _____ (and) vegetables with that. What kind of dressing would you like on your

> salad, French, Russian, _____ (or) Italian? You can have
> _____ (either) French fries _____ (or) a baked
> potato, _____(but) you can't have both.

Complex Sentences

Complex sentences with embedding may prove difficult to process for both LD children and adolescents (Wiig & Roach, 1975). They are formed by relative clause transformations as in "The burglar that the police caught escaped easily." Miller (1973) has reported that relative clauses appear at about the same time as the ability to handle interrogative word questions. The four most common relative pronouns in young children's speech are *what, where, when,* and *that.* It was further observed that *when* was used earlier in relative clauses than in questions. Language disabled youngsters may discern only one expressed idea in sentences with embedding and fail to process the other. In sentences with embedded clauses the components interlock, and one expressed idea is interrupted by the second, requiring recursive processing. The problems may be further compounded by deletions, requiring reconstruction of implied referents, as in the sentence "The new book you would like costs a lot."

The remedial procedures may be designed to include the following:

1. Recognition of complete-incomplete sentences in preparation for processing embedded sentences:
   a. The boys who are playing. (complete/incomplete)
   b. The girls who were playing ball went home. (complete/incomplete)
   c. Wherever you are. (complete/incomplete)
   d. I don't know what you are talking about. (complete/incomplete)
2. Presentation of sentences with relative clauses followed by identification of the component clauses:
   a. The boy who wore a green bathing suit jumped in the water.
      The boy jumped in the water.
      The boy wore a green bathing suit.

Lee, Koenigsknecht, and Mulhern (1975) have provided lesson materials for clinical presentation that emphasize the comprehension and use of syntactic structures by use of storytelling. The materials are developmentally organized and follow a format in which a few lines of the story are read first. The child is then asked to respond to cues or questions concerning the story. The lessons are divided into two parts, levels I and II.

In level I, the lessons emphasize the acquisition of basic sentence structure. The following grammatical forms are introduced: pronoun, main verb, negative, conjunction, secondary verb, interrogative reversal, and wh- question. Level II emphasizes the structures contained in the eight grammatical categories of *Developmental Sentence Scoring* (DDS) (Lee, 1974). The same grammatical forms as found in level I are included, with the addion of indefinite and personal pronouns.

Research has indicated significant increases in both the comprehension and spontaneous use of syntax (Lee, Koenigsknecht, & Mulhern, 1975).

Among receptive language measures which increased significantly from pre- to post-training testing were a measure of sentence recall (Spencer-McGrady Sentence Repetition), and performances on the ITPA *Auditory Reception* subtest, the NSST *Receptive* subtest and the *Oral Commissions* subtest of the DTLA. These findings suggest that the lesson format may prove effective in remediating linguistic processing deficits in high-risk and language and learning disabled children in kindergarten and in the early grades.

References

Asher, J. J. Children's first language as a model for second language learning. *Modern Language Journal*, 1972, **56**, 133-318.

Bangs, T. E. Methodology in auditory training. *Volta Review*, 1954, **56**, 159-164.

Bangs, T. E. *Language and learning disorders of the pre-academic child.* New York: Appleton-Century Crofts, 1968.

Bannatyne, A. D. *Psycholinguistic color system: a reading, writing, spelling and language program.* Urbana, Ill.: Learning Systems Press, 1968.

Bereiter, C., & Hughes, A. *Open Court kindergarten program,* La Salle, Ill.: Open Court, 1970.

Berry, M. F., & Eisenson, J. *Speech disorders: principles and practices.* New York: Appleton-Century Crofts, 1956.

Bever, T. G. The cognitive basis for linguistic structures. In J. R. Hayes (Ed.), *Cognition and the development of language.* New York: John Wiley & Sons, 1970. Pp. 279-352.

Birch, H. G., & Belmont, I. Perceptual analysis and sensory integration in brain-damaged persons. *Journal of Genetic Psychology*, 1964, **105**, 173-79.

Birch, H. G., & Lefford, A. *Intersensory development in children.* Monograph of the Society for Research in Child Development, 1963, **28**, No. 89.

Bracken, D. K., Hays, J. D., & Bridges, C. J. *Listening skills program.* Chicago: Science Research Associates, 1970.

Brown, R. The development of wh- questions in child speech. *Journal of Verbal Learning and Verbal Behavior*, 1968, **7**, Pp. 279-90.

Brown, R., Cazden, C., & Bellugi, U. The child's grammar from I to III. In J. P. Hill (Ed.), *The 1967 Minnesota symposium on child psychology.* Vol. 2. Minneapolis: University of Minnesota Press, 1968. Pp. 28-73.

Chalfant, J. C., & Scheffelin, M. A. Central processing dysfunctions in children: a review of research. *National Institute of Neurological Diseases and Stroke Monograph*, 1969, No. 9.

Chappell, G. E. Generalized auditory agnosia: the first phase of treatment. *Journal of Speech and Hearing Disorders*, 1972, **37**, 152-61.

Chomsky, N. *Syntactic structures.* The Hague: Mouton, 1957.

Clark, E. V. How children describe time and order. In C. A. Ferguson & D. I. Slobin (Eds.), *Studies of child language development.* New York: Holt, Rinehart & Winston, 1973. Pp. 585-606.

Clark, H. H., & Clark, E. V. Semantic distinctions and memory for complex sentences, *Quarterly Journal of Experimental Psychology*, 1968, **20**, 129-38.

de Hirsh, K., Jansky, J., & Langford, L. *Predicting reading failure; a preliminary study.* New York: Harper, 1966.

Durrell, D. D., & Murphy, M. A. The auditory discrimination factor in reading read-iness and reading disability. *Journal of Education*, 1958, **140**, 556-60.

Durrell, D., & Murphy, H. *Speech to print*. New York: Harcourt Brace Jovanovich, 1964.

Fraser, C., Bellugi, U., & Brown, R. Control of grammar in imitation, comprehen-sion, and production. *Journal of Verbal Learning and Verbal Behavior*, 1963, **2**, 121-35.

Gattegno, C. *Words in colour: a new method of teaching the reading and writing of English*. New York: Xerox Corporation, 1963.

Goodglass, H., & Kaplan, E. *The assessment of aphasia and related disorders*. Phila-delphia: Lea & Febiger, 1972.

Hammill, D. D., & Larsen, S. C. The relationship of selected auditory perceptual skills and reading ability. *Journal of Learning Disabilities*, 1974, **7**, 429-35.

Hay, J., & Wingo, E. C. *Reading with phonics*. Philadelphia: Lippincott, 1967.

Holloway, G. F. Auditory-visual integration in language delayed children. *Journal of Learning Disabilities*, 1971, **4**, 204-8.

Inhelder, B., Sinclair, H., & Bovet, M. *Learning and the development of cognition*. Cambridge: Harvard University Press, 1974.

Jakobson, R., Fant, G. M., & Halle, M. *Preliminaries to speech analysis*. Acoustics Laboratory, M.I.T., Technical Report No. 13, 1952.

Johnson, D. J., & Myklebust, H. R. *Learning disabilities: educational principles and practices*. New York: Grune & Stratton, 1967.

Kirshner, A. J. *Training that makes sense*. San Rafael, Calif.: Academic Therapy Publications, 1972.

Lavatelli, C. *Piaget's theory applies to an early childhood curriculum*. Boston: Amer-ican Science & Engineering, 1970.

Lee, L. *Developmental sentence analysis*. Evanston, Ill.: Northwestern University Press, 1974.

Lee, L., Koenigsknecht, R. A., & Mulhern, S. T. *Interactive language development teaching*. Evanston, Ill.: Northwestern University Press, 1975.

Lindamood, C., & Lindamood, P. *Auditory discrimination in depth*. Boston: Teach-ing Resources, 1969.

McGrady, H. J., & Olson, D. A. Visual and auditory learning processes in normal children and children with specific learning disabilities. *Exceptional Chil-dren*, 1970, **36**, 581-89.

Mann, L. Are we fractionating too much? *Academic Therapy*, 1970, **5**, 85-91.

Mann, L., & Phillips, W. A. Fractional practices in special education: a critique. *Ex-ceptional Children*, 1967, **33**, 312-18.

Marslen-Wilson, W. D. Sentence perception as an interactive parallel process. *Science*, 1975, **189**, 226-28.

Miller, W. R. The acquisition of grammatical rules by children. In C. A. Ferguson & D. I. Slobin (Eds.), *Studies of child language development*. New York: Holt, Rinehart & Winston, 1973. Pp. 380-91.

Pitman, J. *Alphabets and reading*. London: Pitman, 1969.

Ritterman, S. I. The role of practice and observation of practice in speech-sound dis-crimination learning. *Journal of Speech and Hearing Research*, 1970, **13**, 178-83.

Saleh, H. J. *Auditory perception*. Hamden, Conn.: Learning Systems, 1970.

Saporta, S. Frequency of consonant clusters. *Language*, 1955, **31**, 25-30.

Savin, H. B., & Perchonock, E. Grammatical structure and the immediate recall of English sentences. *Journal of Verbal Learning and Verbal Behavior*, 1965, **4**, 348-53.

Semel, E. M. *Sound-Order-Sense: a developmental program in auditory perception*. Chicago: Follett Educational Corp., 1970.

Semel, E. M. The effects of auditory perception training on the performance of second graders on tests of auditory perception. Doctoral dissertation, Boston University, 1972.

Semel, E. M. *Semel auditory processing program*. Chicago: Follett Publishing Co., in press.

Semel, E. M., & Wiig, E. H. Comprehension of syntactic structures and critical verbal elements by children with learning disabilities. *Journal of Learning Disabilities*, 1975, **8**, 53-58.

Silvaroli, N. J., & Wheelock, W. H. An investigation of auditory discrimination training for beginning readers. *The Reading Teacher*, 1966, **20**, 247-51.

Stern, C., & Gould, T. *Children discover reading*. Syracuse, N.Y.: L. W. Singer, 1965.

Van Riper, C. *Speech correction: principles and methods*. (4th ed.) Englewood Cliffs, N.J.: Prentice-Hall, 1963.

Vogel, S. A. Syntactic abilities in normal and dyslexic children. *Journal of Learning Disabilities*, 1974, **7**, 47-53.

Warburton, F. W., & Southgate, V. *I.t.a.: an independent evaluation*. London: Newgate Press Limited, 1969.

Wiig, E. H., & Roach, M. A. Immediate recall of semantically varied "sentences" by learning-disabled adolescents. *Perceptual and Motor Skills*, 1975, **40**, 119-25.

Wiig, E. H., & Semel, E. M. Comprehension of linguistic concepts requiring logical operations. *Journal of Speech and Hearing Research*, 1973, **16**, 627-36.

Wiig, E. H., & Semel, E. M. Logico-grammatical sentence comprehension by adolescents with learning disabilities. *Perceptual and Motor Skills*, 1974, **38**, 1331-34.

Wiig, E. H., & Semel, E. M. Productive language abilities in learning disabled adolescents. *Journal of Learning Disabilities*, 1975, **8**, 578-86.

Wiig, E. H., Semel, E. M., & Crouse, M.A. The use of morphology by high-risk and learning disabled children. *Journal of Learning Disabilities*, 1973, **6**, 457-65.

Willette, R., Jackson, B., & Peckins, I. *Auditory perception training*. Chicago: Developmental Learning Materials, 1970.

Winitz, H. *Articulatory acquisition and behavior*. New York: Appleton-Century Crofts, 1969.

Winitz, H. Problem solving and the delaying of speech as strategies in the teaching of language. *American Speech & Hearing Association*, 1973, **15**, 583-86.

Winitz, H., & Preisler, L. Effect of distinctive feature pretraining in phoneme discrimination learning. *Journal of Speech and Hearing Research*, 1967, **10**, 515-30.

7

Remediation of Cognitive Processing Deficits

Overview

This chapter discusses remediation principles and suggests strategies and methods for improving (1) cognitive processing of semantic units and vocabulary, (2) semantic classification, (3) cognitive processing of semantic relations, and (4) cognition of semantic transformation and implications. Procedures are emphasized which respond to areas of cognitive-semantic deficits observed in language and learning disabled school children.

The results of psycholinguistic and cognitive studies of the normal patterns of acquisition of words and concepts are discussed (R. Brown, 1973; Clark, 1968; Clark, 1972; Moorehead & Ingram, 1973; Waryas, 1973). The implications of the findings for the planning of a sequence of remedial intervention are stressed.

Among suggested formats and procedures lending themselves to the remediation of cognitive-semantic processing deficits are (1) same–different judgments of the meaning of word or sentence pairs, (2) correct–incorrect judgments of the concepts or ideas expressed in sentences, (3) selection of words and concepts from a set of alternative choices, (4) sentence completion within given semantic constraints, (5) oral cloze procedures, and (6) responses to yes/no questions regarding the meaning of sentences or paragraphs. Sources of additional discussions of remedial principles and methods as well as of programmed materials for improving cognitive–semantic processing abilities are suggested throughout.

Improving Cognitive Processing of Semantic Units and Vocabulary

Language and learning disabled youngsters may experience problems in the cognitive processing of words and concepts (semantic units). Selected vocabulary deficits may occur within one or more of the vocabulary categories (nouns, verbs, adjectives, pronouns, prepositions, adverbs). Observations suggest that comprehensive difficulties may occur for:

1. Dual or multiple-meaning words such as *building, check, drive, run.*
2. Verbs describing complex actions or movements such as *bouncing, swaying, tumbling, twisting.*
3. Adjectives denoting aspects of space or time (length, height, width, age, distance), affect, or quality, or which require seriation (comparatives, superlatives).
4. Adverbs derived from adjectives such as *quietly, slowly.*
5. Adverbs such as *here* and *there* (situationally-bound definite adverbs) or *somewhere* and *anywhere* (situationally-bound indefinite adverbs).
6. Prepositions denoting a change in direction or condition (directional prepositions), prepositions used to denote time (temporal prepositions), or unusual uses of or grammatically conditioned prepositions.
7. Personal (gender and case), possessive, reflexive, demonstrative, indefinite, and negative pronouns.

The strategies and methods selected for intervention must respond to the deficit areas and reflect the relative levels of difficulty experienced within each problem area. In planning remedial intervention, the educator–clinician must therefore consider: (1) the sequence in which materials are presented and specific difficulties are approached and (2) the stimulus-response combinations.

Within each deficit area, remediation should begin at the level of already established abilities to familiarize the youngster with the educational-clinical patterns to be used and to secure initial success. The subsequent progression should move from areas of strength to ones of weakness and employ materials of gradually increasing difficulty. The repertory of synonyms, antonyms, and multiple-meaning words must also be established in several of the vocabulary categories. Within the *adjective, pronoun,* and *preposition* categories, the materials should be presented in sequences reflecting either theoretically or observationally based hierarchies of difficulty.

Among general procedures and patterns selected for use in intervention are

a. Examples requiring identification of an incorrectly used word in a context (sentence or paragraph):
   The boy *drank* the hamburger.
   Yesterday Mary went to the park. *He* took a blanket to sit on. When she got to the park, Mary looked around to see if any of *their* friends were there.
b. Examples requiring substitution of an incorrect or nonsense word in a context presenting multiple choices for responding:
   The boy *jag* the hamburger (ate/drank).
   The ride on the bus lasted two hours. Bob thought it was too *bic* (short/long).

c. Examples requiring identification of synonyms or antonyms in isolation or in context from a series of multiple choices.
   Big (tall/little)
   The boy turned the light *on* (up/off).
d. Examples requiring substitutions for incorrect or nonsense words in context:
   The boy *jag* the hamburger.
   The girl went to the store. *Zib* bought a new dress.
e. Cloze examples in which deleted target words must be supplied:
   The boy _____ the hamburger.
   The boy washed himself and the girl washed _____.
f. Examples requiring identification of words based on descriptions or definitions:
   You can eat it. It is made of ground beef and served in a bun. It is a _____.
   You can ride it to get from Boston to New York. It rides on tracks. It is a _____.
g. Examples requiring detection and/or description of differences in word meaning (shades of meaning):
   The boy *laughed*. The boys *giggled*. The boys *smiled*.
   In the circus we saw the clowns *balancing, tumbling,* and *leaping*.
h. Examples requiring responses to sentences, paragraphs, or stories, using questions which are aimed at identifying a specific target word or word category.
   The boys ate the hamburger.
      Who ate the hamburgers?
      What did the boys eat?
   The juggler balanced the ball on the pole.
      Who balanced the ball?
      Where was the ball balanced?

Specific procedures may be used for the remediation of difficulties in comprehending certain vocabulary items and categories. The use of both general and specific intervention strategies will be discussed and illustrated below.

Improving Verb Comprehension

Improving the comprehension of verbs may require the use of specific remedial strategies. To enhance the receptive verb repertory and the differentiation between verb meanings, the motor actions associated with specific verbs may have to be established. The language disabled child with verb comprehension problems often benefits from association between a motor act and the verbal label depicting the activity. As an example, the differences in meaning between the verbs *turning, twisting, twirling,* and *sliding* may be better understood if the child experiences the associated activities motorically. Specific activities such as acting out given verbs, labeling motor activities, and following oral commands may be used in remediation to establish the associations.

Certain verbs may cause problems in following oral commands. Examples are *lend, send, bring,* and *ring.* Confusions between these words generally follow patterns that reflect phoneme discrimination difficulties. It may be necessary to provide opportunities for the LD child to discriminate and differentiate between these verbs in minimal sentence pairs without contextual cues to develop efficient processing and adequate comprehension. Examples are

1. Bring the bell—Ring the bell
2. Walk fast—Talk fast

The use of *auxiliaries* and *infinitives* may cause additional problems in interpreting verbs and verb phrases. Establishing the selectional rules for these units may facilitate comprehension of the main verb. Confusions often suggest that the child believes that auxiliaries and infinitives change the meaning of the main verb. The selectional rules for secondary verbs may be established using, among others, (a) correct-incorrect, (b) multiple-choice, and (c) cloze procedures. Examples:

a. Mary is sure that she was go to New York. (correct/incorrect)
   Paul was been at the store. (correct/incorrect)
   Jack has gone to school. (correct/incorrect)
b. Tomorrow, the boy _____ go to the zoo. (has/will)
   Peter's mother said: "You _____ go to the movies." (can/have)
c. Tomorrow, Jane and Bill go to New York. They think they _____ go by bus.
   Father said: "Finish your dinner. I want you _____ _____ all your vegetables."

Improving Adjective Comprehension

The problems that learning disabled children may encounter in comprehending adjectives appear to relate to (1) the saliency of the attribute described, (2) difficulties in analysis and synthesis of adjective sequences, and (3) problems in remembering the linguistic constraints on the order in which adjectives may occur in sequence. The remedial procedures should be designed to (1) develop the meaning of various adjectives and (2) establish knowledge of the structural rules for adjective sequences. The following chart (Table 14) suggests a sequence for the introduction of attributes described by specific adjectives.

Specific procedures that may assist in developing the discrimination and differentiation of adjectives include:

a. Selection of a child based on a description of attributes: Show me a girl with a red skirt and a blue blouse.
b. Linking of specific attributes (adjectives) with target nouns using a multiple-choice example: An apple is _____ (blue/red). A car is _____ (light/heavy).
c. Identification of a selected attribute (color, size, quantity, etc.) in an adjective sequence: The girl had two big red apples.
   What size were they?
   What color?

d. Describing shades of meaning expressed by selected adjectives: The girl was nice. The girl was pleasant. The girl was pretty.

TABLE 14

Suggested Sequence for the Introduction of Adjectives in the Remediation of Language Processing Deficits

Aspect	Adjectives
1. Color	red, blue, green
2. Size	big, small, little
3. Color/Size	big red, small blue
4. Shape	round, square
5. Color/Size/Shape	big red square
6. Length/Height/Width	long, short, thin
7. Age	old, young, new
8. Taste/Smell	sweet, sour, pungent
9. Attractiveness	pretty, ugly, nice
10. Speed	fast, slow
11. Temperature	hot, cold
12. Quality	hard, rough, smooth
13. Affect	happy, sad, angry
14. Distance	near, far, distant

Improving Pronoun Comprehension

The difficulties encountered by learning disabled youngsters in comprehending pronouns appear to reflect problems in acquiring the substitution (selectional) rules for pronominalization. As a result, the remedial procedures should employ a variety of noun-pronoun substitution examples.

Personal Pronouns

Gleason (1955, p. 105) classifies the eight personal pronouns of English in a paradigm of four forms:

Subjective	Objective	Possessive	Possessive-Replacive
I	me	my	mine
we	us	our	ours
you	you	your	yours
he	him	his	his
she	her	her	hers
it	it	its	its
they	them	their	theirs

Research of the normal acquisition of pronouns indicates that third person pronouns such as *he, she,* and *it* appear in spontaneous speech from the age of two years four months (Chipman & deDardel, 1974). Moorehead and Ingram (1973) have related children's pronoun acquisition to linguistic levels in the age range from one year and seven months to three years one month. The acquisition was as follows:

Level	Pronouns
I	I
II	my, it, it, me
III	you, your, she, them
IV	we, he, they, us, you, him, his
V	her, its, her, our

The comprehension of pronouns is further complicated by the fact that the presence or absence of emphatic stress may indicate the reference of pronouns (Maratsos, 1973). Illustrative examples are

1. John hit Harry and then Sarah hit him. (Harry is hit by Sarah)
2. John hit Harry and then Sarah hit *him*. (John is hit by Sarah)

As these examples indicate, the grammatical and semantic roles of the actors are changed as little as possible when the pronound is unstressed. When the pronoun receives emphatic stress, the listener must perceive the change of roles implied.

Maratsos (1973) observed that young children (three, four, and five years) can comprehend unstressed pronouns better than stressed ones. The stressed pronouns were better interpreted with increasing age. Learning disabled children may not discern the changes implied by differences in stress. This suggests that the remedial procedures should incorporate identification and discrimination examples for unstressed-stressed pronouns.

Learning disabled children may also fail to grasp the rules for pronominalization in sentences with two identical noun phrases such as "John came to dinner and he stayed a week." They may not discern that sentences such as "He came to dinner and John stayed a week" violate syntactic rules.

Waryas (1973) emphasizes the interaction between syntactic and semantic features in pronouns. She presents an analysis of pronouns which emphasizes three features: (1) person, (2) number, and (3) case. The pronouns are classified within a communication system as referring to the *speaker*, the *listener*, or *other*. In order to differentiate third person pronouns, the referents which are semantically + *other* must be further specified as + *human*. Those which have human referents must be further specified as + *male*.

After the pronouns have received semantic specification, they must be defined according to the role in the surface structure. This specification results in the identification of (1) subject marking, for example, *I*, (2) reflexive marking, for example, *myself*, (3) possessive marking, for example, *my*, and (4) replacive pronoun, for example, *mine*. When the pronoun contains none of these features, the objective case is chosen.

Waryas (1973) provides the following suggestions for the design of remedial procedures:

1. Semantic features (speaker/listener/other; human/nonhuman; male/female) should be emphasized before syntactic features.

2. Pronominalization of the speaker and listener roles should begin early.
3. Semantic feature differentiation should be emphasized before syntactic case marking.
4. Control of singular forms should be established before plurals.
5. The referents for pronouns should be established first if the child shows confusions in the referents.

The implications of the composite findings for the design of remedial procedures suggest that:

1. The referents for the personal pronouns, *I, we, you, he, she, it, they* (subjective case) should be established first if the youngster shows confusions (Moorehead & Ingram, 1973; Waryas, 1973).
2. Pronominalization of the speaker and listener roles may occur next to establish semantic feature differentiation (Waryas, 1973).
3. Pronouns in the objective case or with possessive marking may be introduced next, emphasizing differentiation of semantic features and presenting singular forms before plural forms (Moorhead & Ingram, 1973; Waryas, 1973).
4. The possessive-replacive pronouns should be introduced last in the sequence (Moorehead & Ingram, 1973).
5. Differentiation of stressed-unstressed forms of pronouns should occur late in the remedial sequence (Maratsos, 1973).

Establishing the referents for personal pronouns may require remediation involving the use of objects in activities or games. As an example, the educator-clinician may give an object to one or more of the children in a group saying:

a. I gave the ball to Joe. Joe has the ball. *He* has the ball.
b. I gave the ball to Ann. Ann has the ball. *She* has the ball.
c. I gave the balls to Jane and Mary. Jane and Mary have the balls. *They* have the balls.

Subsequent activities may require that the youngsters (a) judge whether or not the pronouns used are correct or incorrect, (b) select the appropriate personal pronoun from a set of alternatives, or (c) use pronominalization. Examples:

a. I gave the car to Joe. She has the car now. (correct/incorrect)
   I gave the pencil to Mary. She has the pencil. (correct/incorrect)
   I gave the blocks to Jack and Phyllis. I have the blocks now. (correct/incorrect)
b. I gave the cards to Jane. She/they has the cards now.
   I gave the cards to Bob. She/he has the cards now.
   I gave the bone to the dog. We/it has the bone now.
c. I gave the ring to you, Ellen. Who has the ring?
   I gave the shoes to you, Ann and David. Who has the shoes?

Methods designed to establish comprehension and differentiation of objective, possessive, or possessive-replacive pronouns may use similar activities and examples:

    a. I gave the matches to Bill. The matches now belong to her. (correct/incorrect)

    I gave the penny to Jane. The penny now belongs to it. (correct/incorrect)

    I gave the candy to Bob and Erik. The candy now belongs to them. (correct/incorrect)

    The penny belongs to Mary. The penny is mine. (correct/incorrect)

    The apples belong to Joe and Bob. The apples are theirs. (correct/incorrect)

    b. I gave the paper to Joan. The paper now belongs to him/*her*.

    I gave the crayons to Jerry and Beth. The crayons now belong to us/*them*.

    The pencil belongs to Angel. The pencil is *his*/hers.

    The pencils belong to you and me. The pencils are mine/*ours*.

Same-different judgments, multiple-choice, and cloze procedures may also be used to establish differentiation of the various possessive and possessive-replacive pronouns:

    a. The apple belongs to me.

    The apple is yours. (same/different)

    The pennies belong to them.

    The pennies are theirs. (same/different)

    b. I gave an apple to Jane. Now the apple belongs to *her*/hers.

    I gave the letters to Ann and Jane. The letters are *theirs*/hers.

    c. Jack bought a new car. The car now belongs to _____. _____ old car broke down.

    The boy gave the girl a flower. The flower is now _____.

The differentiation of the meaning of sentences with stressed and unstressed pronouns is most readily established in same-different formats followed by interpretation of differences by the educator-clinician:

1. George yelled at Bob and then Joe yelled at *him*.
2. George yelled at Bob and then Joe yelled at him. (same/different)

    Interpretation:

1. George yelled at Bob and then Joe yelled at George.
2. George yelled at Bob and then Joe yelled at Bob.

Among sources that emphasize intervention strategies to improve comprehension and differentiation of personal pronouns are *Language and Learning Disorders of the Pre-Academic Child* (Bangs, 1968), the *Sound-Order-Sense* (Semel, 1970), and the *Wilson Initial Syntax* programs, (Wilson, 1972) and articles by Gottsleben, Tyack, and Buschini (1974) and Waryas (1973), among others.

Demonstrative Pronouns

The demonstrative pronouns (this, that, these, those) which express differences in the location in space may require remediation based on observation of the implied spatial relationships. Following oral directions with a demonstrative, such as "Give me that book. It is on my desk over there." may facilitate comprehension. Activities designed to establish the referential basis (spatial) for the demonstrative pronouns may use an object. It may be placed in different locations, and a demonstrative may be used to describe the object. A sample activity may be described as follows:

> You and the child have a ball that you are throwing back and forth. It is labeled "this" ball. Put the ball on the other side of the room. "It is over there" and is now labeled "that ball." Better still, use two balls, one near you and one at the other end of the room. The one near you is "this" ball, the one farther away is "that" ball. You may use different objects and position yourself in different places. *This* is nearby, *that* is over there. When the child has mastered the idea, complicate it by moving around yourself to show him how "this" and "that" are interchanged depending upon your location relative to the object. "That" blackboard becomes "this" blackboard when you walk over to it. "This chalk" becomes "that chalk" when you move away from it. Use the plurals also. If you have several balls they are "these balls." They become "those balls" if they are not near. "This" and "that" ball can become "these" balls when you retrieve one and bring it together with the other.

Many LD children have trouble with these pronouns because they sound alike and because they change, depending on where the object is in relation to the speaker.

Improving the Comprehension of Prepositions

The difficulties that language and learning disabled youngsters may encounter in comprehending prepositions reflect confusions between:

1. Spatial aspects denoted by prepositions such as *in* and *on* (definite spatial prepositions) and *at* and *by* (indefinite spatial prepositions).
2. Prepositions such as *at* and *in* which may be used to denote either spatial or temporal aspects.
3. Prepositions used as idioms in sentences such as "She ran *into* her friend."
4. Multiple-meaning prepositions.

Classification of Prepositions

Clark (1968) has discussed prepositions in terms of meanings of (a) direction, (b) position, (c) manner, and (d) time. They may have something animate, inanimate, or abstract as their objects and seem to cluster according to these distinctions. In a related attempt to classify prepositions, Takahaski (1969) discusses the spatial prepositions, *at, to, on,* and *in,* in terms of the dimensions involved.

According to Takahaski (1969), the preposition *at* denotes a *point* (a dimensionless conceptual space) and is conceived by the process of reducing all dimensions. The preposition *to* denotes the first dimension in space, a *line,* which is bound by two points. The preposition *on* denotes two dimensions in space, a *plane* or *surface,* bound by lines. The preposition *in* is considered to denote the fourth dimension in space, a three-dimensional body enclosed by surfaces. In relation to this model, learning disabled youngsters experience fewer difficulties interpreting prepositions denoting two or three dimensions in space, for example, *on* and *in*, which define the spatial aspects. They may experience difficulties with prepositions denoting the first dimension in space or a dimensionless conceptual space, for example, *to* and *at*.

Greene et al. (1961) have provided the following complete list of prepositions that may be used in planning the scope of remediation:

about	at	beyond
above	before	but (except)
across	behind	by
after	below	concerning
against	beneath	down
along	beside	during
among	besides	except
around	between	for
from	on	toward
in	out	under
inside	outside	until
into	over	up
like	past	upon
near	since	with
of	through	within
off	to	without

Fries (1952) reports that among the prepositions, nine (of, in, to, for, at, on, from, with, by) comprise 90% of the prepositions in written materials. It is further reported that there are 250 possible meanings for these nine prepositions. Streng (1972, p. 245) points to the fact that most of the common prepositions may be used as idioms and that there are few patterns to indicate which ones are appropriate. The possible confusions are illustrated by a set of sentences in which prepositions in conjunction with the verb *ran* function as idioms:

Louise ran for the School Board.
Laverne ran into her friend.
Lorraine ran across some old letters.
Lois ran through her lines.

These examples illustrate the complexity involved in processing prepositions. They also suggest why children with abstraction and generalization problems may experience difficulties and suggest the variables that must be considered in planning remediation strategies.

Development of Prepositions

Several observations of the normal developmental patterns for prepositions may be used to suggest a sequence for introducing prepositions. Brown (1973) reports that *in* and *on* are the first prepositions learned. In early language, they always denote spatial aspects; in adult speech *in* and *on* may be used to denote abstract aspects as in the phrase *in time*. Clark (1972, p. 752) reports the following sequence in learning antonym pairs of spatial and temporal prepositions:

in-out	before	above-below
on-off		over-under
up-down	before	above-below
		over-under
in-front	before	ahead-behind
in-back		
in-front	before	first-last
in-back		early-late
		before-after

She also presents data regarding the development of semantically correct usage of prepositions by children in the age range from four to five and one-half years (Table 15).

TABLE 15

Percent Responses by Age Group to Each Semantic Field

Pair	Semantically appropriate				Adult correct				
	Age: I	II	III	Mean	Age:	I	II	III	Mean
Big-small	100	92	100	97		90	90	97	95
Long-short	82	82	95	89		40	57	85	61
Tall-short	80	92	92	88		37	60	82	60
High-low	45	82	87	71		10	35	82	42
Old-young	50	67	87	68		35	50	77	54
Thick-thin	12	37	85	45		7	15	47	23
Wide-narrow	7	20	55	27		0	0	27	9
Deep-shallow	2	15	45	21		2	5	37	14
In front-in back	82	87	95	88		80	87	95	87
Up-down	67	95	100	87		65	87	95	82
In-out	52	87	97	79		52	87	97	79
On-off	50	70	92	71		42	65	87	65
First-last	50	70	97	72		42	57	92	63
Over-under	32	52	80	55		12	35	65	27
Early-late	20	45	90	52		15	30	75	40
Above-below	15	35	82	44		0	7	42	16
Ahead-behind	17	42	65	41		17	30	62	36
Before-after	17	37	72	42		10	22	57	28

SOURCE: Reprinted with permission of publishers from: Clark, E. V. On the child's acquisition of antonyms in two semantic fields. *Journal of Verbal Learning and Verbal Behavior*, 1972, **11**, 750-58.

NOTE: Each percentage point based on 40 data points.

Hunt (1965) investigated the control of prepositions in writing by analyzing written language samples of children in the fourth, eighth, and twelfth grades. He observed that prepositional phrases were the third most frequent modifiers of nouns and that only half the prepositions used in each grade indicated place. Furthermore, the number of prepositional phrases in a sentence correlated with clause length.

For remediation, the findings suggest that:

1. *Definite spatial* prepositions such as *in* and *on* should be introduced and established first followed by *indefinite spatial* prepositions such as *at* and *by*.
2. *Spatial* prepositions which denote temporal aspects such as *in* and *at* may follow next in the sequence.
3. *Instrumental* prepositions such as *with* and *without*, probably the most difficult, should be introduced last.

Boehm (1969, p. 11) provides a sequence of concept presentation that appears applicable to planning remediation strategies for prepositions. The suggested procedural sequence is as follows:

1. Introduction of the concept using concrete materials
2. Specific labeling of the concept
3. Use of the concept in several concrete situations to facilitate generalization
4. Representation of the concept by pictures or photographs

Remedial Procedures

As in the case of the demonstrative pronouns, the differences in location in space denoted by the various spatial prepositions may need to be established through direct physical experiences. This may be accomplished by having the child act out verbal commands requiring him to place a common object or position himself in different definite locations in space:

1. Sit *on/under/behind* your desk.
2. Stand *on/in front of/behind* your chair.
3. Put your pencil *under/on* the desk.
4. Put the chair *in/in front of* the closet.
5. Put the chair *in front of/behind* the desk.
6. Put the pencil *on top of* your book.
7. Put the chalk *between* the book and the pencil.
8. Put the pencil *beneath* the book.

Subsequently, the child may be asked to move in specified directions in space, following verbal commands:

1. Crawl *under* the desk.
2. Jump *over* the book.
3. Walk *outside/inside*.
4. Run *to* my desk.
5. Hide *behind* the bookcase.
6. Hop *in front of* my chair.

The child may also be asked to place objects at various points in space indicated by indefinite prepositions:

1. Put the chair *by*/*near* my desk.
2. Put the chair *against* the wall.
3. Put the chair close *to* your desk.
4. Put the pencil *by* the book.
5. Hold the chalk *above* your head.
6. Push the book *beyond* your reach.

Since children may confuse prepositions sharing speech sounds (phonological features), verbal commands may be used which juxtapose and contrast these prepositions. The commands should include the following prepositions:

a. on—off
b. in—on
c. behind, below, beneath, beside, between
d. above, across, against, around
e. in, inside, into

Associating a location such as a zoo with actions or events that may occur there may further establish the comprehension of spatial prepositions. The following multiple-choice examples require reauditorization of prepositional phrases while listening to and selecting appropriate choices:

1. *at the zoo:*
   a. you can go swimming,
   b. you can catch fish,
   c. you can feed elephants.
2. *on the beach:*
   a. you can see tigers,
   b. you can watch the clouds,
   c. you can play in the sand.

The prepositional phrases introduced above may also be elicited:

1. Where can you build sand castles?
2. Where can you watch the monkeys?

When spatial prepositions are used to denote a point in time, the specific preposition to be used is determined by selectional rules that are usually automatically acquired. These rules may have to be explained to the learning disabled child before he can respond to other intervention strategies. Examples of selectional rules determining the specific prepositions follow.

1. Specific times during the day are indicated by the preposition *at* as in *at two o'clock, at lunch, at noon,* etc.
2. The preposition *on* is used to denote specific days of the week, and *in* and *during* used to indicate the months or seasons of the year.

Several sources discuss educational procedures and present programs for improving the comprehension and expression of prepositions (Bangs, 1968; Johnson & Myklebust, 1967; Semel, 1970, in press; Snider & Symington,

1974; Wilson, 1972). Bangs (1968) suggests concrete situations and activities to improve the young child's (three to four years old) comprehension of prepositions. Johnson and Myklebust (1967) also begin remediation at the concrete level by asking the child to put his hand *on/under* the table and to manipulate a ball by putting it *in/on* a box. At a more abstract level, they suggest using pictures and emphasize that the prepositions must be used in a variety of contexts to facilitate generalization. They also emphasize sentence patterning in which (1) the preposition may be altered while keeping verb and object, (2) the object is changed while verb and preposition are kept constant, and (3) combinations of verb, preposition, or object are changed.

Wilson (1972) presents a program in which the prepositions *in, on, under, in front of, behind, next to,* and *over* are used and compared at both the concrete and abstract level. Different settings and contexts are also provided for teaching the same concept. The program introduced by Snider and Symington (1974) is programmed and introduces only the prepositions *in* and *on*. A series of two-dimensional items are introduced using a discrimination method that requires discrimination between *in* and *on* for all items. The program may be expanded to include other prepositions such as the antonym pairs investigated by Clark (1972).

Among materials which may be used in remediation are the *Preposition Concepts Picture Cards* (E. Brown, 1973), the *Perceptual Concept Charts for Early Learners* (The Instructor Publications), and *Out and In* (Hulbert, 1970).

Antonyms, Synonyms, Homonyms, and Multiple-Meaning Words

The difficulties that may be encountered by learning disabled youngsters in differentiating and comprehending words and concepts are often reflected in multiple-meaning words, synonyms, antonyms, and homonyms. In planning a sequence for remediation of these problems, it is sometimes necessary to begin at a level of established abilities. When the *concept of opposition* is established so that the child can grasp the difference between *empty* and *not empty*, it may be useful to begin remediation with antonyms.

Antonyms

The development of antonym vocabulary comprehension should progress from using concrete, frequent words and concepts to using less frequent and more abstract ones. The vocabulary presented in verbal opposites tests is generally sequenced according to relative frequency, reading level, and along a continuum from concrete to abstract (Baker & Leland, 1959; Botel, 1970; Kreezer & Dallenbach, 1929). These tests may be used as guidelines for selecting and sequencing vocabulary items according to the principles of frequency and level of abstraction.

Synonyms

The important aspect to establish in developing comprehension and use of synonyms is that they are not identical in meaning. They are related by meaning and may convey approximately the same intent. Within the repertory of synonyms, those which change meaning depending upon context seem especially difficult to establish. The word *bold* may serve as a synonym for the word *courageous* in the context "The soldier was courageous" and as a synonym for *shameless* in other contexts. The primary focus in remediation should be to alert language and learning disabled children to these varied interpretations. At times, more than one synonym may be substituted for a word. Often the possible synonyms differ in the degree in which they approximate the meaning of the original word. As an example, an angry man may be described as *furious, outraged, villainous,* or *infuriated.* Although the synonyms differ in shades of meaning, they share a negative connotation. Synonyms having a similar connotation are often used in newscasts, advertising, and sports announcements. They add variety to language and often confuse language disabled youngsters.

Homonyms

Homonyms are words that sound identical but are spelled differently and have widely different meanings. They may belong to the same or to different parts of speech. As examples, the meaning of the homonyms *sail* and *sale* can generally be discerned from the contexts in which they appear. In planning remediation strategies the variables influencing the perception and interpretation of words need to be considered.

The frequency of word usage has been found to be an important factor in determining the ease with which words can be identified on auditory tests (Rosenzweig & Postman, 1957, 1958). In a similar vein, Black (1952) and Charney (1966) reported findings which suggested that context and experience were influencing factors of word recognition. On this basis, Rutberg (1972) hypothesized that homonyms would be interpreted (spelled) according to frequency of usage rules based on the word counts by Thorndike and Lorge (1944). The responses to eight of the twenty homonyms selected differed significantly from the reported frequencies of usage. The words most affected were *peace* (piece), *male* (mail), and *cell* (sell), suggesting that homonym interpretation depends upon word frequency as well as cultural patterns.

Multiple-Meaning Words

Multiple-meaning words are words that may function as different parts of speech depending upon context. Consider the words *run, table, over, go,* and *mark.* They may function as, among others, nouns, verbs, adjectives, and prepositions depending upon the context in which they appear.

Based on clinical experiences in helping children with language comprehension problems, semantic classification and categorization skills must be established before adequate differentiation of word meanings can be expected. Specific remediation strategies for these skills will be discussed in the following section on semantic classification.

Remedial Procedures

The comprehension of antonyms may be established using a variety of remedial formats. Among these are (a) procedures which require correct/incorrect judgments, (b) selection of the appropriate antonym from a set of multiple choices, (c) sentence completion or cloze procedures, and (d) questions focusing on antonyms in sentences and paragraphs. Examples:

a. The sun shines at night. (correct/incorrect)
   Elephants are big. (correct/incorrect)
   Bob said that he was Nancy's sister. (correct/incorrect)
   He drank the coffee till his cup was full. (correct/incorrect)
b. The present made Joe *happy*/sad.
   Trucks are light/*heavy*.
   Lions are tame/*wild*.
   The boy loved his birthday present. He *accepted*/refused it.
c. Lemons are sour. Sugar is _____.
   The father was tall. The little boy was _____.
   Mother said "I sent the letter to you." Bill answered "I never

   _____.

d. The new car was not big.
   What size was the car?
   Bob did not leave in the daytime.
   When did he leave?
   When mother got back to the kitchen the milk was gone. The bowl was no longer full.
   What was the bowl?

The differentiation between synonyms and homonyms is most readily established in formats which use yes/no questions followed by explanation or verification. Examples:

a. Synonyms:
   Sally giggled when she heard the joke.
   Did Sally look sad when she heard the joke?
   What did Sally do?
   Burt was infuriated when the boys teased him.
   Was Burt angry?
b. Homonyms:
   Sally and her mother went to a sale last week.
   Did Sally and her mother go sailing?
   Did they go shopping?
   When the mail arrived the boys ran to get it.
   Did the boys go pick a man up?
   Did they get the letters?

Improving Semantic Classification

The ability to categorize and classify concepts underlies the vocabulary comprehension of antonyms, synonyms, homonyms, and multiple-meaning words. As an example, the differentiation and comprehension of the words *newspaper* and *magazine* depend upon abstracting and contrasting similarities and differences and classifying and reclassifying the concepts according to their various characteristics.

Learning disabled children may have problems abstracting either similarities or differences or both. They may find it difficult to classify and reclassify concepts and have been reported to have particular difficulties with the inclusion aspects of classification (Klees & Lebrun, 1972). Some may persevere in categorizing a word or concept within a specific class and be unable to shift the set to permit the necessary reclassification. Flexibility in relation to classifying reflects flexibility in thinking.

Procedures which may assist in establishing word classification skills may require:

1. Association between the name of a class member with the label for the semantic class, using a multiple-choice format (subordinate–superordinate association):
   Is a lion an animal or a bird?
   Is tag a game or a toy?
2. Association between the label for a semantic class and the name of one or more class members, using a multiple-choice format (superordinate-subordinate association):
   Which is an animal? a table, a dog, or a car.
3. Identification of names of members that do not belong to the class in question (deletion of false subordinates):
   Which of these does not belong? apple, pear, shoe, banana.
4. Selection of names of class members belonging to a specific category from among a list of choices (matching subordinates to a superordinate):
   Listen to these: red, white, and blue. Are they colors, toys, or foods?
5. Categorization of the names of members of different classes according to the appropriate class descriptions (subordinate categorization by function):
   Listen to these: bread and butter, shoes and socks. Which are things you eat? Which are things you wear?
6. Categorization of the names of different class members on the basis of shared attributes (subordinate categorization by attribute):
   Listen to these: candy, lemons, and cookies. Which are sweet? Which are sour?
7. Categorization of names of class members belonging to different classes according to the appropriate class names (subordinate categorization by class label):
   Listen to these: apples, marbles, checkers, oranges. Which are games? Which are fruits?
8. Abstracting and formulating similarities between objects, events, etc.:
   How are apples and oranges alike?
   How are cars and trains alike?

9. Abstracting and formulating differences between objects, events, sea-
sons, ideas, feelings, etc.:
What is the difference between summer and winter?
What is the difference between Halloween and Thanksgiving?

The last two examples require redefinition and recategorization of words
and concepts through abstraction of various characteristics. When they are
preceded by the classification procedures, they may assist in developing or
enhancing semantic transformation abilities.

It may be necessary to develop basic classification abilities in some language and learning disabled children. Inhelder, Sinclair, and Bovet (1974)
have described nonverbal training procedures for class inclusion and seriation using a series of logical exercises to establish the cognitive operations
necessary to establish inclusive relationships. They observed that many children progressed simultaneously on class inclusion and conservation tasks de-
spite the fact that only class inclusion was emphasized in training, suggesting
that common reasoning strategies had been developed. The relationship between these nonverbal reasoning strategies and verbal classification is discussed in relationship to Kohnstamm's work (Kohnstamm, 1967). It is suggested that difficulties in the mental operations basic to class inclusion may
explain why subjects may use adjectives such as *long, short, thin,* and *thick*
but may not be able to describe contrasts such as *long but thin* or *short but
thick*. They state that "Lack of lexical knowledge can no more explain such
behavior than lack of perceptual discrimination. The real difficulty lies in the
mental operations necessary to establish compensatory or inclusive relationships" (Inhelder, Sinclair, & Bovet, 1974, p. 197).

Among educational programs, Lavatelli (1970) introduces an early childhood curriculum based on Piagetian principles. The program may be used
with learning disabled children in the early grades to establish the logical operations basic to cognitive processing of spoken language.

Improving Cognitive Processing of Semantic Relations

Processing sentences expressing logical relationships between words or
phrases seems difficult for many LD youngsters (Wiig & Semel, 1973,
1974b). Our language contains several types of sentences and sentence structures that express logical relations between concepts. Among them are comparative sentences and sentences with *if . . . then* structures. The processes
involved in perceiving and interpreting sentences that require logical operations can be illustrated using the example of a verbal analogy, a semantic relation (Guilford, 1967).

Consider the verbal analogy "Trees have leaves. Flowers have (petals)." In
order to complete this analogy the logical relationship between *trees* and
leaves, a whole-part relationship, must be discerned. This logical relationship
must be repeated to complete the second relationship in the analogy. It is also
necessary to (1) know the composition of a flower, (2) have the word *petal*

available in long-term memory store, and (3) have a firm verbal association between the word *flower* and the names for its various parts. The relationships between *trees, leaves, flowers,* and *petals* can also be expressed in a part-whole analogy, "Leaves grow on trees. Petals grow on (flowers)." In this analogy the part-whole relationship expressed initially must be extended to complete it.

The two verbal analogies presented above may be expressed in different constructions in which the verbs do not facilitate abstraction of the logical relationships. The relationships between *trees, flowers, petals,* and *leaves* may be stated in sentences such as (1) "Trees are to leaves as flowers are to (petals)" (a whole-part analogy) or (2) "Leaves are to trees as petals are to (flowers)" (a part-whole analogy). The latter constructions are more difficult, but they are frequently used in teaching. As an example, the teacher may use an analogy to demonstrate that it is possible to live in Chicago, Illinois, and North America at the same time. The explanation may take the forms "Chicago is part of Illinois, and Illinois is part of North America" or "Chicago is to Illinois as Illinois is to North America." Perceiving and interpreting logical relationships is basic to the cognitive processing of auditory language.

Linguistic concepts such as "If it rains, then I'll wear a raincoat" and "She introduced me to her uncle" also require logical operations for interpretation. In order to understand the former sentence, the cause-effect relationship must be discerned; in the latter case, the familial relationship must be understood. There are a variety of linguistic concepts learning disabled youngsters need to understand, among them:

1. Sentences expressing comparative relationships: Elephants are bigger than tigers.
2. Sentences expressing passive relationships: John was brought by Mary.
3. Sentences expressing spatial relationships: Peter was walking between Burt and Fred.
4. Sentences expressing temporal-sequential events and relationships: Lunch will be served before noon.
5. Sentences expressing familial relationships: George is my wife's uncle.
6. Sentences with cause-effect relationships, using concepts such as *if . . . then, because, so,* and *therefore.*
7. Sentences expressing inclusion-exclusion, using concepts such as *all, none, some, any, all except, all but, not,* and *neither-nor.*

Improving Processing of Verbal Analogies

Remediation strategies designed to establish verbal analogies must consider the type and level of difficulty of the analogy. Materials should be designed to proceed from a relatively easy to a relatively difficult level. Among variables to consider are

1. The type of analogy required (whole-part, part-whole, antonym, etc.).
2. The relative level of difficulty of the required analogy.
3. The relative level of difficulty of the analogy format.

Verbal analogies may express one or more of the following relationships between the first two words:

1. Whole-part relationship: A *dog* is to *hair* as a *bird* is to *feathers*.
2. Part-whole relationship: A *key* is to a *door* as a *dial* is to a *telephone*.
3. Part-part relationship: A *nail* is to *hair* as a *talon* is to *feathers*.
4. Action to object relationship: *Driving* is to a *car* as *flying* is to a *plane*.
5. Object to action relationship: A *steak* is to *broiling* as a *cake* is to *baking*.
6. Purpose relationship: A *bat* is to a *baseball* as a *racket* is to *tennis*.
7. Cause-effect relationship: *Lightning* is to *thunder* as *fire* is to *smoke*.
8. Spatial relationship: The *United States of America* is to *Canada* as *South America* is to *North America*.
9. Temporal relationship: *Morning* is to *breakfast* as *noon* is to *lunch*.
10. Sequential relationship: *April* is to *May* as *June* is to *July*.
11. Numerical relationship, sequential or nonsequential: *Fourteen* is to *seven* as *twenty* is to *ten*.
12. Familial relationship: A *brother* is to a *sister* as an *uncle* is to an *aunt*.
13. Degree relationship: *Inches* are to *feet* as *yards* are to *miles*.
14. Antonym relationship: *Big* is to *little* as *night* is to *day*.
15. Synonym relationship: *Laugh* is to *giggle* as *crying* is to *sobbing*.
16. Grammatical relationship: *Boy* is to *boys* as *child* is to *children*.

The sequence in which the various analogy types are introduced depends upon the relative ease with which these relationships can be perceived by the youngster. The sequence can be abstracted from knowledge of previous success in establishing semantic classification and transformation. On this basis:

1. Whole-part analogies should be introduced before part-whole ones.
2. Antonym should be introduced before synonym analogies.
3. Action-object relationships should be introduced before object-action ones.
4. Sequential relationships (temporal, e.g., March, April, May, or spatial, e.g., big, bigger, biggest) should be introduced before temporal or spatial relationships which are not in sequence.
5. All other relationships should be introduced before grammatical relationships are presented.

In terms of relative difficulty of possible formats, ones such as "Leaves grow on trees. Petals grow on flowers." are easier than formats such as "A leaf is to a tree as a petal is to a flower," which are more complex linguistically.

Procedures requiring (a) correct/incorrect judgments, (b) selection of appropriate target words from sets of alternatives, and (c) sentence completion lend themselves readily to intervention:

a. A dog has paws. A boy has hair. (correct/incorrect) (whole-part relationship)

A boy can be a brother. A girl can be an uncle. (correct/incorrect) (antonym relationship)

You bake a cake. You broil a hamburger. (correct/incorrect) (action–object relationship)

We can swim in the summer. We can ski in the mountains. (correct/incorrect) (temporal relationship)

b. A doorknob belongs on a door. A dial belongs on a window/*phone*. (part-whole relationship)

You can drive a car. You can fly a car/*kite*. (action-object relationship)

You use a racket to play tennis. You use a bat to play football/*baseball*. (purpose relationship)

Monday comes before Tuesday. Saturday comes before *Sunday*/Friday. (temporal-sequential relationship)

c. A dog has a mouth. A bird has a _____. (whole-part relationship)

An egg can be fried. An apple can be _____. (object-action relationship)

Thunder comes after lightning. Smoke comes after _____. (cause–effect relationship)

A horse is big but an elephant is bigger. A butterfly is small but a mosquito is _____. (grammatical and spatial relationship)

Improving Processing of Linguistic Concepts

Among the linguistic concepts requiring logical operations for interpretation are five sentence types (logico-grammatical sentences) that have been reported to cause difficulty for youngsters with learning disabilities (Wiig & Semel, 1973, 1974b). In order of difficulty, these are (1) comparative sentences, (2) passive sentences, (3) sentences which express spatial relationships, (4) sentences which contain sequential events, and (5) sentences with familial relationships. Although the general remediation principles discussed earlier are applicable, in addition, each sentence category has specific characteristics that influence presentation sequence.

Comparative Relationships

Within the comparative relationships, observations and research suggest that the relative levels of difficulty are determined by the following factors:

1. Sentences that compare only two elements such as "Apples are bigger than cherries" are easier to process than sentences that compare three or more elements such as "Apples are bigger than cherries and cherries are bigger than raisins" or "Are apples bigger than cherries and watermelons?"

2. Sentences and questions that express a true relationship such as "Are elephants bigger than tigers" are easier to process than sentences that express a false relationship, "Are tigers bigger than elephants?"

3. Sentences that express a positive comparison such as *bigger than* or *taller than* are easier to process than those which give negative comparisons such as *smaller than* or *shorter than*.

It follows that remediation should progress from using positively stated, true statements comparing only two concepts (Apples are bigger than cherries) to negatively stated, false questions comparing more than two concepts (Are elephants smaller than tigers and lions?).

Passive Relationships

Within the passive relationships, reversible passive sentences with proper nouns such as "Mary was pushed by Jane" are more difficult than irreversible passives such as "The car was driven by John." Intervention procedures should therefore be designed to gradually reduce the semantic cues that may facilitate processing. A substitution procedure may be used in which a declarative sentence is given first. Then a passive sentence is substituted which is either correct or incorrect. An illustrative sequence is as follows:

1. The man drives the car.
2. The car is driven by the man. (irreversible passive)
3. The boy walked the dog.
4. The dog was walked by the boy. (irreversible passive)
5. The boy brought the girl.
6. The girl was brought by the boy. (reversible passive)
7. The girl brought the boy.
8. The boy was brought by the girl. (reversible passive)
9. The boy brought Mary.
10. Mary was brought by the boy. (reversible passive with one proper noun)
11. Mary brought John.
12. John was brought by Mary. (reversible passive with two proper nouns)

The comprehension of passive sentences depends heavily upon knowledge of the syntactic rules for passive transformation. Therefore, remediation may also utilize strategies relevant to improving linguistic processing.

Spatial Relationships

The comprehension of spatial relationships requires knowledge of the meaning of the various prepositions and prepositional phrases. The intervention strategies should therefore follow in sequence directly after the meanings of the various prepositions and prepositional phrases have been established. Spatial relationships in which two elements are compared as in "Jack walked in front of Jill" should be introduced before relationships requiring comparison among more than two elements as in "Jane swam between Betty and Ann. Who was in the middle?"

Temporal-Sequential Relationships

Sentences expressing sequential events are easier to process and interpret when the events occur in their logical sequence. It is easier to interpret and respond to the question "Does February come before March" than "Does March come after February?" It is also easier to interpret a correct sequence such as "Does summer come before fall" than "Does fall come before summer?'' These factors must be accounted for in sequencing the materials for remediation. Some LD youngsters may not be able to sequence temporal events correctly or consistently. It may therefore be necessary to establish automatic sequences for major temporal events, such as days of the week, months of the year, or holidays, before progressing to procedures designed to improve the comprehension of sentences expressing sequential events or temporal relationships.

Familial Relationships

Familial relationships may pose several problems for the learning disabled youngster. The family structure must be related to differences in age; the structure of the intact family must be perceived accurately; if the family is not intact, the child must be able to adapt to this lack of experience. Finally, the child must substitute proper names by using the appropriate labels for individual family members.

Analysis of kinship terms has resulted in two models which may be used to describe a hierarchy in familial relationship terms (Romney & D'Andrade, 1964; Wallace & Atkins, 1960). These models are similar in that both agree that *sex* and *generation* are significant dimensions. They differ in that Wallace and Atkins (1960) introduce the dimension *linearity* in their theoretical model while Romney and D'Andrade (1964) introduce the component *reciprocity (father-son, aunt-uncle)*.

The data reported by Romney and D'Andrade (1964) further indicated that the most salient kinship terms for high school students were *father* and *mother; son* and *daughter* were low in saliency. Wiig and Semel (1974a) observed that grade-school children acquired control of the terms *grandmother* and *grandfather* first, followed by the terms *uncle* and *aunt. Brother* and *sister* were often substituted for the kinship term *cousin*, which does not contain the component *sex* and was developed last.

In remediation, the labels for direct family members (father, mother, sister, brother) should be established before labels for grandparents (grandmother, grandfather), and for relatives (uncle, aunt, cousin). Pictures of various members of the child's own family may be used to develop knowledge of family structure, familial relationships, and labels for family members. In developing knowledge of family structure, a family tree may be helpful.

Remedial Procedures

Wiig and Semel (1973) used parts of the *Sound-Order-Sense* program focusing on improving the comprehension of linguistic concepts (comparative, passive, spatial, temporal-sequential, and familial relationships) (Semel, 1970) for intensive language stimulation. They reported significant improvements by a group of language disabled transition-class (nonpromoted first grade) children, suggesting that logical processing deficits may respond to intervention. The intervention program progressed as follows:

The program consisted of four phases. Each phase contained representative samples from (1) the *Sound* subsection for discrimination and identification of phonemes in words and sentences, (2) the *Order* subsection for discrimination and identification of suprasegmentals (sentence intonation patterns) and relationships between sequential events, (3) the *Sense* subsection for recognition of comparative and spatial relationships, and (4) the *Activity Cards* for identi-

fication and formulation of inflectional and derivational affixes, passive constructions, and possessive relationships. Each subsection was of similar length
and duration. Responses to the first three phases were nonverbal and based on
following directions to simultaneous auditory and visual input. The last phase
required following directions, problem solving, and verbal formulation. [p. 631]

A variety of intervention strategies for improving the interpretation of linguistic concepts of inclusion-exclusion (all, none, some, any, all except, all
but, not, neither . . . nor, etc.) and cause-effect (if . . . then) have been described by Bereiter and Engelmann (1966). They suggest that comprehension of these concepts may be established by using sentence patterns chosen
on the basis of the rules of inference that apply to them. The procedures are
accompanied by illustrations to form the associations necessary for problem
solving. The basic procedure uses a *five-element model* consisting of either
five circles, squares, or rectangles, and so forth. The rationale for choosing
this model is to provide presentations that are refined, simplified and dra-
matic. Each linguistic concept is defined to the child, using the five-element
model. Subsequently, the child answers questions that include the specific
linguistic concept used in reference to the model. The procedures outlined to
establish the linguistic concept *if . . . then* will serve to illustrate the design.

In the first step, the *five-element model* (squares) is introduced and the
concept, size, is defined by demonstration and association. The educator
points to the big squares saying "What can I say about these squares that I
cannot say about any of the other squares?" When the concept that they are
big is firmly established, the first part of the linguistic concept is introduced
using the format "If squares are big, _____." The children must provide the
reference to the color shared by the big squares (white). Next, the educator
uses color as the basis for reference in the format "If squares are red, what
else can I say about them?"

After the basic *if . . . then* concept has been established, the children are
asked to solve basic *if . . . then* problems using similar question formats. Subsequently, this basic concept is extended with appropriate changes in the
model to include negation (If a square is *not* big it is [little]) or (*If* a square is
not big it is not [red]). The last step in the remediation sequence transfers the
use of the acquired linguistic concepts to everyday language and situations.
As an example, the *if . . . then* concept may be used in a concrete everyday
situation using examples such as "If you put the books on the shelf, I'll let you
read the comic strips. You put the books on the shelf. What will happen?"

The basic procedures described by Bereiter and Engelmann (1966) depend
heavily on classification and categorization of the parts of the five-element
model. The interpretation of some cause-effect relationships such as "If Su-
san is planning a picnic and it rains then she can (postpone it/have it in-
side/etc.)" and "If Peter saves fifty dollars then he can buy (a car/a bike/ice
skates/etc.)" may depend upon other abilities such as (1) seriation according
to relative values or other characteristics, (2) knowledge of the potential implications, (3) anticipation of a variety of possible outcomes, and (4) moral
judgment.

Inhelder, Sinclair, and Bovet (1974, pp. 101-4) describe verbal training
procedures for comparative terms which may be used in intervention. They
report differences in the use of descriptive and comparative terms between

children who have acquired the principle of conservation and those who have not. Conserving children were observed to use comparative terms such as *more-less* in a clay-modeling situation while nonconserving children used descriptive terms such as *a lot-a little*. Conserving children also used antonyms such as *long/short, thick/thin* to describe differences in length and width. Nonconserving children used undifferentiated terms, for example, *big/little, thick/little*. Conserving children were able to express two comparisons in one sentence; for example, "This pencil is long but thin, the other is short but fat"; nonconservers expressed the differences in four-part structures; for example, "This pencil is long, that one is short, this one is thin, that one is fat." The authors conclude that "there seems to be a clear parallel between the structuring of the cognitive operations and the acquisition of the terms necessary for their expression" (p. 115). This relationship suggests a need to consider cognitive training procedures in the early stages of intervention for language disabled children with significant delays in the acquisition of linguistic concepts.

Improving the Cognition of Semantic Transformation

Our language is rich in idioms, proverbs, and metaphors. If these are taken literally, they may be meaningless or the interpretation may be erroneous. In order to understand the meaning of figurative language, changes in meaning, significance, and use must be discerned and the concrete word meanings must be translated into generalized, abstract concepts. This ability reflects the cognition of semantic transformation (Guilford, 1967). The processes involved are similar to those required in interpreting multiple-meaning words, which must be accurately categorized and reclassified, semantically and grammatically, in order to arrive at the various possible meanings. Although multiple-meaning words have referential bases (they refer to objects, actions, events, or ideas), the words constituting the elements of idioms, proverbs, and metaphors must be translated into nonreferential, abstract, and generalized concepts. The abstract meaning of the various idioms, proverbs, and metaphors may therefore have to be established separately with little transfer occurring from item to item.

Learning disabled youngsters may experience problems in translating and interpreting figurative language. They need to acquire the meaning of many common proverbs, metaphors, and idioms in order to recognize and understand commonly used figurative speech. The list of proverbs and other figurative language is exhaustive, and each example cannot be taught individually. The purpose of intervention is therefore to establish understanding of commonly used figurative speech and recognition of novel figurative statements.

The ability to categorize, reclassify, recategorize, define, and redefine multiple—meaning words is basic to planning intervention strategies to improve the comprehension of figurative language. Procedures to improve word categorization and reclassification have been discussed previously in the section on semantic classes. These strategies may be used to lead into the methods, materials, and sequences designed to improve the interpretation of figurative speech.

Idioms

Idioms frequently employ multiple-meaning words that may be known to the LD child. Several idioms tend to use the same words in various combinations. Parts of the body, as an example, seem to be featured in a large number of idioms. As an illustration, the body part, *eye,* is used in variety of idioms such as *sharp eyes, eyes popped, eyes danced, to have eyes for, to eye it,* etc. Intervention strategies may utilize methods which accentuate the humor of comparing concrete and literal interpretations of idioms. Consider the idioms "He hit the roof" and "I'm all tied up at the office." Illustrations of the literal, concrete and of the general, abstract interpretations may be presented side-by-side as is shown in Figure 6. In remediation, the youngster may be required to identify a set of pictures (literal and abstract interpretations) for each of a series of idioms said by the educator. This procedure may be varied to present only illustrations of the abstract interpretations for the identification.

Other formats appropriate for intervention may present the spoken idiom and two multiple choices:

1. Bill caught a cold.
    a. Bill was able to catch a cold with his hands.
    b. Bill became sick with a cold.
2. The advertising business is a real jungle.
    a. The advertising business is very competitive.
    b. The advertising business has trees and wild animals in it.

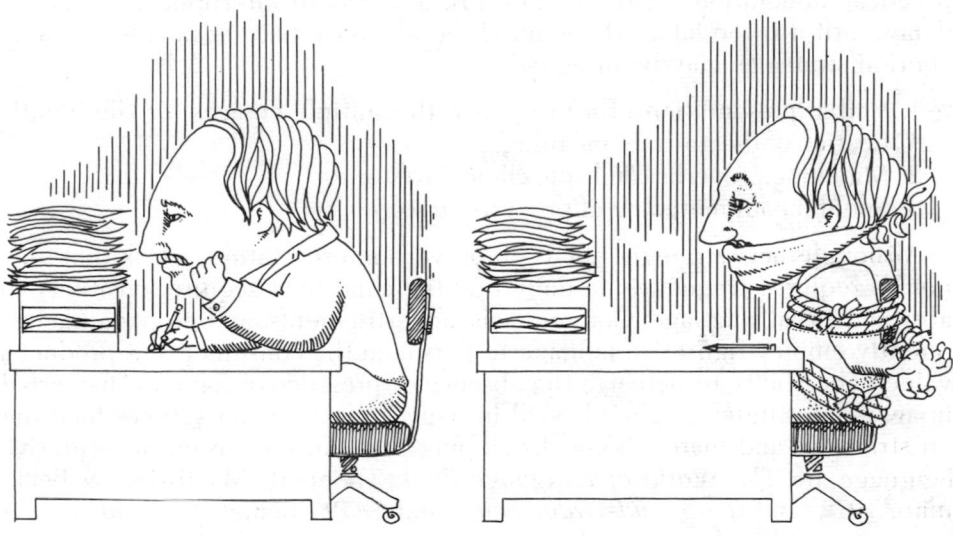

FIGURE 6. Illustration of the literal and abstract interpretation of
the idiom "I'm all tied up at the office."

Metaphors

Metaphors such as "It was as white as snow" express comparisons between the actual subject and a descriptive image. The two things being compared are widely different but share some common, highlighed aspect. Metaphors and similes are often differentiated. Although the images created by the two are the same, the *simile* features the verb *like* as in "Bob eats like a bird." Metaphors and similes should be introduced in remediation with an explanation of the principles involved. Subsequent remediation procedures may use multiple-choice formats:

1. Sally is as busy as a beaver.
   a. Sally is not very busy.
   b. Sally is very busy.
2. When Bill got the award, he was pleased as punch.
   a. Upon receiving the award, Bill looked like a bowl of punch.
   b. Upon receiving the award, Bill was very happy.

Sentence pairs may also be presented, and the youngster may be required to identify words that are repeated and ones that create an image rather than describe a fact:
1. They drank punch. They were pleased as punch.
2. They worked like beavers. They liked the beavers.

Proverbs and Platitudes

Proverbs and platitudes share the imagery of metaphors. In addition, they contain moral advice discerned only when the generalized, abstract meaning is understood. The proverb "Strike while the iron is hot" may be interpreted at a lower level to mean "Don't let the iron get cold before you strike," a practical admonition. At the higher abstract level of interpretation, "Don't delay until it is too late," the general moral advice becomes evident. Intervention strategies may be designed for:

1. Verbal presentation of a proverb with multiple choices for the identification of the abstract meaning.
2. Matching proverbs (multiple choice) to stories.
3. Spontaneous matching of proverbs to stories.

Although these strategies focus on proverb interpretation, a task that may not be required frequently in daily life, the child may acquire sensitivity to abstract verbal language. Commercials, advertisements, and propaganda frequently employ figurative langage to persuade the consumer of a product's value. The ability to perceive the absence or presence of logic in the verbal imagery constitutes a valuable skill in daily living. Among sources focusing on strategies and materials for developing the comprehension of figurative language are *The World of Language Books* (Bennett, Mysliwiec, & Beckman, 1972) and the *Sound-Order-Sense* and *SAPP* (Semel, 1970, in press).

Improving the Cognition of Semantic Implications

The ability to discern implied cause-effect relationships and predict consequences and outcomes reflects the cognition of semantic implications (Guilford, 1967). Learning disabled youngsters may demonstrate problems in perceiving the implications of verbal statements; a need for intervention is therefore indicated. In order for a child to grasp the total meaning of a monologue, dialogue, or conversation, he must interpret each concept presented and discern the inferences and implications that were not expressed.

Interpretation of unspoken cause-effect relationships requires knowledge of the relationships between specific causes and their potential consequences and between specific consequences and their possible causes. If the child is told that it is going to rain, the potential consequences may be that he will get wet or that he must stay inside. If the child were told that his family needed to have the car fixed, the possible causes may be numerous.

When the child has formed associations between a variety of causes and outcomes, he must be taught to discern that causes or effects are not always discussed but may be implied. This ability may be developed by using materials of increasing length and complexity. Intervention may be initiated with sentences and progress to use of paragraphs and complex stories. The procedures may require:

1. Detection of inconsistencies and absurdities in sentences:
   a. He hit the baseball with a racket.
   b. The drive to work was almost thirty miles. After four years, Mr. Adams decided to buy a new bicycle and save money.
   c. It was raining so hard yesterday that Phil took off his shirt to get a suntan.
2. Detection of inconsistencies and absurdities in paragraphs and stories:
   a. It was a beautiful summer day and George decided to go swimming. He put on his bathing suit and drove into the warm water of the lake. After half an hour of swimming, he dried himself off on the shore and lay in the hot summer sun. Then he looked at the water and said, "Gee, I think I'll go ice skating!"
3. Interpretation of ambiguous sentences with multiple choices provided:
   a. Shooting stars are exciting. (Let's get our guns and shoot stars. Let's watch the stars shoot through the sky.)
4. Correction of inconsistencies and absurdities in sentences:
   a. Charlie drank the hamburger.
   b. Brian liked the book so much he burned it.
   c. Ted was going to Europe and didn't know whether to go by boat or bus.
5. Predicting and choosing outcomes of short stories:
   a. John was hanging a picture on the wall. He tried to use a thumbtack. The thumbtack bent against the wall. What could he do?
      1. Try to use tape.
      2. Use another thumbtack.
      3. Not try to hang the picture.
6. Interpreting propaganda and giving appropriate responses to questions:
   a. There is a party on the beach and everyone is drinking soda. One young man says "I've come alive since I have joined the soda pop crowd! Drink soda pop!"
      1. Did the young man really come alive?
      2. What did he join since he started drinking soda pop?
      3. Do you think he is telling the truth?

Understanding the implied meaning of a message may depend upon adequate perception of sentence intonation features (pitch, intensity, duration, rate, juncture). The sentence "Give that to me!" can have a variety of meanings depending upon prosodic differences. "Give that to *me*" means that *I* want what you have. "*Give* that to me" means that I don't want to come and get it, I want it given to me. "Give *that* to me" means that I want the particular object. "Give that to me?" means that I am asking if it is possible that I will be given the particular thing. Learning disabled children may experience problems in perceiving prosodic features and differences in sentences (Vogel, 1974), suggesting a need for intervention.

The intervention procedures may emphasize sentences differing only at the suprasegmental level. The responses may require (a) identification of the stressed word or phrase in oral commands, (b) same-different judgments, or (c) verbal interpretation of differences:

- a. Give the pencil to *me*. (beginning/middle/end)
  Bring *the book* to Jane. (beginning/middle/end)
  Run to the blackboard. (beginning/middle/end)
  Place *the blue pencil* on the big table. (beginning/middle/end)
- b. *Yesterday* Mrs. Jones went to the hospital.
  Yesterday Mrs. Jones went *to the hospital*. (same/different)
  Tomorrow Paul *must* go to school.
  Tomorrow Paul must go to *school*. (same/different)
- c. When I say, "*Run* to the door," what do I want you to be sure to do?
  When I tell you, "Last year we *drove* to Los Angeles," what do I want you to be sure to know?
  When I say, "I can't *read* the paper *in the dark*," what do I want you to do for me?"

Mishler (1972) has discussed the implications of teacher strategies for language and cognition. Analysis of verbal interactions in teaching suggest that the teacher may determine the cognitive style of the group through language usage. The illustration and discussion of verbal interactions and of the cognitive strategies available to the teacher through language may provide guidelines for improving cognitive processing abilities in the classroom.

The Peabody Language Development Kits (Dunn & Smith, 1965, 1966, 1967; Dunn, Horton, & Smith, 1968) provide an excellent source for materials, strategies, and activities designed to develop perception, conceptualization, and expression. At the lower levels, the development of labeling language, linguistic structure and logical thinking is emphasized (Kit P and Level #1). At the higher levels the emphasis is on cognition and convergent and divergent production. The materials and procedures have been found effective in producing gains in overall oral language as well as in specific language abilities, as measured by the *Illinois Test of Psycholinguistic Abilities* (Dunn, Horton, & Smith, 1968). The kits have been used with efficacy with a variety of populations, ranging from trainable (TMR) and educable mentally retarded (EMR) children to slow-learning and disadvantaged children, suggesting general applicability. Van Hattum (1969) has warned that the PDLK should not be used as a "cookbook." The educator-clinician should tailor the program to the assets and deficits of each individual child, a comment concurring with the intent of this text.

References

Baker, H. J., & Leland, B. *Detroit tests of learning aptitude.* Indianapolis: Bobbs-Merrill, 1959.

Bangs, T. E. *Language and learning disorders of the pre-academic child.* New York: Appleton-Century Crofts, 1968.

Bennett, R. A., Mysliwiec, N., & Beckman, B. *The world of language books.* Teacher's ed. Chicago: Follett Publishing Co., 1972.

Bereiter, C., & Englemann, S. *Teaching disadvantaged children in the preschool.* Englewood Cliffs, N.J.: Prentice-Hall, 1966.

Black, J. W. Accompaniments of word intelligibility. *Journal of Speech and Hearing Disorders,* 1952, **17**, 409-18.

Boehm, A. *The Boehm test of basic concepts.* (Manual) New York: Psychological Corp., 1969.

Botel, M. *Botel reading inventory.* Chicago: Follett Educational Corp., 1970.

Brown, E. *Preposition concepts picture cards.* Boston: Teaching Resources Corp., 1973.

Brown, R. *A first language: the early stages.* Cambridge, Mass.: University Press, 1973.

Charney, R. Information in multidimensional sounds. *Journal of Acoustical Society of America,* 1966, **40**, 447.

Chipman, H. H., & deDardel, C. Developmental study of the comprehension and production of the pronoun "it." *Journal of Psycholinguistic Research,* 1974, **3**, 91-99.

Clark, E. V. On the child's acquisition of antonyms in two semantic fields. *Journal of Verbal Learning and Verbal Behavior,* 1972, **11**, 750-58.

Clark, H. H. On the use and meaning of prepositions. *Journal of Verbal Learning and Verbal Behavior,* 1968, 7, 421-31.

Dunn, L. M., Horton, K. B., & Smith, F. O. *Peabody language development kit:* (Level # P) Circle Pines, Minn.: American Guidance Service, 1968.

Dunn, L. M., & Smith, F. O. (Eds.) *Peabody language development kit. (Level #1)* Circle Pines, Minn.: American Guidance Service, 1965.

Dunn, L. M., & Smith, F. O. (Eds.) *Peabody language development kit. (Level #2)* Circle Pines, Minn.: American Guidance Service, 1966.

Dunn, L. M., & Smith, F. O. (Eds.) *Peabody language development kit.* (Level #3) Circle Pines, Minn.: American Guidance Service, 1967.

Fries, C. C. *The structure of English: an introduction to the construction of English sentences.* New York: Harcourt Brace Jovanovich, 1952.

Gleason, H. A. *An introduction to descriptive linguistics.* New York: Holt, Rinehart & Winston, 1955.

Gottsleben, R., Tyack, D., & Buschini, G. Three case studies in language training: applied linguistics. *Journal of Speech and Hearing Disorders*, 1974, **39**, 213-23.

Greene, H. A., Loomis, K. A., Davis, P. C., & Biedenharn, N. W. *The new building better English*. New York: Harper & Row, 1961.

Guilford, J. P. *The nature of human intelligence*. New York: McGraw-Hill, 1967.

Hulbert, E. *Out and in*. New York: Scholastic Book Services, 1970.

Hunt, K. *Grammatical structures written at three grade levels*. Champaign, Ill.: National Council of Teachers of English, 1965.

Inhelder, B., Sinclair, H., & Bovet, M. *Learning and the development of cognition*. Cambridge: Harvard University Press, 1974.

Johnson, D. J., & Myklebust, H. R. *Learning disabilities: educational principles and practices*. New York: Grune & Stratton, 1967.

Klees, M., & Lebrun, A. Analysis of the figurative and operative processes of thought of 40 dyslexic children. *Journal of Learning Disabilities*, 1972, **5**, 389-96.

Kohnstamm, G. A. *Teaching children to solve a Piagetian problem of class inclusion*. The Hague: Mouton, 1967.

Kreezer, G., & Dallenbach, K. M. Learning the relation of opposition. *American Journal of Psychology*, 1929, **41**, 432-41.

Lavatelli, C. *Piaget's theory applies to an early childhood curriculum*. Boston: American Science & Engineering, 1970.

Maratsos, M. B. The effects of stress on the understanding of pronominal co—reference in children. *Journal of Psycholinguistic Research*, 1973, **2**, 1-8.

Mishler, E. G. Implications of teacher strategies for language and cognition: observations in first-grade classrooms. In C. B. Cazden, V. P. Johns, & D. Hymes (Eds.), *Functions of language in the classroom*. New York: Teachers College Press, 1972. Pp. 267-98.

Moorehead, D. M., & Ingram, D. The development of base syntax in normal and linguistically deviant children. *Journal of Speech and Hearing Research*, 1973, **16**, 330-52.

Romney, A. K., & D'Andrade, R. G. Cognitive aspects of English kin terms. In A. K. Romney & R. G. D'Andrade (Eds.), *Transcultural studies in cognition. American Anthropologist*, 1964, **66**, 3:2, 146-70.

Rozenzweig, M. R., & Postman, L. Intelligibility as a function of frequency of usage. *Journal of Experimental Psychology*, 1957, **54**, 412-22.

Rozenzweig, M. R., & Postman, L. Frequency of usage and the perception of words. *Science*, 1958, **127**, 263-66.

Rutberg, B. The written response to the oral presentation of homonyms. Master's thesis, Boston University, 1972.

Semel, E. M. *Sound-Order-Sense: a developmental program in auditory perception*. Chicago: Follett Educational Corp., 1970.

Semel, E. M. *Semel auditory processing program*. Chicago: Follett Publishing Co., in press.

Snider, L., & Symington, N. Programmed approach to training "in" and "on." *DCCD Bulletin*, 1974, **11**, 8-19.

Streng, A. *Syntax, speech and hearing: applied linguistics for teachers of children with language and hearing disabilities*. New York; Grune & Stratton, 1972.

Takahaski, G. Perception of space and the function of certain English prepositions. *Language Learning*, 1969, **19**, 217-33.

Thorndike, E., & Lorge, I. *The teacher's word book of 30,000 words.* New York: Teacher's College, Columbia University, 1944.

Van Hattum, R. F. New dimensions for the speech and hearing program in the schools: language and the retarded child. Paper presented at the California State Department of Education, San Diego, 1969.

Vogel, S. A. Syntactic abilities in normal and dyslexic children. *Journal of Learning Disabilities*, 1974, **7**, 47-53.

Wallace, A. F., & Atkins, J. The meaning of kinship terms. *American Anthropologist*, 1960, **62**, 58-79.

Waryas, C. I. Psycholinguistic research in language intervention: the pronoun system. *Journal of Psycholinguistic Research*, 1973, **2**, 221-37.

Wiig, E. H., & Semel, E. M. Comprehension of linguistic concepts requiring logical operations. *Journal of Speech and Hearing Research*, 1973, **16**, 627-36.

Wiig, E. H., & Semel, E. M. Development of comprehension of logico-grammatical sentences by grade school children. *Perceptual and Motor Skills*, 1974, **38**, 171-76. (a)

Wiig, E. H., & Semel, E. M. Logico-grammatical sentence comprehension by adolescents with learning disabilities. *Perceptual and Motor Skills*, 1974, **38**, 1331-34. (b)

Wilson, M. *The Wilson initial syntax program.* Cambridge, Mass.: Educators Publishing Service, 1972.

8

Deficits in Language Formation and Production

Overview

Descriptions of clinical observations of language production and sentence formation deficits associated with learning disabilities are presented as a background for subsequent reviews of research of normal and deviant expressive language characteristics. The normal developmental sequences reported by, among others, Berko (1958), Brown (1973), Cazden (1972), Chomsky (1969), and Menyuk (1969) for the acquisition of morphology and syntax are reviewed as a basis for discussions of the characteristics and bases of linguistic deficits reported in language and learning disabled children and adolescents. Observations of deficits in sentence formation are also related to factors and characteristics of expressive language reported in normal school children and adults (Caroll, 1960; Hass & Wepman, 1974; Jones & Wepman, 1961).

The consensus of the available data on morphological and syntactic abilities of learning disabled children and adolescents indicates that we can expect deficits in a large proportion of this population. Deficits can be expected in those LD youngsters who exhibit discrepancies of fifteen or more points between verbal and performance IQs with the verbal being lower. The results of at least one study suggest that (a) between 75% and 85% of learning disabled youngsters may experience significant delays in the acquisition of syntax (Semel & Wiig, 1975), (b) the language deficits may persist into adolescence (Wiig & Semel, 1975b), and (c) deficits in language processing relate significantly to academic achievement and to written syntax (London, 1974; Semel & Wiig, 1975).

The chapter further presents evidence of word finding difficulties (dysnomia) and deficits in convergent and divergent language production in learning disabilities. The bases and characteristics of these deficits are discussed in relationship to studies of word finding deficits in adult aphasics (Geschwind, 1972; Goldstein, 1948; Luria, 1966, 1973) and of word substitutions in normal adults (Fromkin, 1973).

Characteristics

Observations suggest that the verbal expression and production problems associated with learning disabilities are subtle, explaining why they are frequently overlooked in educational management and have received relatively little attention in research. We can observe and analyze some of the oral language problems as they are reflected in surface structure by listening to the LD youngster in a variety of situations.

Learning disabled children and adolescents characteristically substitute and use an unnecessarily large number of words in their oral language production. They produce grammatically incorrect and incomplete sentences and use only a small number of prepositional phrases, structures expressing comparative, spatial, and temporal relationships, and optional transformations. The bases for these expressive language problems have been suggested to relate to word finding and retrieval deficits and to deficits in sentence formulation, conceptualization, symbolization, and verbal (motor) encoding (Bannatyne, 1971; Johnson, 1968; Johnson & Myklebust, 1967; Myklebust, 1964; Wiig & Semel, 1975a, 1975b).

It has been shown that learning disabled youngsters generally have adequate receptive vocabulary levels (Strauss & Lehtinen, 1947); however in spontaneous speech some of them appear to overuse a limited, concrete vocabulary and a restricted set of syntactic structures. At times, some learning disabled children jump from one topic to the next with total abandon when they engage in conversation. Sentences may be left incomplete, and the topics selected for discussion may lack a logical progression. Their language may sound appropriate when they speak to parents, siblings, or peers. It frequently becomes inconsistent in structure and logic when learning disabled youngsters speak with authority figures or describe abstract concepts, feelings, and ideas.

Closer examination of some learning disabled youngsters' attempts to communicate abstract ideas or address authority figures suggests that word selection and retrieval and sentence formulation abilities decrease. As a result, they may overuse certain adjectives such as *nice, pretty, lovely,* or *great* and may be inclined to use extravagant exaggeration in phrases in which adjectives and adverbs with contrasting meanings are juxtapositioned, such as *awfully pretty* and *terribly nice*. The adjectives selected are usually limited in number, tend to be concrete, and of high frequency. They generally do not denote subtle differences in quality or quantity and often indicate a preference for expressing color, size, or affect.

At the syntactic level, LD children frequently produce agrammatical sentences in which elements of several transformations may be combined or reversed as in "The man was stole the chicken" and "Do I want ice cream?" for "I do want ice cream." They may also respond to questions with another question followed by the answer, as in answering a question such as "When is dinner ready?" with the sequence "When is dinner ready? Around six o'clock." They frequently use fillers such as *and then, now, um,* and *let's see.* They may substitute nouns, verbs, adjectives, and adverbs and seem to have special problems in recalling proper names. Sometimes they appear to use a large number of words in an attempt to describe a concept whose name eludes them. They may use functional definitions such as "You know, the thing you cut bread with" to indicate a noun. In their efforts to find specific words, they may digress and never arrive at the point of a story. When the learning disabled child substitutes words, they generally belong to the same grammatical or semantic categories as the intended words.

The tendency for learning disabled children to echo verbal stimuli vocally and subvocally or to shadow (by mouthing) a speaker may be observed in both social and educational settings and interactions. This habit may relate to problems in processing language and reflect attempts to cope. When listening to a story, some learning disabled children may repeat each word in a sentence immediately after it has been spoken. Some children will repeat only the last words of an occasional complex phrase as in echoing the words *on the roof* when hearing "When the cat saw the dog it jumped upon the roof."

The tendency to echo or shadow may manifest itself at the nonverbal level. Learning disabled children are often observed to shadow a speaker by mouthing or they respond incessantly by nodding their heads and smiling. The nonverbal responses may become more pronounced when the learning disabled child experiences comprehension problems, suggesting that they may serve to reinforce a sense of security or to reward the speaker for his verbal attention. The learning disabled child may reauditorize and rehearse the verbal stimuli vocally or subvocally to gain time for auditory processing and interpretation.

Characteristic oral language problems in learning disabilities may be grouped into two major categories, linguistic and semantic. Within the linguistic domain, we can observe problems at the phonological, morphological, and syntactic levels. Within the semantic domain, difficulties occur in convergent as well as in divergent production of spoken language. The following sections will discuss each of the deficit areas in further detail.

Sentence Formulation: Morphology and Syntax

The internalization of linguistic rules (phonological, morphological, and syntactic) permits the child to generate novel sentences that he may never have heard in actuality. The syntactic rules specify the word order of sentences, and the morphological rules specify word inflections and markers. Although word order is of primary importance in generating sentences, word inflections provide both semantic information, indicating number and tense, and grammatical information by marking words as members of form classes. Learning disabled children and adolescents have been recognized to exhibit deficits or delays in the acquisition and use of both morphology and syntax (Bakwin, 1965; Doehring, 1968; Hallgren, 1950; Ingram, 1960; Johnson & Myklebust, 1967; Orton, 1937; Rabinovitch, 1959; Semel & Wiig, 1975; Vogel, 1974; Wiig, Semel, & Crouse, 1973; Zangwill, 1960).

Some investigators report that the oral syntax of learning disabled children does not differ significantly from that of academic achievers during spontaneous conversation, but that differences exist on structured linguistic tasks such as sentence repetition, completion, and transformation (Rosenthal, 1970; Vogel, 1974). This observation suggests that LD children are able to compensate for linguistic deficits when the semantic and/or linguistic constraints are minimal; however, when either or both constraints are imposed, their linguistic abilities prove inadequate. Johnson and Myklebust (1967) suggest that the learning disabled child is not able to retain the linguistic structure of sentences he hears; as a result, he does not have the linguistic patterns necessary to generate appropriately ordered sentences.

The acquisition of morphology and syntax has been the focus of extensive study by, among others, Berko (1958), Bloom (1973), Brown (1973), Cazden (1972), Chomsky (1964, 1969), and McNeill (1970). Chomsky (1964) proposes a language acquisition model in which the child formulates an internalized grammar (set of rules) from the linguistic input provided by his auditory environment. The child then uses the rules to generate original sentences. As he matures, the internalized rules are expanded to generate new hypotheses about the grammar of the linguistic community until his rules match those of the environment. The internalized language structure is the product of innate structure, genetic course of maturation, and experience, and represents linguistic competence. Chomsky states that in the course of language acquisition "reinforcement, casual observations, and natural inquisitiveness (coupled with a strong tendency to imitate) are important factors as in the remarkable capacity of the child to generalize, hypothesize and process information in a variety of very special and apparently highly complex ways" (1964, p. 563).

Normal Acquisition of Syntax

The normal acquisition and use of syntactic structures, operations, and transformations has received considerable attention by, among others, Menyuk (1969), Chomsky (1969), and Hass and Wepman (1974). Investigations of the acquisition of syntax during the preschool years and first grade has yielded evidence of developmental trends in the use of sentence types.

Menyuk (1969) reported that the normal child uses all the classes in base-structure rules by age three. This indicates that the young child handles the functional relationships between subject (S), predicate (P), and object (O) that are implicit in the base-structure string. It also indicates that the classes defined by these functional relationships, that is, S → NP (noun phrase); P → VP (verb phrase); O → NP and VP, are well understood. Menyuk also reported that during the period preceding age three, the order of development of various sentence types was as follows:

1. Joining of elements to make sentences.
2. Development of subject + predicate sentences.
3. Expansion of the VP to include an auxiliary verb and copula.
4. Embedding of an element within a sentence and attachment of the element to the verb.
5. Permutation of elements within a string (auxiliary/modal and tense markers).

Although children younger than three were observed to produce completely well-formed declarative, negative, and question sentences, they exhibited deviations in the use of base rules. The deviations reflected violations of the rules determining what can appear in a certain context and redundancies within classes. The deviations were interpreted by Menyuk to indicate that a symbol was further expanded to insure understanding by the listener or to provide greater definition.

Menyuk (1969) further reports on the observed order of usage of syntactic operations which underlies the formulation of completely grammatical structures. The reported order of usage was as follows: (1) addition, (2) deletion, (3) substitution, (4) permutation, (5) embedding, and (6) nesting.

First graders were also observed to formulate sentences that deviated from complete grammaticalness. Their agrammatical productions were characterized by redundancies resulting from reiteration of a particular class. Menyuk cites the response, "He'll might get in jail," as an example of reiteration of a modal (auxiliary verb) within the verb phrase.

Analysis of the formulation of various sentence types by first graders indicated that the expansion of basic structures and addition of new structures has not been completed by age seven. The data reported on the correct usage of the various sentence types by first graders are summarized in Table 16. Menyuk concludes that the deviations observed in first graders represent more or less complete approximations to completed rules.

TABLE 16

Summary of the Percentages of 1st Graders Who Produced Well-Formed
Sentence Types as Reported by Menyuk (1969)

Percentages	Sentence Types
100	Infinitival complement
100	Adjectivie, nominal-compound, and possessives
97	Adverb inversion
95	"and" conjunction
90	Imperative sentences
89	Conjunction deletion
89	Separation with verb + particle construction
87	Relative clauses
69	Reflexive structure
66	Substitution and embedding
64	Passive construction
41	Pronominalization
35	"cause" (because) conjunction
29	Nominalization
20	Participal complement
20	"if" conjunction
19	"so" conjunction

Aspects of the acquisition of syntax by five- to ten-year-olds were investigated by Chomsky (1969). She assessed the interpretation of four constructions, (1) ask/tell, (2) promise/tell, (3) easy to see, and (4) pronominalization, all of which share the feature that the grammatical relations expressed are not explicit at the surface-structure level. Chomsky summarizes her findings to reflect developmental trends for each of the constructions.

Pronominalization was acquired earliest and was interpreted correctly by all children at or above age 5½ but with consistent failure before then. *Easy to see* was interpreted correctly by all children at age 8½ and above, and the developmental pattern suggested a potential learning period of from three to four years. The construction *promise/tell* was interpreted correctly by all 9-year-olds and showed a mixed pattern of acquisition in 6, 7, and 8-year-olds. For the construction *ask/tell* there was considerable variation in the age of acquisition, and the general pattern suggested a gradual improvement with age up to 10. Chomsky comments that the significance of the findings related to the unexpectedly late acquisition of some syntactic structures. Unfortunately, the possible relationships to cognitive and logical growth were not explored.

In a recent study, Hass and Wepman (1974) analyzed the spoken syntax of 180 school children, ranging in age from five to thirteen years. They chose three variables for their analysis: (1) part-of-speech usage, (2) syntactic elaboration, and (3) constructional variety, that is, mean number of embedded clause components per sentence, mean length of noun phrase, and mean number of markers per finite verb. A principal components' factor analysis revealed the following factors: (1) fluency, (2) embeddedness, (3) finite verb structure, (4) NP structure, and (5) qualified speech. Of these, only the factor *embeddedness* clearly related to variables that changed with age. It suggested a dimension of surface-structure elaboration and tapped relatively more complicated noun phrase and sentence structure, but was independent of total words and proportion of words. The remaining factors were considered to reflect stylistic variations.

The consensus of the investigations of the acquisition of syntax by normal children points to increasing usage of complex transformation and to the emergence of embeddedness as an indicator of relative syntactic maturity. At the same time, the findings suggest that stylistic variations emerge early and that the cognitive and logical bases for the acquisition of certain syntactic structures warrant further attention.

Normal Acquisition of Morphology

Berko (1958) investigated four- to seven-year-olds' knowledge of morphology (word-formation rules) in an ingenious research design in which inflectional and derivational morphemes were applied to nonsense words associated with nonsense pictures. As an example of the design, she tested the noun plural in the example illustrated in Figure 7.

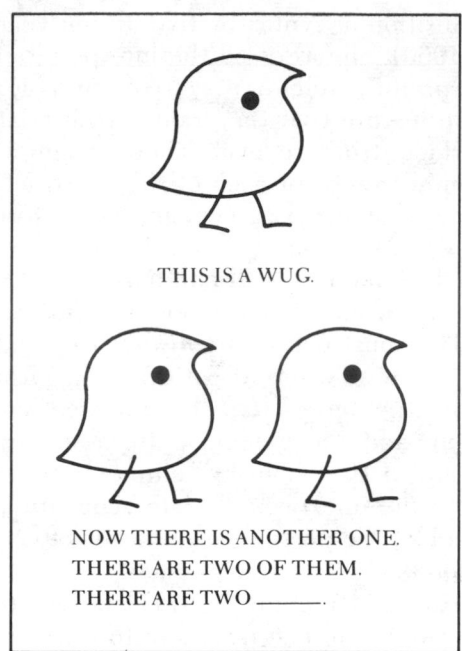

THIS IS A WUG.

NOW THERE IS ANOTHER ONE.
THERE ARE TWO OF THEM.
THERE ARE TWO _____.

FIGURE 7. The plural allomorph in /-z/.

SOURCE: Reprinted with permission of author from: Berko, J. The child's learning of English morphology. *Word*, 158, **14**, 150-77.

Berko's design was dictated by her wish to insure that the child's knowledge of morphology was tapped rather than his rote memory of the inflections and derivations of actual words. Comparison of the responses made by preschoolers (ages 4 to 5) and first graders (ages 5½ to 7) indicated that the knowledge of morphology evolved in an orderly fashion. Analysis of the acquisition of inflections further indicated that the children first learned a general rule and later acquired more specific ones. They were best able to apply inflectional endings that were regular, highly frequent, and that had the fewest variants.

Berko further observed that the boys and girls exhibited similar knowledge of morphology and suggested that the learning of morphological rules is related to intelligence since "this type of inner patterning is clearly a cognitive process." The differences in the responses by preschoolers and first graders were significant for about 50% of the test items. First graders demonstrated improvements suggesting perfection of the knowledge of rules for simple plurals and possessives and for the progressive tense. Later studies using Berko's experimental test of morphology have substantiated the order of acquisition of morphological rules by normal and by EMR children (Newfield & Schlanger, 1968; Wiig, Semel, & Crouse, 1973).

Several studies have explored the acquisition of morphemes as evidenced in spontaneous speech and considered the variables that determine the order of acquisition (Anisfeld & Gordon, 1968; Brown, 1973; Cazden, 1972; deVilliers & deVilliers, 1973; Menyuk, 1963a, 1963b, 1964). Brown established the mean order of acquisition of fourteen morphemes from the spontaneous speech samples of three children, Adam, Eve, and Sarah. He observed a developmental sequence as follows: (1) represent progressive, (2) *in* and *on*, (3) regular plural, (4) past tense irregular, (5) possessive, (6) uncontractible copula, (7) articles, (8) past regular, (9) third person irregular, (10) uncontractible auxiliary, (11) contractible copula, and (12) contractible auxiliary. Brown comments that "when the effects of allomorphic variation are partialled out, Berko's data support the order we found except in the case of the third class of allomorph" (Brown, 1973, p. 292). Brown concludes that both semantic and grammatical complexity determined the order of acquisition and that it was not related to the frequency order of morphemes in parental speech.

In a related study, deVilliers and deVilliers (1973) obtained cross-sectional data from twenty-four children, ranging in age from sixteen to forty months, on the acquisition of the morphemes studied by Brown. Their data showed significant positive correlations with Brown's order and with Mean Length of Utterance (MLU). They also concluded that semantic and grammatical complexity determined the order of acquisition.

Studies of the knowledge of general and specific morphological rules of school-age children give evidence of improved abilities proceeding from the application of general rules to increasing differentiation of rules (Bryant & Anisfeld, 1969; Koziol, 1973; Menyuk, 1963a). Menyuk (1963a, 1963b, 1964) established that significantly more children at nursery school than at grade school level omitted the irregular past form of verbs and substituted regular past forms. She also observed that kindergarten children exhibited uniquely childish forms at the morphological level (Menyuk, 1964). These occurred in third person singular and plural of the present tense of verbs, past tense of verbs, singular and plural of nouns, possessive pronouns, and adjectives.

Menyuk (1963b) analyzed the use of alternate restricted rules, that is, rules producing structures that are not completely well-formed. She observed that, as children matured, the use of restricted rules tended to decline from 38% at age three to 13% at age seven and there was also a trend suggesting increasing differentiation of rules.

Koziol (1973) investigated the development of noun plural rules during the primary grades. The result indicated that the period of major learning on a recognition task occurred between kindergarten and the first grade. Production of the plural forms of regular nouns appeared to be delayed by approximately one grade level, and production of irregular nouns was delayed by two to three grade levels. The children also experienced problems until the third grade in applying the plural allomorphs to words with final *sk* and *st* clusters.

Deficits in Morphology in Learning Disabilities

The acquisition and use of morphology by children with learning disabilities has not been investigated extensively. Two studies by Vogel (1974) and Wiig,

Semel, and Crouse (1973) seem to provide the sources for specific knowledge of the morphological deficits that may be associated with learning disabilities.

Vogel (1974) assessed learning disabled children's knowledge of morphological rules using the *Exploratory Test of Grammar* (Berry, 1969). The results of the investigation indicated that dyslexic children with reading comprehension difficulties performed significantly poorer on the test of morphology than their academically achieving controls. A stepwise discriminant analysis of the data further indicated that knowledge of morphology was among the three measures that best differentiated between achieving and learning disabled children. The error patterns were unfortunately not analyzed by Vogel, and qualitative differences in the acquisition of morphology by dyslexic children remained unexplored.

Wiig, Semel, and Crouse (1973) investigated quantitative and qualitative differences in the use of morphology by high-risk and learning disabled children and normally developing age peers. Their findings indicated that the high-risk and learning disabled children exhibited significantly poorer knowledge of morphology than their controls, suggesting delays in the acquisition and internalization of morphological rules.

Comparison of the percentages of correct responses to items and morphological categories showed that the normal children performed significantly better than the high-risk children (Table 17). The largest relative differences were observed for progressive, third singular, and past tense of verbs. The group differences in the ranked percentages of correct responses to the various morphological categories suggested varying delays in the acquisition of rules for the different categories by the high-risk children. The developmental pattern for the high-risk children also differed from the patterns observed for normal preschoolers (Berko, 1958) and for older EMR children (Newfield & Schlanger, 1968), suggesting differences in the cognitive processes that form the bases for the acquisition of morphological rules.

TABLE 17

Percentages of correct responses by item and morphological category for ten high-risk and ten normal children

Item	High-risk	Normal
Plural		
glasses	10	100
wugs	50	100
luns	40	100
tors	30	100
heafs	30	80
cras	40	90
tasses	0	60
gutches	0	30
kazhes	0	40

TABLE 17 (Continued)

Item	High-risk	Normal
nizzes	10	60
Mean:	21	76
Progressive		
zibbing	10	100
Past tense		
binged	0	70
glinged	0	80
ricked	10	70
melted	0	80
spowed	10	70
motted	0	50
bodded	0	60
rang	0	0
Mean:	2.5	60
Third singular		
loodges	0	70
nazzes	10	60
Mean:	5	65
Singular possessive		
wug's	40	90
bik's	30	80
niz's	20	80
Mean:	30	83
Plural possessive		
wugs'	60	100
biks'	50	100
nizzes'	70	100
Mean:	60	100
Adjectival inflection		
quirkier	0	20
quirkiest	0	10
Mean:	0	15
Compounding		
wughouse	10	30
Derivation		
zibber	0	0
wuglet	0	0
quirky	0	0

SOURCE: Reprinted with permission of publishers from: Wiig, E. H., Semel, E. M., and Crouse, M.A. The use of morphology by high-risk and learning disabled children. *Journal of Learning Disabilities*, 1973, **6**, 457-65.

The LD children also applied the morphological rules tested at a quantitatively lower level than their academically achieving controls. The greatest relative differences between the learning disabled and achieving children in the percentages of correct responses to morphological categories were observed for third person singular of verbs, possessives, and adjectival inflections (Table 18). This finding paralleled the observations for high-risk children and suggests a continuum of morphological deficits in the two populations.

TABLE 18

Percentages of correct responses by item and morphological category for twelve LD and twelve achieving children

Item	Learning disabled	Achievers
Plural		
glasses	58	100
wugs	92	100
luns	82	92
tors	75	92
heafs	75	82
cras	67	75
tasses	17	67
gutches	42	58
kazhes	33	67
nizzes	33	67
Mean:	57	80
Progressive		
zibbing	67	100
Past tense		
binged	42	82
glinged	67	82
ricked	50	67
melted	92	92
spowed	67	75
motted	33	67
bodded	17	75
rang	33	50
Mean:	50	74
Third singular		
loodges	58	92
nazzes	42	82
Mean:	50	87
Singular possessive		
wug's	67	92
bik's	42	100
niz's	33	82

TABLE 18 (Continued)

Item	Learning disabled	Achievers
Mean:	47	91
Plural possessive		
wugs'	42	100
biks'	42	92
nizzes'	75	100
Mean:	53	97
Adjectival inflection		
quirkier	8	67
quirkiest	33	75
Mean:	21	71
Compounding		
wughouse	67	58
Derivation		
zibber	25	42
wuglet	0	8
quirky	0	8

SOURCE: Reprinted with permission of publishers from: Wiig, E. H., Semel, E. M., and Crouse, M.A. The use of morphology by high-risk and learning disabled children. *Journal of Learning Disabilities,* 1973, **6**, 457-65.

There were other similarities in the responses made by the high-risk and learning disabled children which appear of diagnostic and therapeutic significance. Both groups exhibited varying delays in the acquistion of morphological rules, suggesting qualitative as well as quantitative deficits. High-risk and learning disabled children also demonstrated less predictable, idiosyncratic patterns of difficulty than their controls. In a similar vein, their responses indicated a lack of transfer of the phonological conditioning rules across morphological categories, suggesting deficits in abstraction and generalization. In contrast, the normal and academically achieving children demonstrated this transfer of the rules. This finding agrees with observations for normal preschool and first grade children by Berko (1958).

Clinical observations of the spontaneous use of rules for forming noun plurals and past tenses of irregular verbs suggest that the delays in the acquisition and use of morphology persist throughout the primary grades. Learning disabled third, fourth, and fifth graders frequently substitute regular past tense forms of verbs for the irregular past forms. They do not show the significant developmental trends observed when normal nursery school and first grade children were compared (Menyuk, 1963a, 1963b, 1964). They also seem to experience persisting problems in forming the plural of irregular nouns and in applying plural allomorphs to nouns which end in *st* and *sk* clusters, rules which should have been firmly established by the third grade

(Koziol, 1973). There remains a need to investigate which morphological deficits persist into adolescence in association with learning disabilities.

Deficits in Syntax in Learning Disabilities

The acquisition of syntax by children with learning disabilities remains to be subjected to rigorous study even though recent investigations have focused on this aspect of development (Rabinovitch, 1959: Semel & Wiig, 1975; Vogel, 1974; Wiig & Semel, 1975b).

Vogel (1974) evaluated and compared syntactic and morphological abilities of twenty dyslexic and twenty normal children ranging in age from seven years four months to eight years five months. The expressive abilities assessed were expression of syntax as measured by the *Northwestern Syntax Screening Test* (NSST) (Lee, 1969). The results of the comparison showed that the dyslexic and normal children did not differ significantly in their expressive syntactic abilities as measured by the *Northwestern Syntax Screening Test.*

This finding contrasts with the results of an investigation of the comprehension and expression of syntactic structures by Semel and Wiig (1975). They administered the NSST (Lee, 1971) to thirty-four learning disabled children and seventeen academically achieving controls, ranging in age from seven to eleven years. Their findings suggested that learning disabled children demonstrate significant delays in the comprehension and use of syntactic structures. Of the learning disabled children, 56% scored below the tenth percentile and 62% below the twenty-fifth percentile established for children their ages or younger on the *Expressive* subtest, and the LD children performed significantly poorer as a group than their academically achieving age peers. There was also a significant positive relationship (r = .78) between performances on the *Receptive* and *Expressive* subtests of the NSST. Analysis of the syntactic structures causing difficulties in expression indicated that close to 20% of the total errors occurred on an item that required repetition of direct and indirect objects in sequence. The remaining errors occurred in response to items that required (1) expressive use of the demonstratives *this* and *that,* (2) formulation of declaratives and interrogatives with *is* and *has,* (3) formulation of *will throw, is throwing, jumps,* and *jumped,* (4) expressive use of direct quotes with distinction between *who* and *what,* (5) formulation of passive sentences with identical nouns, *boy was pulled by the girl* and *girl was pulled by the boy,* and (6) formulation of direct and indirect objects in sequence, *brings the boy the girl* and *brings the girl the boy.*

Vogel (1974) reported that the dyslexic children of her study demonstrated delays in the use of syntax in spoken language as measured by *Developmental Sentence Scores* (Lee & Canter, 1971). Unfortunately, she did not discuss the characteristics of the structures which were either absent or which deviated from normal in the dyslexic speech samples.

In an attempt to assess the nature of the deviations in the use of syntax by children with learning disabilities, Slegman (1974) analyzed the spontaneous speech samples of four dyslexic children, three boys and one girl, ranging in age from ten years eight months to twelve years four months and with WISC full-scale IQs ranging from 99 to 113 (*M* = 103). All of those children exhibited discrepancies between verbal and performance IQs ranging from twelve to twenty-five points ($M = 19.25$), the verbal IQs being consistently poorest. They demonstrated specific modality deficits as indicated by the results of extensive psychological and educational evaluation. Their academic achievement scores on the *Stanford Achievement Tests* ranged from 3.0 to 4.7 ($M = 3.6$).

Of the four children, two boys and one girl scored below the fiftieth percentile according to the norms established using the *Developmental Sentence Scores* for children ranging in age from 6½ years to 6 years 11 months, suggesting delays in their use of syntax of from five to six years. The fourth youngster at age 11 years 8 months still used deviant structures even though he scored above the norms for 6-year-olds. This youngster exhibited deviations from grammaticalness in 25% of his sentences. These deviations were similar to those reported in first graders by Menyuk (1969) and were characterized by redundancies in otherwise well-formed sentences with reiteration of a class. The predominant deviation occurred as a result of reiteration of *who/what* in relative clauses as in the sentences "was trying to figure out *what who* shot this man" and "he wouldn't care *who what* happened." The second deviation occurred as a result of reiteration of the verb in the verb phrase as in "The man *was stole* the chickens." This boy also used verb tenses inconsistently, used incorrect past tenses of irregular verbs, and used the progressive tense incorrectly as in "and then the guys *going* after them."

The three learning disabled youngsters who scored below the fiftieth percentile when compared to normal six-year-olds used predominantly simple declarative sentences, and their sentences did not express ideas in a logical or correct sequence. They experienced problems in formulating conjunctions and violated the rules for deletion as in "They came back into the house, saw that the porridge was aten from the little bear. And the chair was broken, went to their bedroom and saw Goldilocks." When complex sentences were attempted the results were agrammatical as in "While that, the bears were coming back." There was evidence of frequent word-finding problems, and indefinites were used abundantly. Most of their morphological and syntactic errors occurred in the verb category. They incorrectly combined present and past tenses as in "All she *does is drank* the wine" and formed irregular verbs incorrectly as in "the porridge *was aten*" and "he *stoled* the poem." The possessive of nouns and pronouns also presented difficulties for these children as evidenced by sentences such as "Then she went to the *mama's bear's beds*" and "it made *him* stomach feel so painful." Although these observations must be considered tentative and suggestive only, they support previous observations of morphological and syntactic deficits (Wiig, Semel, & Crouse, 1973; Semel & Wiig, 1975).

There is evidence suggesting that syntactic deficits in oral language persist into adolescence (Wiig & Semel, 1975b). Learning disabled adolescents were observed to formulate significantly more agrammatical and incomplete sentences on a sentence production task in which a stimulus word was to be incorporated into a sentence than did their achieving age peers (Table 19).

Their agrammatical sentences were formulated in response to the stimulus words *after* and *belongs*. All but 4 of their grammatical sentences were simple declarative, and 68 of the 182 sentences were started with *I*. Three sentences contained a subordinate clause and only 1 was an interrogative. The academic achievers produced a total of 27 sentences with coordinated and subordinated classes, 2 interrogative sentences, and 2 negative sentences. Only 32 sentences were started with *I*.

TABLE 19

Comparison of Sentence Production Measures for 32 Learning Disabled and 32 Academically Achieving Adolescents

	Mean	SD	χ^2
Errors			
Learning Disabled	0.59	0.76	
Achievers	0		
Mean Word Length			
Learning Disabled	4.80	0.99	4.13*
Achievers	6.05	1.49	
Mean Response Delay (Sec.)			
Learning Disabled	3.12	2.45	4.13*
Achievers	1.70	0.87	

SOURCE: Reprinted with permission of publishers from: Wiig, E. H., and Semel, E. M. Productive language abilities in learning disabled adolescents. *Journal of Learning Disabilities*, 1975, **8**, 578-86.

NOTE: χ^2 = chi square; *p = < .05.

In an unpublished study, London (1974) compared fifteen learning disabled children's performances on the *Picture Story Language Test* (Myklebust, 1965) and on the *Northwestern Syntax Screening Test* (Lee, 1971). The ages of the children ranged from seven years three months to ten years four months (M = eight years four months). The results indicated that the performances on the *Expressive* subtest of the NSST (Lee, 1971) correlated positively and significantly with the syntax quotient on the *Picture Story Language Test* (r = .55) and with chronological age (r = .46). The multiple correlation obtained with the latter measures was r = .80, indicating that spoken syntax can be adequately predicted from knowledge of written syntax and age. In a related study, Semel and Wiig (1975) reported that expressive syntactic ability of learning disabled children as measured by the *Northwestern Syntax Screening Test* correlated positively and significantly with WISC full-scale MA (mental age) (r = .67) and measures of mathematical achievement (r = .50), reading comprehension (r = .53) and general information (r = .60) on the *Peabody Individual Achievement Test* (Dunn & Markwardt, 1970).

Relationship of Deficits to Factors in Expressive Language

Characteristics of the expressive language of adults, especially as they are reflected in differences in surface structure, have been related to a variety of variables. Gleser, Gottschalk, and John (1959) observed a direct relationship between surface-structure differences and differences in IQ. Other investigators have reported relationships between surface structure and vocational interests (Fehrer et al., 1948), leveling versus sharpening cognitive style (Livant, 1962), active versus passive behavioral stance (Dobb, 1958), and level of need achievement (Zatzkis, 1949). Similar relationships should be indicated within a population of learning disabled adolescents and young adults. It does, however, appear as if some of the differences in surface structure observed between LD children and adolescents and their academically achieving age peers reflect basic differences in conceptualization, symbolization, sentence formulation, and verbal encoding. These differences can be related to the central dimensions of individual syntactic differences that have been identified through factor analysis by Caroll (1960) and Jones and Wepman (1961).

Caroll (1960) labeled five factors in prose style and identified the indexes which loaded most highly on each of the factors. An overview of the factors and indexes is presented in Table 20. In relation to these factors, the spoken language of learning disabled youngsters seems characterized by *Personal Affect* with a preponderance of pronouns and personal pronouns and relatively short words and sentences. Their spoken language seems singularly lacking in the features which are associated with *Ornamentation* and *Characterization*. Their sentences tend to lack in the variety of descriptive adjectives, contain a low proportion of nouns with Latin suffixes, lack dependent clauses, and contain a low proportion of intransitive and a high proportion of transitive and copulative verbs.

TABLE 20

Overview of Factors and Indexes Identified in Prose Style
by Caroll (1960)

Factor	Factor Name	Indexes
I	Personal Affect	• Many pronouns and personal pronouns • Few syllables
II	Ornamentation	• Long sentences, clauses, and paragraphs • Wide variation in sentence length • Frequent use of dependent clauses • High proportion of nouns with Latin suffixes • Many descriptive adjectives • Few unmodified common nouns preceded by "the" • Low proportion of verbs denoting physical action

TABLE 20 (Continued)

Factor	Factor Name	Indexes
III	Abstraction	• High proportion of noun clauses • Low proportion of numerical expressions • Low number of determining adjectives, pronouns, and participles
IV	Seriousness	• High number of determiners • High proportion of indefinite and quantifying determining adjectives • Low proportion of indefinite articles
V	Characterization	• High proportion of copulative and intransitive verbs • High proportion of adjective clauses • Low proportion of transitive verbs and few proper nouns

Jones and Wepman (1961) have reported six factors characterizing the syntax of adult spoken prose when it was scored for parts-of-speech and related aspects. The factors and the indexes are summarized in Table 21. When analyzed according to the factors identified by Jones and Wepman (1961), the spoken language of learning disabled children and adolescents is characterized by a lack of descriptive *Specificity* and *Richness of Vocabulary*. There also seems to be an abundance of features characteristic of Factors IV, V, and VI. These features relate to the abundance of interjections, indefinite pronouns, and conjunctions, the lack of adjectives, and the frequency of filled pauses and word repetitions.

TABLE 21
Overview of Factors and Indexes Identified in Adult Spoken Prose by Jones and Wepman (1961)

Factor	Factor Name	Indexes
I	Specificity	• Many articles, uncommon and common nouns, uncommon adjectives, and prepositions • Few personal pronouns in the nominative case, common verbs, adverbs, and indefinite pronouns
II	Richness of Vocabulary	• Many uncommon verbs, adjectives, and nouns • Few common verbs and indefinites
III	Pronominal Prepositional Phrases	• Many prepositions and personal pronouns in objective case
IV	Phrases like "Well, it is"	• Many interjections, indefinite pronouns, and auxiliaries
V	Effort to Maintain Conversation	• Many conjunctions, relatives, and total words • Few common adjectives
VI	Hesitancy	• Many filled pauses and repeated words

Convergent Language Production

Language is generally produced within a set of limits or constraints. In spontaneous conversation, a speaker generally has the freedom to select vocabulary items and linguistic structure from his own thoughts, ideas, and feelings. The constraints are relatively minimal although the speaker would not be allowed to choose vocabulary which violated the social situation or to produce agrammatical sentences. As a result, the speaker is controlled by both semantic (selectional) and linguistic constraints which determine his verbal behavior.

Linguistic constraints determine the structural aspects or the surface structure of a message. As an example, when we begin a sentence with the semantic unit *Yesterday* we have imposed linguistic constraints which dictate that the verb must be expressed in the past tense or in a form which reflects the past in time.

Semantic constraints, on the other hand, determine the meaning to be expressed and the words which will best express that meaning. The characteristics of the objects or events we want to describe impose semantic (selectional) constraints within which we must choose our words. When we are asked to name a pictured object such as a *red ball* or to give a verbal opposite for a word such as *night*, semantic constraints have been imposed which control our word selection. We must retrieve and use words which are appropriate for the specific context or which best describe the attributes we want to emphasize. Take the example of the picture of the red ball. If we were asked to name the object, we would respond "ball." If we were told to name the color, our response would be "red." In this type of situation, the speaker functions under rather rigid semantic constraints since there may be only one word that will satisfy the demands. The ability to retrieve a specific word or word sequence to satisfy a set of semantic constraints has been called convergent semantic production ability (Guilford, 1967).

Efficient convergent language production depends heavily upon adequate long-term memory store and efficient retrieval from long-term memory. Convergent semantic production abilities develop into adolescence (Guilford, 1967) and they are tapped in a variety of tests for intelligence, learning aptitude, and psycholinguistic ability (Baker & Leland, 1959; Kirk, McCarthy, & Kirk, 1968; Wechsler, 1949, 1955). Convergent semantic production often presents problems for the LD youngster.

Learning disabled children may demonstrate reductions in verbal fluency or dysnomia. This problem is reflected by reduced accuracy and speed of verbal associations and availability of verbal labels (Bannatyne, 1971; Johnson & Myklebust, 1967; Kass, 1962; Lerner, 1971; Orton, 1937; Rabinovitch, 1959). Johnson and Myklebust describe the problem of dysnomia as being "a deficit primarily in reauditorization and word selection" (1967, p. 114). They maintain that the learning disabled child with dysnomia understands and recognizes the target word but is unable to retrieve it on demand. They note that problems of reauditorization have been referred to as word-finding difficulty or dysnomia. When the learning disabled child searches for a target word, he may resort to gesture. Johnson and Myklebust (1967, p. 1150) describe this phenomenon in a learning disabled girl who, searching for the word *crash* to describe an accident, doubled her fists, hit them together, and covered her ears indicating the loud noise made on impact.

Dysnomia: Characteristics and Bases

Anomia, dysnomia (a less severe form of anomia), amnesic aphasia, and word-finding difficulty have been described extensively in the literature on adult aphasia (Geschwind, 1972; Goldstein, 1948; Schuell & Jenkins, 1972; Schuell, Jenkins, & Jimenez-Pabon, 1964). Geschwind (1972) defines anomia as "the inability of the patient (aphasic) to name things shown to him " or failure to name on confrontation. He identifies four types of naming errors and differentiates anomia from word finding, that is, "finding of words in the flow of speech." In classical anomia the difficulty tends to be general, relate to both sound and meaning, and to cross modalities. In disconnection anomia, errors occur only in a specific modality. As an example, a patient may name a visually presented object correctly, but, when blindfolded, be unable to name the same object when placed in either hand.

Spreen (1968), among others, has discussed the relationship between frequency of word usage and naming difficulty in aphasia. Wiig and Globus (1971) established relationships between the ease with which aphasics identify words and associative strength and logical relationship.

Word-finding difficulties have also been observed in normal adults, but they are lesser in degree than in aphasics (Brown & McNeill, 1970; Fromkin, 1973). Brown and McNeill (1970) suggest that "suffix-chunking" plays a role in word recall. They also noted that the subjects were able to determine the number of syllables in a target word even though they were unable to retrieve it. Sounds and phonemes were observed to aid recall. As an example, Brown's subjects produced the following phonologically related words while searching for the word *sampan:* saipan, siam, sarong, sanching, and sympoon. First and last phonemes were more easily recalled than middle sounds. They suggest that attention to the initial phoneme is strongest and is followed by attention to the final and last to the medial sounds. Lerner (1971) postulates a similar basis for dysnomia in learning disabilities. She describes dysnomia as "a deficiency in remembering and expressing what words sound like" (1971, p. 151).

Fromkin (1973) describes phonologically, morphologically, and semantically based "slips of the tongue." She uses the response "There's a small Chinese . . . I mean Japanese restaurant" to illustrate a semantically based error. Another example of a semantic error is described in the substitution of *dachshund* for *Volkswagen*. This error is considered to result from the erroneous selection of a word with the shared semantic features, +small, +animate, +German, since the lexical entry for Volkswagen could have been *Beetle* or *Bug*. Fromkin also notes errors resulting from transpositions of morpheme units as in using *ambigual* for *ambiguous, motionly* for *motionless,* and *intervenient* for *intervening,* error types which are not uncommon among learning disabled youngsters.

Word-Finding Deficits in Learning Disabilities

Attempts to investigate the nature and extent of word-finding problems in learning disabilities are limited; therefore, the results of the three studies presently available must be considered preliminary in nature. The ability of LD youngsters to name pictures in a confrontation-naming task requiring convergent production of semantic units has been explored by Denckla (1974), Jansky and deHirsch (1972), and Wiig and Semel (1975b). The basis for Jansky's interest in learning disabled children's ability to name pictures is related in the comment that "reading, like picture naming, requires ready elicitation of spoken equivalents." (Jansky & deHirsch, 1972). They demonstrated that the performances by kindergarteners on a *Picture-Naming Test* were the most powerful predictors of reading failure. The picture-naming ability measures correlated positively and significantly (r = .53) with reading achievement at the end of second grade.

Denckla (1974) further explored the picture-naming competence of dyslexic and nondyslexic children with minimal brain dysfunction, ranging in age from eight to ten years. The working hypothesis was that dyslexic and nondyslexic children would show dissociated patterns of difficulty on a picture-naming task analogous to patterns reported for left- and right-hemisphere and bilaterally-damanged adults (Newcombe et al., 1971). In the effort to determine patterns in word-naming difficulty for pictured objects, Denckla (1974) analyzed and compared the total scores, error categories, and response latencies.

The results of the investigation indicated that dyslexic children made significantly more errors in naming pictured objects than their normal controls. Dyslexic and nondyslexic MBD (minimal brain dysfunction) children were best differentiated by the significantly higher number of errors made by the dyslexics on words which were of low frequency of usage. In the group of twenty dyslexics, Denckla (1974) further reported that total picture-naming scores did not correlate significantly with WISC full-scale or verbal IQ, but correlated significantly with reading age (r = .46), supporting previous observations by Jansky and deHirsch (1972).

When the types of the naming errors on the ten most difficult items were analyzed, the errors made by the dyslexic children were characterized by circumlocution (41% of total), for example, responding to a picture of a stethoscope with "thing which doctor uses to listen to your heart." In contrast, the nondyslexic MBD children gave a relatively high proportion of wrong names (61% of total), for example, calling a tuning fork a "magnet." The quality of naming error also differed between the two groups: nondyslexic children produced wrong names that were remote and not related by association to the intended name; for example, naming a picture of dice "Swiss cheese" and calling a metronome a "paint set"; dyslexic children gave wrong names which were phonetically ("staxaphone" for xylophone) or semantically ("telescope" for stethoscope) related to the correct names. Denkla concludes that the nondyslexic MBD children exhibited evidence of "visual object agnosia" or the visual-perceptual deficits observed by Poppelreuter (1917) and that their errors suggested figure-ground or part-whole confusions.

Dyslexic children also demonstrated significantly longer response latencies for the more difficult items than both the normal controls and the nondyslexic MBD children (Denckla, 1974). Based on the low, total correct naming scores and the relatively long response latencies, the dyslexic children were considered to display subtle dysphasia similar to residual aphasia in adults (Newcombe et al., 1971). Their errors were considered to be clearly related to deficits in the process of retrieval since correct circumlocutions and associative paraphasia responses predominated.

Wiig and Semel (1975b) have observed similar picture-naming deficits in adolescents with learning disabilities. They used the *Visual Confrontation Naming* subtest of the *Boston VA Aphasia* test (Goodglass & Kaplan, 1972) to assess and compare the speed and accuracy with which thirty-two academically achieving and a like number of LD adolescents retrieved verbal labels in response to pictorial presentations of objects, letters, geometric forms, actions, numbers, and colors. The learning disabled adolescents made significantly more naming errors (Mean = 3.38) than their academically achieving controls (Mean = 0.84) (Table 22). Analysis of the quality of their errors indicated that associative word substitutions predominated (70.5% of total) followed by omissions (27.4% of total) and perseverations, that is, immediate repetitions of a previous response (2.1% of total). When the learning disabled adolescents omitted a verbal label, they pointed to the pictorial stimulus, paused, and moved to the next item, suggesting either inability to activate an encoding response or an attempt to avoid failure.

TABLE 22

Summary of Confrontation Naming Performances by 32 Learning
Disabled and 32 Academically Achieving Adolescents

	Mean	SD	χ^2
Errors			
Learning Disabled	3.38	2.60	9.57**
Achievers	0.84	1.09	
Total Response Time (Sec.)			
Learning Disabled	53.34	12.06	4.13*
Achievers	43.78	7.49	

SOURCE: Reprinted with permission of publishers from: Wiig, E. H., and Semel, E. M. Productive language abilities in learning disabled adolescents. *Journal of Learning Disabilities*, 1975, **8**. 578 – 86.

NOTE: *p < .05;   **p < .01.

The learning disabled adolescents also demonstrated significantly longer response latencies with a mean duration for the total naming task of 53.3 seconds than the achievers with a mean duration of 43.8 seconds. The findings concur with the observations reported for younger dyslexic children by Denckla (1974). They suggest that anomia and verbal paraphasia associated with learning disabilities may persist into adolescence. They also support the views that specific learning disabilities may be placed in the "aphaseological context" (Alajouanine, Lhermitte, de Ribaucourt-Ducarne, 1960; Benson & Geschwind, 1969; Nielsen, 1946).

Wiig and Semel (1975b) also assessed learning disabled adolescents' ability to retrieve and name antonyms using the *Verbal Opposites* subtest of the *Detroit Tests of Learning Aptitude* (Baker & Leland, 1959). [The total response

time to ceiling, that is, five items failed in succession, was measured to evaluate the speed of responding. Therefore, testing was always started with the
first item.] Learning disabled adolescents scored significantly lower on the
Verbal Opposites test and used significantly longer time to respond to each
item than did achieving adolescents (Table 23).

TABLE 23

Summary of Verbal Opposites Test Performances by 32 Learning
Disabled and 32 Academically Achieving Adolescents

	Mean	SD	χ^2
Age Scores (Raw Scores)			
Learning Disabled	11-1	1-9	13.13**
	(44.5)	(6.81)	
Achievers	14-6	1-7	
	(58.0)	(5.79)	
Mean Response Time per Item (Sec.)			
Learning Disabled	4.8	1.89	5.70*
Achievers	3.9	0.62	

SOURCE: Reprinted with permission of publishers from: Wiig, E. H., and Semel,
E. M. Productive language abilities in learning disabled adolescents. *Journal of
Learning Disabilities*, 1975, **8**, 578 – 86.

NOTE: *p < .05;   **p < .001.

These findings indicate significant reductions in the ability of learning disabled adolescents to retrieve accurate verbal opposites and in the speed of retrieval and suggest reduced ability for convergent production of semantic
units and relations (Guilford, 1967). They also suggest that learning disabled
adolescents and adults with acquired aphasia share similar quantitative reductions in the speed of retrieval of verbal labels. Luria (1973, p. 158) reports
mean response lags of similar durations (ranging from two and one-half to fifteen seconds) for adults with acquired left parieto-temporal lesions. Goldstein (1974) observed similar reductions in learning disabled adolescents'
ability to formulate and produce verbal analogies using the *Verbal Association* subtest of the ITPA (Kirk, McCarthy, & Kirk, 1968), confirming the suggestion that the convergent production ability for semantic relations may be
reduced in learning disabilities.

The quality of the errors made by the LD adolescents on the *Verbal Opposites* subtest concurred with previous observations of dysnomia in dyslexic
children (Denckla, 1974; Kolers, 1972). The learning disabled adolescents
made word substitutions which were within the same general semantic category as the intended words. As an example, the responses to a relatively easy
stimulus word, *brother,* (fourth item) were frequently *son* instead of *sister*.
This type of response suggests ability to identify the abstract category to
which a stimulus word belongs, but inability to retrieve the exact opposite.

Verbal paraphasias (word substitutions) similar to those exhibited by the
LD adolescents are a characteristic of adult aphasics with left temporal, parieto-occipital, or parieto-occipital-temporal lesions (Goldstein, 1948; Good-

glass & Kaplan, 1972; Luria, 1966, 1973). Luria (1973) has suggested that verbal paraphasias result from an inability to discover a required dominant word from within a set of related words of equal probability. Goldstein (1948) has suggested that verbal paraphasias reflect figure-ground problems. The consistent observation across age levels of anomia and verbal paraphasia as an aspect of dyslexia and learning disabilities (Bannatyne, 1971; Denckla, 1974; Kolers, 1972; Wiig & Semel, 1974) strengthens the position that the convergent language production deficits in learning disabilities reflect subtle aphasia.

Wiig and Semel (1975b) observed that word-finding and retrieval deficits of learning disabled adolescents observed on the *Visual Confrontation Naming* and *Verbal Opposites* subtests were substantiated by ratings of speech characteristics in conversation. They rated the spontaneous conversations of thirty-two learning disabled and thirty-two academically achieving adolescents for (1) *Melodic Line* (i.e., sentence intonation pattern which normally extends over an entire sentence), (2) *Phrase Length* (i.e., the number of words in the longest uninterrupted run of words), (3) *Verbal Agility* (i.e., ease and accuracy of phoneme sequence articulation), (4) *Grammatical Form* (i.e., sentence structure), (5) *Paraphasia in Running Speech* (i.e., word substitutions and insertions of semantically erroneous words and circumlocation, (6) *Word Finding* (i.e., the capacity to evoke concept names and provide informational content) (Goodglass & Kaplan, 1972).

The ratings indicated that all academically achieving adolescents exhibited normal speech characteristics. In comparison, the learning disabled adolescents scored close to normal on all characteristics other than *Phrase Length* and *Grammatical Form* (Table 24).

TABLE 24
Ratings of Speech Characteristics in Conversation by 32
Learning Disabled and 32 Academically Achieving Adolescents

Speech Characteristic	Learning Disabled		Achievers	
	Mean	Range	Mean	Range
Melodic Line	6.34	4 - 7	7	-
Phrase Length	5.22	3 - 7	7	-
Articulatory Agility	6.34	3 - 7	7	-
Grammatical Form	4.94	4 - 7	7	-
Paraphasia in Running Speech	6.13	2 - 7	7	-
Word Finding	4.22	2 - 7	4*	-

SOURCE: Reprinted with permission of publishers from: Wiig, E. H., and Semel, E. M. Productive language abilities in learning disabled adolescents. *Journal of Learning Disabilities*, 1975, **8**, 578 – 86.

NOTE: 4* denotes 'information proportional to fluency.'

The longest phrases used by the learning disabled adolescents contained an average of five words, and with a few exceptions the sentences used by them were the simple declarative type. The academic achievers used structurally varied sentences, and the longest phrases contained an average of eleven words. Five of the learning disabled adolscents rated consistently low on the speech characteristics. Other qualitative differences included the use of atypical intonation patterns. Formulation of simple declarative sentences with word substitutions, circumlocutions, and an excess of low information words such as pronouns and indefinite words (something, somebody, sometime, somewhere) were common among the LD adolescents. They also demonstrated the lowest scores on the *Verbal Opposites, Visual Confrontation Naming, Controlled Association,* and *Word Definition* subtests.

Word Definition Deficits

Wiig and Semel (1975b) also assessed the word definition abilities of thirty-two learning disabled and a like number of academically achieving adolescents. The subjects were asked to define the words *robin, apple, return, different, bridge, continue, history, material, decide,* and *opinion* (Schuell, 1965). The learning disabled adolescents gave significantly fewer correct definitions than their academically achieving controls. They frequently described a function to define a noun. As examples, *apple* and *history* were often defined as something you eat and something you learn in school, respectively. They also named a noun derivation such as "decision" to define a relatively abstract verb such as *decide*. The five relatively abstract words *bridge, history, material, decide,* and *opinion* were defined incorrectly by twenty-two of the learning disabled adolescents but by only two of the academically achieving controls.

The word definitions given by the learning disabled adolescents to the stimulus words suggested abstraction of limited, concrete aspects of the concept, but abstract general aspects were overlooked. These deficits may reflect reductions in the cognition and convergent production of semantic units and transformations (Guilford, 1967).

Divergent Language Production Abilities

A person's expressive language abilities are judged in part by the facility with which he can produce a variety of vocabulary items and sentence structures to describe an event or an idea. In relation to the Structure-of-Intellect model (Guilford, 1967), the ability to provide a variety of verbal responses to a stimulus situation characterizes divergent production ability.

Divergent semantic production abilities reflect the speaker's creativity and flexibility in the use of language. It reflects how well a person can provide variety in word selection and syntactic structure, expand on a subject or topic, and focus and refocus the listener's attention on attributes and characteristics of objects, events, feelings, and ideas. A person with superior divergent language production abilities would be able to describe the fog in a variety of ways ranging from the prosaic "The fog is grey" to the poetic "The fog rolled in, isolating everyone in his own sphere of existence, creating echoes of loneliness."

In educational and academic settings, divergent language abilities are rewarded in subject areas such as English composition, history, and foreign languages. In relation to factors that have been found to account for individual differences in style or syntax, the ability to produce a variety in vocabulary and sentence structure characterize the factors *Ornamentation* (Caroll, 1960), descriptive *Specificity*, and *Richness of Vocabulary* (Jones & Wepman, 1961).

Divergent production abilities have been established by Guilford (1967) for:

1. semantic units (e.g., naming of class members based on knowledge of class names or properties)
2. semantic classes (e.g., giving unusual uses for objects or materials)
3. semantic relations (e.g., controlled associations and multiple analogies)
4. semantic systems (e.g., construction of a variety of sentences following given rules and constraints)
5. semantic transformations (e.g., remote associations, puns)
6. semantic implications (e.g., planning, elaboration)

Developmental studies of divergent production abilities indicate that children in the early grades who score high on tests of divergent production are evaluated to express wild, silly, and sometimes naughty ideas (Torrance, 1962a). In later grades (five and six) these children are considered to have "good" ideas even though their ideas may be so unusual that they cannot be evaluated by ordinary criteria and standards. Torrance (1962b) has also reported low correlations between traditional intelligence test scores (Stanford-Binet, Kuhlman-Anderson, Otis, California Tests of Mental Maturity) and composite divergent production test scores of elementary school children. This finding has been substantiated with both high school and graduate students (Torrance, 1962b, Yamamoto, 1964).

Clinical observations suggest that divergent production abilities may constitute an area of relative strength in the learning disabled child and adolescent. They frequently demonstrate unusual solutions to nonverbal and verbal problems and may show extraordinary creativity in specific areas (nonverbal, symbolic, or semantic) as reflected by the fluency (speed and accuracy), flexibility, originality, and elaboration of their divergent productions. This facility frequently masks underlying language deficits. Their ability for divergent semantic productions seems, however, to be limited by specific deficits related to the speed and accuracy with which they can retrieve a multitude of semantic units, systems, and relations. In addition, associative errors, paraphasias, and perseverations seem to interfere with their divergent language production abilities. These reductions in divergent language production abilities have been discussed by Bannatyne (1971), Johnson and Myklebust (1967), Lerner (1971), and Orton (1937), among others.

Deficits in Divergent Production of Semantic and Linguistic Units

Wiig and Semel (1975b) investigated and compared the speed and accuracy with which thirty-two learning disabled and the same number of academically achieving adolescents named the members of the semantic classes *Foods*, *Animals*, and *Toys* in a controlled association task. The task was adapted from the *Boston VA Aphasia* test (Goodglass & Kaplan, 1972) and required retrieval and naming of as many class members as possible within a period of sixty seconds. The classes *Foods*, *Animals*, and *Toys* were chosen to provide a range of possibilities for spontaneous grouping (associative clustering) of class members, a strategy reported to consistently facilitate recall (Bousfield, Cohen, & Whitmarsh, 1958; Gerjuoy & Spitz, 1966). The choice of the classes was determined by a pilot study which indicated that academically achieving adolescents consistently named most class members for the class *Foods*, second most for the class *Animals*, and least for the class *Toys*. Similarly, associative clustering tendencies were most evident for *Foods*, less evident for *Animals*, and least evident for *Toys*.

The study indicated that the learning disabled adolescents produced significantly fewer names for *Foods* than the academically achieving controls but that their performances were similar for *Animals* and *Toys*. The results are summarized in Table 25. The responses by the learning disabled adolescents to the class *Foods* indicated that they did not employ obvious grouping strategies to facilitate recall. They tended to name foods at random, shifting from one category, such as meats, to the next. In contrast, the academic achievers used associative clustering strategies. They grouped foods either by category (fruits, vegetables, meats, etc.) or in relationship to meals (breakfast, lunch, dinner). Both groups demonstrated similar grouping strategies for animals but named toys randomly. Animals were categorized on the basis of their being tame or wild, pets or farm animals. This categorization strategy is frequently employed in early education and may have become fairly automatic for both groups.

The learning disabled adolescents were also distinguished by their immediate or delayed repetitions of items. When naming *Foods*, twelve LD adolescents gave one or more immediate or delayed repetitions while only three academic achievers gave one delayed repetition. When naming *Animals*, fourteen learning disabled adolescents gave two or more immediate or delayed repetitions of the names of class members while only one achiever repeated an item in a delayed repetition. When naming *Toys*, five learning disabled adolescents produced perseverative responses (i.e., immediate repetitions), but none of the academic achievers repeated any responses.

The findings of the study suggest that the learning disabled adolescents exhibited delays in the acquisition of associative strategies to facilitate the retrieval and recall for the divergent production of semantic units and relations in controlled associations (Guilford, 1967). Based on previous observations that learning disabled children and adolescents tend to score within normal limits on tests of receptive vocabulary (Semel & Wiig, 1975; Strauss & Kephart, 1955; Strauss & Lehtinen, 1947; Wiig & Semel, 1973, 1974b), we can-

TABLE 25

Summary of Test Performances on a Controlled Association Test by 32 Learning
Disabled and 32 Academically Achieving Adolescents

Test	Mean	Range	SD	χ^2
Foods (No. in 60 sec.)				
Learning Disabled	18.66	8–28	4.46	
Achievers	23.16	14–30	4.60	5.70°
Animals (No. in 60 sec.)				
Learning Disabled	18.00	8–26	3.90	
Achievers	18.75	13–28	3.43	0.95
Toys (No. in 60 sec.)				
Learning Disabled	11.09	5–19	3.07	
Achievers	13.03	5–23	4.44	0.95

SOURCE: Reprinted with permission of publishers from: Wiig, E. H., and Semel,
E. M. Productive language abilities in learning disabled adolescents. *Journal of
Learning Disabilities*, 1975, **8**, 578-86.
NOTE: *p < .05.

not assume that the learning disabled adolescents did not have as large a
vocabulary of food items stored in long-term memory as the academic
achievers. We must conclude that the deficits observed in the divergent
production of semantic units and relations reflect difficulties in the retrieval
of associated concepts and semantic units from long-term memory. The
data also suggest that the lack of efficient associative clustering strategies
placed the learning disabled adolescents at a disadvantage.

The findings also give reason to suspect that the LD adolescents experienced problems in applying criteria for their selections from long-term
memory, since they repeated the names of group members twice more frequently then their academically achieving age peers. The immediate and delayed repetitive responses may also reflect short-term memory deficits similar
to those observed in processing spoken language. Learning disabled adolescents may not be able to hold class members in short-term memory and remember which ones they have named. This interpretation is supported by
the fact that the academic achievers named class members in a series in
which the intervals between responses were relatively short while the intervals between each series were noticeably longer. In contrast, the learning disabled adolescents tended to recall names of class members one at a time
rather than in series. This contrast suggests that academic achievers recalled
"conceptual chunks," a strategy that would facilitate retrieval and recollection of the items named (Simon & Chase, 1973).

The finding that learning disabled adolescents differed significantly from
academic achievers in their ability to produce controlled associations (Wiig &

Semel, 1975b) contrasts with previous observations of syntactic (sequential) - paradigmatic (in-class) association abilities of learning disabled children (Bartel, Grill, & Bartel, 1973). Their results indicated that learning disabled children develop linguistic categorization rules at expected ages. The data do not conflict when it is considered that semantic and linguistic categorization may not reflect the same cognitive processes.

Bartel, Grill, and Bartel (1973) demonstrated that both learning disabled and academically achieving children gave most paradigmatic responses, that is, responses within a grammatical class such as nouns, verbs, etc., to stimuli from the form-class *nouns* and least to stimulus words from the form-class *prepositions*. Their findings concurred with previous observations by Brown and Berko (1960), Deese (1962a, 1962b), and Entwistle, Forsyth, and Muuss (1964). There were no significant differences in the proportions of syntactic-paradigmatic responses by the normal and learning disabled children, indicating similarities in linguistic competence and in the acquisition of linguistic strategies for categorization of words. The authors stress that the association task did not test the effects of memory. They suggest that the linguistic deficits associated with learning disabilities may reflect memory problems that prevent the learning disabled child from performing in accordance with his linguistic competence.

There are suggestions that learning disabled adolescents also experience difficulties in the divergent production of semantic systems. Wiig and Semel (1975b) observed that LD adolescents retrieved a predominance of relatively short, simple declarative sentence structures in response to the stimulus words *coat, new, want, have, after,* and *belongs*. In contrast, academic achievers produced a variety of relatively longer syntactic structures, reflecting their superiority in formulating semantic systems and syntactic structures. These observations have been discussed in the section dealing with deficits in convergent language production.

Clinical observations indicate that learning disabled children and adolescents may experience problems in divergent production of semantic transformations and implications. They demonstrate difficulties in formulating alternative responses to metaphors such as "It rained like cats and dogs," and proverbs such as "A stitch in time saves nine," and in formulating alternative titles for a story. They may also demonstrate problems in explaining cause-effect relationships and in completing stories such as *The Little Red Hen* in which the implications of actions must be verbalized. These observations suggest areas for future investigations.

Relationships between Auditory Language Processing and Oral Language Production in Learning Disabilities

A recent investigation has focused on assessing the relationships between auditory language processing and oral language production abilities of adolescents with learning disabilities (Wiig, Lapointe, & Semel, 1975). Various language processing and production measures were obtained from thirty-two learning disabled adolescents, ranging in age from twelve years five months to sixteen years four months. The tests administered to the group were (1) the *Peabody Picture Vocabulary Test* (Dunn, 1959), (2) the *Northwestern Syntax Screening Test* (Lee, 1971), (3) the *Visual Reception, Visual Association,* and *Auditory Association* subtests of the *Illinois Test of Psycholinguistic Ability* (Kirk, McCarthy, & Kirk, 1968), (4) the *Token Test* (DeRenzi & Vignolo, 1962), (5) the *Wiig-Semel Test of Linguistic Concepts* (Wiig & Semel, 1974a), (6) the *Newcombe-Marshall Sentence Repetition Test* (Newcombe & Marshall, 1967), (7) the *Verbal Opposites* subtest of the *Detroit Tests of Learning Aptitude* (Baker & Leland, 1959), (8) the *Visual Confrontation Naming* and *Controlled Association* subtests of the *Boston Diagnostic Test* (Goodglass & Kaplan, 1972), and (9) the *Producing Sentences* and *Defining Words* subtests of the *Minnesota Test for the Differential Diagnosis of Aphasia* (Schuell, 1965). A summary of the performances on the various tests is presented in Table 26.

TABLE 26

Summary of Performances on Tests of Language Processing and Production by 32 Learning Disabled Adolescents

Test	Mean	SD	Range
Newcombe-Marshall (Score)	13.8	3.13	8 −20
Wiig-Semel (Score)	40.4	4.81	31 −47
Token Test Part V (Score)	22.0	2.40	17 −26
Token Test Total (Score)	58.8	4.55	44 −65
NSST Receptive (Score)	36.6	2.56	29 −40
NSST Expressive (Score)	34.7	3.93	23 −40
PPVT (MA)	14.3	1.20	11.1−18.0
ITPA Auditory Assoc. (Score)	35.7	2.57	29 −40
ITPA Visual Reception (Score)	33.1	3.69	29 −40
ITPA Visual Assoc. (Score)	31.8	4.84	19 −40
DTLA Verbal Opposites (Age)	11.0	1.84	4.6−15.0
DTLA Verbal Opposites (Sec. per item)	4.5	0.81	3.2− 6.8
Confrontation Naming (Score)	32.3	2.99	24 −36
Confrontation Naming (Total time sec.)	54.1	12.24	32 −85
Controlled Assoc. Foods (No./min.)	18.9	4.08	11 −28
Controlled Assoc. Animals (No./min.)	18.1	3.75	10 −26
Controlled Assoc. Toys (No./min.)	11.1	3.11	5 −19
Sentence Production (Correct)	5.5	0.79	3 − 6
Sentence Production (Mean length)	4.8	0.96	3.1− 7.5
Sentence Production (Delay in sec.)	3.1	2.45	0.5−12.6
Word Definition (Correct)	4.7	1.71	2 − 8

SOURCE: Wiig, E.H., Lapointe, C., and Semel, E.M. Relationships among language processing and production abilities of learning disabled adolescents. Paper presented at the Annual Convention of the American Speech and Hearing Association, Washington, D.C., 1975.

A summary of the significant correlation coefficients (Kendalls' tau) obtained between the various language measures and measures of age and intellectual ability is presented in Table 27.

In summary, the findings indicate that

1. Performances on all of the auditory language processing tests with the exception of the *Newcombe-Marshall Sentence Repetition Test*, which depends heavily on short-term auditory memory, correlated positively and significantly with WISC verbal scale IQ. Among the language production measures, only the measure of accuracy in confrontation—naming correlated significantly and positively with WISC verbal scale IQ.
2. Among the language processing test performances, the performances on the *Auditory Association, Visual Reception,* and *Visual Association* subtests of the ITPA correlated positively and significantly with each other and with language processing tests tapping cognitive and logical growth in the syntactic and semantic domains (PPVT, NSST, Wiig-Semel test).
3. Performances on the *Token Test* correlated positively and significantly with measures of verbal cognitive abilities (WISC verbal IQ) and with measures of expressive syntactic abilities (NSST).
4. Among the language production tests, performances that were timed and assessed speed of retrieval generally correlated negatively with measures of accuracy in language processing (PPVT and NSST) and with measures of accuracy in oral language production (Verbal Opposites, Confrontation Naming, Sentence Production, Controlled Associations), suggesting that longer response delays were predictive of inaccurate responses.
5. Among the oral language production tests, all measures of speed of production correlated positively with each other, suggesting that reduced speed of production on one task is associated with reduced speed of production and retrieval on another.
6. Performances on the *Controlled Association* subtests correlated positively with each other as did several of the measures of divergent and convergent semantic production abilities (Verbal Opposites, Confrontation Naming, Sentence Production, Verbal Associations).

The composite findings suggest a basis for the separation of and possible independence between the auditory language processing and oral language production abilities of learning disabled adolescents. They suggest that the sum of the liabilities in language comprehension and expression remains constant in this population; that is, if a learning disabled adolescent demonstrates a deficit in auditory language processing it will generally be counterbalanced by assets or adequate performances in oral language production. The performances of the learning disabled adolescents fall within a narrow performance band, and the profile of language abilities is uneven.

TABLE 27

Kendall's Rank Correlations (Tau) Between Measures of Language Processing and Production

Variables	1	2	3	4	5	6	7	8	9	10	11	12	13	14	15	16	17	18	19	20
1. Age (CA)																				
2. Newcombe-Marshall																				
3. Wiig-Semel	-.27																			
4. Token V.	-.31	.26	.28																	
5. Token T.	-.27		.36	.77																
6. NSST Rec.			.32																	
7. NSST Exp.			.28	.37	.44	.47														
8. PPVT (MA)						.30	.33													
9. Aud. Assoc.			.27			.31		.31												
10. Vis. Assoc.	-.25		.28			.27	.26	.21	.33											
11. Vis. Rec.	-.32		.47			.29	.23		.33	.50										
12. WISC Verb. IQ	-.26		.43	.31	.33	.38	.39	.26	.42	.38	.31									
13. Verb. Opp. Age							.42													
14. Verb. Opp. (Sec./Item)					.24															
15. Con. Nam. (Correct)	-.22	-.24	.21							.27		.28	.31							
16. Con. Nam. (Time)						-.29		-.22					-.23		-.26					

TABLE 27 (Continued)

Variables	1	2	3	4	5	6	7	8	9	10	11	12	13	14	15	16	17	18	19	20
17. Con. Assoc. (Foods)									.26							-.28				
18. Con. Assoc. (Animals)								.32	.33			.30				-.38	.47			
19. Con. Assoc. (Toys)									.21					-.29			.24	.37		
20. Sen. Prod. (Correct)		-.33								.28				-.23	.36				.33	
21. Sen. Prod. (Length)															.29				.22	.53
22. Sen. Prod. (Delay)									.32	.23				.29						.22
23. Word Def. (Correct)													.42		.35		.24		.26	

SOURCE: Wiig, E. H., Lapointe, C., and Semel, E. M. Relationships among language processing and production abilities of learning disabled adolescents. Paper presented at the Annual Convention of the American Speech and Hearing Association, Washington, D.C., 1975.

NOTE: Tau ≥ .21 p ≤ .05; Tau ≥ .29 p ≤ .01; Tau ≥ .39 p ≤ .001.

225

References

Alajouanine, T., Lhermitte, F., & de Ribaucourt-Ducarne, B. Les alexies agnosiques et aphasiques. In *Les grandes activites du lobe occipital*. Paris: Masson et Cie, 1960.

Anisfeld, M., & Gordon, M. On the psychophonological structure of English inflectional rules. *Journal of Verbal Learning and Verbal Behavior*, 1968, **7**, 973-79.

Baker, H. J., & Leland, B. *Detroit tests of learning aptitude*. Indianapolis: Test Division of Bobbs-Merrill, 1959.

Bakwin, H. Learning problems and school phobia. *Pediatric Clinics of North America*, 1965, **12**, 995-1014.

Bannatyne, A. *Language, reading, and learning disabilities*. Springfield, Ill.: Charles C Thomas, 1971.

Bartel, N. R., Grill, J. J., & Bartel, H. W. The syntactic-paradigmatic shift in learning disabled and normal children. *Journal of Learning Disabilities*, 1973, **6**, 59-64.

Benson, D. F., & Geschwind, N. The alexias. In P. J. Vinken & G. W. Bruyn (Eds.), *Disorders of speech, perception and symbolic behavior*. Vol. 4. *Handbook of clinical neurology*. Amsterdam: North-Holland Publishing Co., 1969. Pp. 112-40.

Berko, J. The child's learning of English morphology. *Word*, 1958, **14**, 150-77.

Berry, M. F. *Language disorders of children: the bases and diagnoses*. New York: Appleton-Century Crofts, 1969.

Bloom, L. *Language development: form and function in emerging grammars*. Cambridge: M.I.T. Press, 1970.

Bousfield, W., Cohen, B., & Whitmarsh, G. Associative clustering of words of different taxonomic frequencies of occurrence. *Psychological Reports*, 1958, **4**, 39-44.

Brown, R. *A first language: the early stages*. Cambridge: Harvard University Press, 1973.

Brown, R., & Berko, J. Word association and the acquisition of grammar. *Child Development*, 1960, **31**, 1-14.

Brown, R., & McNeill, D. The "tip of the tongue" phenomenon. In R. Brown (Ed.), *Psycholinguistics*. New York: Free Press, 1970. Pp. 274-301.

Bryant, B., & Anisfeld, M. Feedback versus non-feedback in testing children's knowledge of English pluralization rules. *Journal of Experimental Psychology*, 1969, **8**, 250-55.

Caroll, J. B. Vectors of prose style. In T. A. Sebeok (Ed.), *Style in language*. New York: John Wiley & Sons, 1960. Pp. 283-92.

Cazden, D. Child language and education. New York; Holt, Rinehart & Winston, 1972.

Chomsky, C. *The acquisition of syntax in children from 5 to 10.* Cambridge: M.I.T. Press, 1969.

Chomsky, N. A review of B. F. Skinner's *Verbal Behavior.* In J. Fodor & J. Katz (Eds.), *The structure of language.* Englewood Cliffs, N.J.: Prentice-Hall, 1964. Pp. 547-78.

Deese, J. *The structure of association in language and thought.* Baltimore: Johns Hopkins Press, 1962. (a)

Deese, J. Form class and the determiners of association. *Journal of Verbal Learning and Verbal Behavior,* 1962, **1,** 79-84. (b)

Denckla, M. B. Naming of pictured objects by dyslexic and non-dyslexic "MBD" children. Paper presented at the Academy of Aphasia, 1974.

De Renzi, E., & Vignolo, L. A. The token test: a sensitive test to detect receptive disturbances in aphasics. *Brain,* 1962, **85,** 665-78.

de Villiers, J. G., & de Villiers, P. A. A cross-sectional study of the acquisition of grammatical morphemes in child speech. *Journal of Psycholinguistic Research,* 1973, **2,** 267-78.

Dobb, L. W. Behavior and grammatical style. *Journal of Abnormal (Social) Psychology,* 1958, **56,** 398-401.

Doehring, D. G. *Patterns of impairment in specific reading disability.* Bloomington: Indiana University Press, 1968.

Dunn, L. M. *Peabody picture vocabulary test.* Circle Pines, Minn.: American Guidance Service, 1959.

Dunn, L. M., & Markwardt, F. C. *Peabody individual achievement test.* Circle Pines, Minn.: American Guidance Service, 1970.

Entwistle, D., Forsyth, D., & Muuss, R. The syntactic-paradigmatic shift in children's word association. *Journal of Verbal Learning and Verbal Behavior,* 1964, **3,** 19-29.

Fehrer, E., Cofer, C. N., Tuthill, C. E., & Gresham, M. An exploratory study of relationships between certain written language measures and vocational interests. *Journal of General Psychology,* 1948, **39,** 49-72.

Fromkin, V. A. Slips of the tongue. *Scientific American,* 1973, **229,** 110-17.

Gerjuoy, I., & Spitz, H. Associative clustering in free recall: intellectual and developmental variables. *American Journal of Mental Deficiency,* 1966, **70,** 918-27.

Geschwind, N. The varieties of naming errors. In M. T. Sarno (Ed.), *Aphasia: selected readings.* New York: Appleton-Century Crofts, 1972. Pp. 46-55.

Gleser, G. C., Gottschalk, L. A., & John, W. The relationship of sex and intelligence to choice of words. *Journal of Clinical Psychology,* 1959, **15,** 182-91.

Goldstein, G. Analogous reasoning abilities of learning disabled adolescents. Unpublished master's thesis, Boston University, 1974.

Goldstein, K. *Language and language disturbances.* New York: Grune & Stratton, 1948.

Goodglass, H., & Kaplan, E. Boston diagnostic aphasia examination. Philadelphia: Lea & Febiger, 1972.

Guilford, J. P. *The nature of human intelligence.* New York: McGraw-Hill, 1967.

Hallgren, B. Specific dyslexia (congenital word-blindness): a clinical and genetic study. *Acta Psychiatrica et Neurologica,* Copenhagen, 1950, Supplement No. 65, 1-287.

Hass, W. A., & Wepman, J. M., Dimensions of individual difference in the spoken syntax of school children. *Journal of Speech and Hearing Research*, 1974, **17**, 455-69.

Ingram, T. T. Pediatric aspects of specific developmental dysphasia, dyslexia, and dysgraphia. *Cerebral Palsy Bulletin*, 1960, **2**, 254-67.

Jansky, J., & de Hirsch, K. *Preventing reading failure: prediction, diagnosis, intervention*. New York: Harper & Row, 1972.

Johnson, D. J. The language continuum. *Bulletin of the Orton Society*, 1968, **18**, 1-11.

Johnson, D. J., & Myklebust, H. R. *Learning disabilities: educational principles and practices*. New York: Grune & Stratton, 1967.

Jones, L. V., & Wepman, J. M. Dimensions of language performance in aphasia. *Journal of Speech and Hearing Research*, 1961, **4**, 220-32.

Kass, C. Some psychological correlates of severe reading disability (dyslexia). Unpublished doctoral dissertation, University of Illinois, 1962.

Kirk, S. A., McCarthy, J. J., & Kirk, W. D. *Illinois test of psycholinguistic ability:* (Rev. ed.) Urbana: University of Illinois Press, 1968.

Kolers, P. A. Experiments in reading. *Scientific American*, 1972, **227** (1), 84-91.

Koziol, S. The development of noun plural rules during the primary grades. *Research in the Teaching of English*, 1973, **7** (1), 30-50.

Lee, L. *Northwestern syntax screening test*. Evanston, Ill.: Northwestern University Press, 1969, 1971.

Lee, L. L., & Canter, S. Developmental sentence scoring: a clinical procedure for estimating syntactic development in children's spontaneous speech. *Journal of Speech and Hearing Disorders*, 1971, **36**, 315-37.

Lerner, J. *Children with learning disabilities*. Boston: Houghton Mifflin Co., 1971.

Livant, W. P. Grammer in the story reproductions of levelers and sharpeners. *Bulletin of the Menninger Clinic*, 1962, **26**, 283-87.

London, P. M. A study of expressive language patterns of learning disabled children. Unpublished research, Boston University, 1974.

Luria, A. R. *Higher cortical functions in man*. New York: Basic Books, 1966.

Luria, A. R. *The working brain*. New York: Basic Books, 1973.

McNeill, D. *The acquisition of language: the study of developmental psycholinguistics*. New York: Harper & Row, 1970.

Menyuk, P. Alternation of rules in children's grammar. *Journal of Verbal Learning and Verbal Behavior*, 1963, **3**, 480-88. (a)

Menyuk, P. Syntactic structures in the language of the child. *Child Development*, 1963, **34**, 407-22. (b)

Menyuk, P. Syntactic rules used by children from preschool through first grade. *Child Development*, 1964, **35**, 533-46.

Menyuk, P. *Sentences children use*. Cambridge: M.I.T. Press, 1969.

Myklebust, H. R. Learning disorders: psychoneurological disturbances in childhood. *Rehabilitation Literature*, 1964, **25**, 354-60.

Myklebust, H. R. *Development and disorders of written language*. Vol. I. *Picture story language test*. New York: Grune & Stratton, 1965.

Newcombe, F., & Marshall, J. C. Immediate recall of sentences by subjects with unilateral cerebral lesions. *Neuropsychologia*, 1967, **5**, 329-34.

Newcombe, F., Oldfield, R. C., Ratcliff, G. G., & Wingfield, A. Recognition and naming of object-drawings by men with focal brain wounds. *Journal of Neurology, Neurosurgery and Psychiatry,* 1971, **34**, 329-40.

Newfield, M. U., & Schlanger, B. B. The acquisition of morphology by normal and educable mentally retarded children. *Journal of Speech and Hearing Research,* 1968, **4**, 693-706.

Nielsen, J. M. *Agnosia, apraxia, aphasia: their value in cerebral localization.* New York: Hoeber, 1946.

Orton, S. T. *Reading, writing and speech problems in children.* New York: Norton, 1937.

Poppelreuter, W. A. *Die psychischen Schädigungen durch Kopfschuss im Kriege 1914/16.* Vol. 1. Die Störungen der niederen und höheren Sehleistungen durch Verletzungen des Okzipitalhirns. Leipzig: Voss, 1917.

Rabinovitch, R. D. Reading and learning disabilities. Vol. 2. In S. Arieti (Ed.), *American Handbook of Psychiatry.* New York: Basic Books, 1959. Pp. 857-70.

Rosenthal, J. H. A preliminary psycholinguistic study of children with learning disabilities. *Journal of Learning Disabilities,* 1970, **3**, 391-95.

Schuell, H. *Minnesota test for differential diagnosis of aphasia.* Minneapolis: University of Minnesota Press, 1965.

Schuell, H., & Jenkins, J. J. Reduction of vocabulary in aphasia. In M. T. Sarno (Ed.), *Aphasia: selected readings.* New York: Appleton-Century Crofts, 1972. Pp. 1-18.

Schuell, H., Jenkins, J. J., & Jimenez-Pabon, E. J. *Aphasia in adults.* New York: Harper & Row, 1964.

Semel, E. M., & Wiig, E. H. Comprehension of syntactic structures and critical verbal elements by children with learning disabilities. *Journal of Learning Disabilities,* 1975, **8**, 53-58.

Simon, H. A., & Chase, W. G. Skill in chess. *American Scientist,* 1973, **61**, 394-403.

Slegman, D. Sentence formulation deficits of learning disabled children. Unpublished clinical paper (research), Boston University, 1974.

Spreen, O. Psycholinguistic aspects of aphasia. *Journal of Speech and Hearing Research,* 1968, **11**, 467-80.

Strauss, A. A., & Kephart, N. D., *Psychopathology and education of the brain-injured child: progress in theory and clinic.* Vol. 2 New York: Grune & Stratton, 1955.

Strauss, A. A., & Lehtinen, L. E. *Psychopathology and education of the brain-injured child.* Vol. 1. New York: Grune & Stratton, 1947.

Torrance, E. P. Developing creative thinking through school experiences. In S. J. Parnes and H. F. Harding (Eds.), *A source book for creative thinking.* New York: Charles Scribner's Sons, 1962. Pp. 31-47. (a)

Torrance, E. P. *Guiding creative talent.* Englewood Cliffs, N.J.: Prentice-Hall, 1962. (b)

Vogel, S. A. Syntactic abilities in normal and dyslexic children. *Journal of Learning Disabilities,* 1974, **7**, 47-53.

Wechsler, D. *Wechsler intelligence scale for children.* New York: Psychological Corp., 1949.

Wechsler, D. *Wechsler adult intelligence scale.* New York: Psychological Corp., 1955.

Wiig, E. H., & Globus, D. Aphasic word identification as a function of logical relationship and association strength. *Journal of Speech and Hearing Research*, 1971, **14**, 195-204.

Wiig, E. H., Lapointe, C., & Semel, E. M. Relationships among language processing and production abilities of learning disabled adolescents. Paper presented at the Annual Convention of the American Speech and Hearing Association, Washington, D.C., 1975.

Wiig, E. H., & Semel, E. M. Comprehension of linguistic concepts requiring logical operations by learning-disabled children. *Journal of Speech and Hearing Research*, 1973, **16**, 627-36.

Wiig, E. H., & Semel, E. M. Development of comprehension of logico-grammatical sentences by grade school children. *Perceptual and Motor Skills*, 1974, **38**, 171-76. (a)

Wiig, E. H., & Semel, E. M. Logico-grammatical sentence comprehension by learning disabled adolescents. *Perceptual and Motor Skills*, 1974, **38**, 1331-34. (b)

Wiig, E. H., & Semel, E. M. Language production deficits in learning disabled adolescents. Paper presented at the Second International Scientific Conference on Learning Disabilities, Brussels, 1975. (a)

Wiig, E. H., & Semel, E. M. Productive language abilities in learning disabled adolescents. *Journal of Learning Disabilities*, 1975, **8**, 578-86. (b)

Wiig, E. H., Semel, E. M., & Crouse, M. A. The use of morphology by high-risk and learning disabled children. *Journal of Learning Disabilities*, 1973, **6**, 457-65.

Yamamoto, K. Evaluation of some creative measures in a high school with peer nominations as criteria. *Journal of Psychology*, 1964, **58**, 285-93.

Zangwill, O. *Cerebral dominance and its relation to psychological function*. London: Henderson Trust, 1960.

Zatzkis, J. The effect of need for achievement on linguistic behavior. Master's thesis, Wesleyan University, 1949.

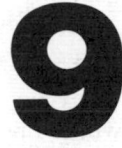

Assessing Language Production Abilities

Overview

This chapter introduces a review of selected diagnostic methods and tests for assessing: (1) short-term memory for verbal materials (digits, words, and sentences), (2) convergent production of language, (3) divergent production of language, and (4) productive control of linguistic structure. The need for assessing each ability area independently is presented against the background of research evidence of language production deficits of school-age children and adolescents.

The discussions of the tests and subtests emphasize the processes involved in responding to each test. Error patterns are discussed and the implications for diagnosis and remediation are presented. The reviews also stress the sensitivity of each test in identifying language production deficits in language and learning disabled youngsters. The need to utilize more than a single test or subtest to corroborate and determine the bases for specific language production deficits and to provide appropriate educational or clinical management is emphasized.

The majority of the tests appropriate for evaluating short-term memory for verbal materials and convergent and divergent language production abilities are subtests of extensive test batteries for the assessment of intellectual or psycholinguistic abilities or learning aptitude. The authors recognize that the diagnostician must exhibit caution and judgment in selecting and using subtests of comprehensive tests such as the *Wechsler Intelligence Scale for Children* or the *Stanford-Binet Intelligence Scale* to evaluate the status of specific language production abilities.

Tests designed to evaluate the productive control of linguistic structure are generally appropriate for only a narrow age range. The sentence repetition test designed by Newcombe and Marshall (1967) which varies the syntactic complexity and the syntactic and semantic constraints of sentences is an exception. The limited number of tests currently available for assessing language production abilities during adolescence suggests an area for future test development.

Assessing Auditory Memory and Recall

Children and adolescents with learning disabilities have been reported to exhibit evidence of reductions in short-term auditory memory (Aten & Davis, 1968; Johnson & Myklebust, 1967; Lerner, 1971; McCarthy & McCarthy, 1969; Zigmond, 1969). The short-term auditory memory abilities of the school-age child or adolescent with a suspected language disability may be assessed using materials such as a digit series, or a series of unrelated words or sentences.

The rationale for assessing the immediate memory for verbal materials (digits and words) is that a minimum auditory retention span seems to be required for adequate intellectual functioning as well as for the adequate development of linguistic skills. Furthermore, deficits in rote memory are considered to have diagnostic significance as indicators of organic as well as of functional disorganization. Whimby and Fischhof (1969) and Whimby and Ryan (1969) have established direct relationships between poor digit memory span and poor mental addition and logical problem-solving abilities in college students.

The short-term auditory memory abilities may be evaluated using one or more of the following tests: (1) the *Digit Span* subtest of the *Wechsler Intelligence Scale for Children* (Wechsler, 1949); (2) the *Repeating Digits* and *Repeating Digits Reversed* subtests of the *Stanford-Binet Intelligence Scale* (Terman & Merrill, 1960); (3) the *Auditory Sequential Memory* subtest of the *Illinois Test of Psycholinguistic Ability* (Kirk, McCarthy, & Kirk, 1968); (4) the *Auditory Attention Span for Unrelated Words* subtest of the *Detroit Tests of Learning Aptitude* (Baker & Leland, 1959); (5) the *Auditory Attention Span for Related Syllables* subtest of the *Detroit Tests of Learning Aptitude* (Baker & Leland, 1959); (6) the *Repeat Words* and *Repeat Sentences* subtests of the *Meeting Street School Screening Test* (Hainsworth & Siqueland, 1969); and (7) the *Stanford-Binet Intelligence Scale: Memory for Sentences* subtest (Terman & Merrill, 1960).

WISC: Digit Span

The *Digit Span* subtest of the *Wechsler Intelligence Scale for Children* (Wechsler, 1949) evaluates the auditory memory span for digits. It contains two parts, one which requires repetition of a series of heard digits forward; the other, backward. Each subtest contains seven items, each containing an alternate set of digits if the first series is missed or invalidated. The digits forward series range in length from three through nine digits while the digits backward series range in length from two through eight digits. All items are presented orally at a rate of one digit per second. In comparison, the *Auditory Sequential Memory* subtest of the ITPA (Kirk, McCarthy, & Kirk, 1968) specifies that the digits must be presented at a rate of two per second. This faster rate of presentation is considered to be more sensitive to short-term auditory memory deficits.

The WISC series of digits are composed so that digits are never repeated within a series. This feature also contrasts with the design of the *Auditory Sequential Memory* subtest of the ITPA in which digits may occur more than once in a series. This difference may influence the immediate auditory recall since series which contain same stimuli are easier to recall than series with different stimuli.

The "digits forward" series is considered to measure a "more passive auditory immediate recall type . . . while digits backwards are examples of the more active auditory recall items" (Glasser & Zimmerman, 1967, p. 99). In the digits backward series it is necessary to shift the set from the concrete and abstract and formulate the reversed sequence. According to the Guilford Structure-of-Intellect Model, the factor *Memory Span* is tapped by the digit forward series and *Memory for Symbol Patterns* is tapped by the digits backward.

Memory span for digits has been observed to correlate poorly with other measures of intelligence. Cohen (1959) has reported that factor analysis indicated that the *Digit Span* subtest does not measure general intelligence, memory or "freedom from distractibility." The reliability of the subtest was also lower than for any other subtest of the WISC. Cronbach (1970) has commented on this limitation in the statement that "digit span has low correlations with other parts of the Wechsler, with school marks, and with other learning measures" (p. 294).

In a related study, Aten and Davis (1968) observed that digit spans obtained with a presentation rate of one digit per second did not differentiate learning disabled children from matched controls while retention of unrelated consonant-vowel-consonant nouns indicated memory-span deficits in the learning disabled children. These observations suggest that the diagnostician should exhibit caution in diagnosing short-term auditory memory deficits on the basis of performances on the *Digit Span* subtest of the WISC alone.

Glasser and Zimmerman (1967) provide further discussion of the advantages and limitations of the *Digit Span* subtest. Among advantages they cite that it may serve as a rapid check on verbal memory and attention. They caution that the results are vulnerable to inconsistencies in concentration and attention and manifest anxiety. The diagnostic value of the subtest for children with language disabilities seems to relate to identifying discrepancies between digit forward and backward memories. Wide discrepancies (more than two digits) between the two in favor of digits forward suggest "concrete thinking" and inability to shift response set and perform the mental abstractions necessary to perform the digit reversal. In this vein, clinical observations suggest that LD youngsters with language problems often show significant problems in recalling the digits backward series.

The normative data for the *Digit Span* subtest cover the age range from 5½ through 15½ years; however, the subtest is most sensitive to developmental changes at the lower age levels (5½ through 7½). At higher age levels, the same average score may be expected at several age levels; for example, a score of ten is expected between the ages of 11½ through 13½. The subtest may be expected to be equally limited in sensitivity when used with language disabled youngsters, suggesting that the comparison of the performances of the digits forward and backward series may be of greatest diagnostic value.

Stanford-Binet: Repeating Digits

The *Stanford-Binet Intelligence Scale* (Terman & Merrill, 1960) contains *Repeating Digits* (forward) subtests at several age levels. At year II-6, the child is required to repeat three series of two digits each. At year III, three series of three digits each are presented for repetition. At year VII, the number of digits has been increased to five for each of the three series and at year X to six digits per series.

The digits are said by the examiner with uniform emphasis at a rate of one per second. This rate of presentation is the same as for the WISC *Digit Span* subtest (Wechsler, 1949), but slower than the rate of presentation (two digits per second) used on the ITPA *Auditory Sequential Memory* subtest (Kirk, McCarthy, & Kirk, 1968). The digit series contain no repetitions of digits, agreeing with the format of the WISC *Digit Span* subtest. The digit series must be repeated without error and in correct order after a single presentation.

Repeating Digits Reversed subtests are introduced at four age levels. At year VII, three series of three digits each must be repeated backwards. At year IX, the number of digits in each series is increased to four and at year XII to five digits. At the Superior Adult Level I, three series of digits are presented, each containing six digits. Digits forward and digits reversed items are only presented concurrently at year VII. This format limits the possibility of comparing digits forward and backward performances for diagnostic interpretation of discrepancies.

ITPA: Auditory Sequential Memory

This subtest of the ITPA (Kirk, McCarthy, & Kirk, 1968) also evaluates the ability to recall a sequence of digits. The subtest has twenty-eight items, containing from two to eight digits. The digits are read by the examiner at half-second intervals, a rate considered sensitive to auditory memory deficits. The child must recall and repeat the digits in the exact sequence in which they were presented. The fact that digits may occur more than once may facilitate recall. This format differs from the formats of the digit span subtests of the WISC and *Stanford-Binet* in which digits are not repeated in a series.

Normative data are provided for the age range from two years to ten years three months. Five-month stability coefficients range between .75 and .89 and split-half correlations between .74 and .95, with an increase in the internal consistency a function of age. The test provides information regarding the number of units that the child can store in short-term memory for immediate recall. Sequencing difficulties may be suggested by analysis of the error patterns. The performances on the subtest cannot be translated directly to predict performances on measures of immediate sentence recall (McCarthy & McCarthy, 1969). Learning disabled children may perform relatively better (at higher age levels) on tests of sentence recall since linguistic structure and semantic interpretation may facilitate recall.

DTLA: Auditory Attention Span

The *Auditory Attention Span for Unrelated Words* subtest of the *Detroit Tests of Learning Aptitude* (Baker & Leland, 1959) evaluates short-term auditory memory abilities for unstructured, unrelated words. The subtest contains two sets of items (set *a* and set *b*). Each set consists of seven word groups, increasing in length from two to eight words. The examiner says the words in each set at a rate of one word per second. The child must repeat the word group, retaining the word order. The responses are scored to reflect the number of words recalled on all the items (simple score) and the relative number of words recalled per word group for the total test (weighted score). Normative data are provided for the age range from three to nineteen years.

The *Auditory Attention Span for Related Syllables* of the *Detroit Tests of Learning Aptitude* (Baker & Leland, 1958) evaluates the immediate recall of forty-three sentences. The sentences range in length from five (six syllables) to twenty-two words (twenty-seven syllables). The sentences are not controlled for syntactic complexity, a factor known to influence sentence recall. The sentences are read aloud by the examiner and the subject is requested to recall the sentences verbatim. Repetitions with more than three errors (omissions, substitutions, or additions) are counted as incorrect. Each correct repetition is scored on a point scale to reflect the number of errors.

Norms are provided for the age range from three to nineteen years. Five-month stability correlations for the total test are reported at .68 for a sample of 792 children, ranging in age from seven to twelve years. Correlations between subtest performances are reported to range between .2 to .4.

Johnson and Myklebust (1967) have commented that some learning disabled children may perform better on the memory subtest for *Unrelated Words* than on the memory subtest for *Related Syllables* (sentences). They interpret this observation to indicate that syntactical deficits interfere with the ability to retain meaning and structure simultaneously. Clinical observations indicate that LD children and adolescents who exhibit this memory pattern demonstrate problems in linguistic processing (syntax) as well as in cognitive processing (linguistic concepts).

McCarthy and McCarthy (1969) have reported conflicting observations. They observed that even though learning disabled children may not recall series of words, letters, or nonsense syllables adequately, many can reproduce the words in meaningful sentences. Accordingly, linguistic structure and semantic interpretation appear to facilitate auditory memory and recall for these youngsters. Clinical observations support that some learning disabled children demonstrate this pattern in the recall of verbal materials. The relationship to the syntactic and cognitive processing abilities remains to be established.

Meeting Street: Repeat Words and Sentences

The *Repeat Words* subtest of the *Meeting Street School Screening Test* (Hainsworth & Siqueland, 1969) assesses the child's ability to recall and repeat unknown and familiar sound sequences and to retain their correct form, sequence and rhythm, reflecting short-term auditory memory. The subtest contains eleven items, six of which are phonetically marked for correct pronunciation. Of these six, four are nonsense words and two are real words that may be unfamiliar to the examiner. An example of a nonsense item is *kaka-kada kat*. Of the five real-word items, two are single words such as *musicology* and two contain sequences of three words such as *quack duck quack*. A correct answer, a verbatim repetition of the stimulus, is given a ½ point value, for a possible total of 5½.

Normative data are not available for the individual subtests of the test battery. Total test scores may be converted to scaled scores, and five normative percentile tables are provided for the age range from five years to seven years five months. Test-retest reliability coefficients range from .75 to .85, indicating adequate consistency of the test results over time.

Analysis of error responses permits identification of sequencing problems at the phonological, morphological, and suprasegmental (stress levels). The perception and recall of suprasegmentals and prosody is not generally tapped by tests of word recall, suggesting that this subtest may add to the differentiation of problems in short-term auditory memory.

The *Repeat Sentences* subtest of the *Meeting Street School Screening Test* (Hainsworth & Siqueland, 1969) evaluates the immediate recall of two sentences. The first sentence, "Please pass the meat and peas," contains six words and the second sentence, "Joan and Jane had a chocolate sundae after the movie yesterday," contains eleven words. The repetitions are scored to reflect the number of words that are recalled in correct sequence. The resulting raw scores are subsequently converted into scores from zero to five.

The test manual provides normative data for the total test battery for the age range between five years and seven years five months. There are no norms for the individual subtests. As a result, the interpretation of performances on the *Repeat Sentences* subtest is so limited that it should only be administered as part of the total screening test.

Stanford-Binet: Memory for Sentences

The *Stanford-Binet Intelligence Scale* (Terman & Merrill, 1960) assesses short-term auditory memory for sentences of different lengths at three age levels. At year IV, two sentences are introduced for immediate recall. The sentences contain nine and ten words respectively and both are active—declarative. Both sentences contain a prepositional phrase and the verb of the verb phrase is elaborated in both sentences, for example, *are going to buy* and *likes to feed*.

The two sentences introduced at year XI contain fifteen and sixteen words respectively. Both contain two prepositional phrases in sequence, and one sentence begins with the prepositional phrase *At the summer camp.* These aspects may introduce problems in the immediate recall of the sentences for learning disabled youngsters. At year XIII, the two sentences contain fifteen words each. The structure of these sentences has, however, increased in complexity, a factor which may influence recall. One of the sentences ends with a relative clause, beginning with *which.* The other begins with a noun possessive.

The Stanford-Binet sentences may be used to screen the short-term auditory memory abilities for structured verbal materials of youngsters of the appropriate ages. The recall of the sentences must be verbatim; omissions, substitutions, additions, or changes in word order are scored as errors. Learning disabled youngsters who fail the items may be given additional sentence repetition tests to assess the effects of syntactic structure or semantic consistency on sentence recall. Several of the available sentence repetition tests are reviewed in this chapter in the section on assessing the productive control of linguistic structure.

Assessing Convergent Language Production Abilities

The ability to identify, retrieve, and formulate words or concepts that satisfy the semantic constraints imposed by a context reflects a person's convergent language production abilities (Guilford, 1967). Learning disabled children have been reported to experience difficulties in finding and retrieving words and concepts from long-term memory store, that is, they may exhibit dysnomia (Bannatyne, 1971; Denckla, 1974; Johnson & Myklebust, 1967). These difficulties have been observed to persist into adolescence (Wiig & Semel, 1975).

Difficulties in identifying, retrieving, and formulating words when semantic constraints are introduced may be assessed using one or more of the following tests: (1) the *Visual Confrontation Naming* subtest of the *Boston Diagnostic Aphasia Examination* (Goodglass & Kaplan, 1972); (2) the *Verbal Scale* of the *McCarthy Scales of Children's Abilities* (McCarthy, 1970); (3) the *Verbal Opposites* subtest of the *Detroit Tests of Learning Aptitude* (Baker & Leland, 1959); (4) the *Stanford-Binet Intelligence Scale: Opposite Analogies* (Terman & Merrill, 1960); and (5) the *Auditory Association* subtest of the *Illinois Test of Psycholinguistic Ability* (Kirk, McCarthy, & Kirk, 1968).

Boston Diagnostic: Visual Confrontation Naming

The *Visual Confrontation Naming* subtest of the *Boston Diagnostic Aphasia Examination* (Goodglass & Kaplan, 1972) requires retrieval of verbal labels in response to pictorial presentations, that is, convergent production of semantic units. The pictures represent objects (chair, key, glove, feather, hammock, cactus), letters (H, T, R, L, S, G), geometric forms (square, triangle), actions (running, sleeping, drinking, smoking, falling, dripping), numbers (7, 15, 700, 1936, 42, 7000), and colors (red, brown, pink, blue, gray, purple). The examiner points to each picture, and the person examined must name each item in the order indicated. The scoring form provides space to record the approximate response lag in seconds. Each response is assigned a point score reflecting the delay in responding. Responses given within a period from zero to three seconds receive three points. Responses within three to ten seconds receive two points, responses within ten to thirty seconds receive one point, and failure to respond receives zero points. Articulation and paraphasias may also be noted. The paraphasias are classified as:

1. Neologistic distortion, that is, "introduction of extraneous phonemes or transposition of phonemes so that less than half of the intended word is discernible as an intact unit" (p. 31). (palala for banana)
2. Literal paraphasia, that is, substitution or transposition of phonemes so that more than half the word is intact. (banala for banana)
3. Verbal paraphasia, that is, substitution of an inappropriate word or perseveration of a previously used word.
4. Other, that is, circumlocutions, neologistic jargon, irrelevant speech, and so forth.

The raw score obtained on the subtest is converted into a z-score to permit comparison of performances on the various subtests and obtain a profile of aphasia subscores.

An adaptation of the *Visual Confrontation Naming* subtest has been administered to a group of LD adolescents (Wiig & Semel, 1975). In this adaptation the adolescents were required to name the pictorial stimuli in rapid succession; errors were then recorded and the total response time was measured in seconds. Comparison of the performances by learning disabled and academically achieving adolescents indicated that the LD adolescents made significantly more errors (substitutions and omissions) in naming and used significantly longer time to complete the task. Their errors were (1) word substitutions, (2) omissions, and (3) perseverative responses. The academic achievers made only word substitution errors. These findings suggest that the *Visual Confrontation Naming* subtest may assist in identifying deficits in the accuracy and speed of the convergent production of semantic units by learning disabled adolescents.

The *Visual Confrontation Naming* subtest may be administered and scored in the format described by Goodglass and Kaplan (1972). Similarities among the performances of adult aphasics and adolescents or young adults with learning disabilities would suggest difficulties in word finding. It may also be administered using the adapted format (Wiig & Semel, 1975). The data indicate that academically achieving adolescents ranging from twelve years five months to sixteen years four months may be expected to make an average of 0.84 errors (Range 0 to 4; SD = 1.09) and use, on the average, forty-four seconds (Range 27 to 69; SD = 7.49) to complete the tast. In comparison, learning disabled adolescents in the same age range produced an average of 3.38 errors (Range 0 to 11) and used, on the average, fifty-three seconds (Range 32 to 85) to complete the task. Performances outside the zero to four range by academic achievers or outside of two standard deviations above the mean for the academic achievers may be interpreted to indicate word-finding deficits.

The *Verbal Scale* of the *McCarthy Scales of Children's Abilities* (McCarthy, 1970) contains five subtests: (1) *Pictorial Memory*, (2) *Word Knowledge*, (3) *Verbal Memory*, (4) *Verbal Fluency*, and (5) *Opposite Analogies*. The last three assess abilities related to oral language production. The *Verbal Scale* is described to "assess the child's ability to express himself verbally, and also to assess the maturity of his verbal concepts" (p. 3). The subtests and items tap, among others, short- and long-term memory, divergent production of semantic units (Verbal Fluency), and convergent production of semantic relations (Opposite Analogies).

The *Verbal Memory* subtest assesses the immediate recall (short-term memory) of words and sentences and the recall of a paragraph. The subtest contains two parts: part I evaluates recall of words and sentences, and part II assesses the recall of a story.

Part I of the subtest contains six items. The two initial items assess the recall of series of three concrete, one-syllable words, for example, *toy—chair—light*. The next two items contain a series of four, abstract, two-syllable words, for example, *around—because—under—never*. The last two items consist of sentences with seven and nine key words, respectively. The responses are scored to reflect the number of words (items one to four) and key words (items five and six) that are recalled.

Part II contains a story in an eight-sentence paragraph. The sentences reflect a variety of syntactic structures (*and* conjunctions, direct quote, pronominalization, etc.). Scoring is based on the ideas recalled by the child and therefore reflects semantic interpretation (long-term memory) rather than linguistic coding (short-term memory).

The *Verbal Fluency* subtest requires retrieval of as many class members as possible within a twenty-second time period for the classes: (1) things to eat, (2) animals, (3) things to wear, and (4) things to ride. It provides a variation of a controlled association task. The subtest assesses speed and accuracy of retrieval, spontaneous grouping abilities (associative clustering), and divergent production of semantic classes. Characteristic qualities in responding such as rigidity, perseveration, bluffing, showing off, flexibility and originality may be noted.

The *Opposite Analogies* subtest assesses the ability to perceive and formulate verbal analogies which reflect opposition, that is, convergent production of semantic relations. The subtest contains nine items, eight requiring knowledge and recall of the opposites of adjectives (hot, big, fast, soft, sour, light, thick, and rough) and one requiring knowledge of the opposite of the preposition *up* (I throw the ball *up*, and then it comes _____). The administration manual provides examples of acceptable and unacceptable responses.

The test manual give norms for the age range from 2½ through 8½ years. The normative data relate to performances on all of the subtests which constitute the *Verbal Scale*. No norms are provided for individual subtests, a limiting factor in interpreting reductions differentially and in interpreting the performances for clinical-educational planning. The *Verbal Scale* has been reported to be highly consistent in test-retest situations with reliability coefficients ranging from .84 to .92. It may be used to identify deficits in language production in children in the early grades.

DTLA: Verbal Opposites

The *Verbal Opposites* subtest of the *Detroit Tests of Learning Aptitude* (Baker & Leland, 1959) requires retrieval and formulation of antonyms. It contains ninety-six stimulus items arranged in order of increasing difficulty. The examiner says the stimulus words and the child is instructed to "say a word that means just the opposite" in response. The examiner is instructed to pause for a few seconds after each word to allow for delays in responding. Older children may be started at a basal level at which a series of items are completed successfully. Ceiling is established when five items are failed in succession.

Each correct response is credited one point. The test manual provides a list of the acceptable, exact opposite responses to the stimulus words. Only one antonym is credited for all but three of the items, but colloquial terms or slang words may be credited. Responses indicating that the relation of opposition is understood, for example, "not complex" or "unpassive," are not credited and the youngster is reminded that he must give the *opposite* each time. The task accordingly requires knowledge of a wide vocabulary of antonyms and ability to retrieve a specific antonym within the imposed semantic constraints, reflecting convergent production for semantic classes (Guilford, 1967).

Normative data are available at three-month intervals for the age range from five years three months to nineteen years. Performances on the *Verbal Opposites* subtest have been reported to correlate positively (.68) with performances on the *Verbal Absurdities* subtest. High test-retest reliability coefficients have been reported for the total test over a five-month interval (.96); however, with a test-retest interval of from two to three years, the reliability coefficients dropped to .68.

Wiig and Semel (1975) have reported that LD adolescents demonstrate significant reductions in both the speed and accuracy with which they recall verbal opposites. In the experiment, all adolescents were required to begin with the first item *(boy)*. The individual records indicated that word substitution errors, for example, synonym substitution (son for brother) or associated antonym substitution (daughter in response to brother), were frequent on the easier items. Error responses occurred throughout, but ceiling was often reached at a level appropriate for the chronological age. The learning disabled adolescents also took a significantly longer time to respond, indicating reduced speed of retrieval. The combined findings suggest that the *Verbal Opposites* subtest may assist in identifying convergent production deficits for semantic classes, verbal paraphasias, and dysnomia in children and adolescents with language and learning disabilities.

Stanford-Binet: Opposite Analogies

The *Stanford-Binet Intelligence Scale* (Terman & Merrill, 1960) introduces *Opposite Analogies* subtests at years IV, VI, and VII. At year IV, the subtest contains five items and at years VI and VII four items each. Scoring standards are introduced for each of the subtests and items. An example of an item at year VII is "The point of a cane is blunt; the point of a knife is _____." The *Opposite Analogies* subtests are easy to administer and scoring is objective. These subtests may be used for screening purposes for children at the appropriate age levels. They do not provide estimates of the relative delay in the acquisition of the ability to discern and formulate verbal analogies. Accordingly, additional assessment of the convergent production abilities for semantic relations seems indicated for children who fail an age-appropriate *Opposite Analogies* subtest.

ITPA: Auditory Association

The *Auditory Association* subtest of the *Illinois Test of Psycholinguistic Ability* (Kirk, McCarthy, & Kirk, 1968) evaluates the ability to discern verbal analogies and to formulate appropriate responses. This task is dependent upon convergent production abilities for semantic relations (Guilford, 1967). An example of an item is "Grass is green; sugar is _____." Failure to perform adequately on the subtest may be attributed to either (1) reductions in the available vocabulary of verbal associations, (2) difficulties in discerning the logical relationships expressed between the critical words in the analogy, or (3) reductions in the accuracy of recall of the target words from long-term memory store. Accordingly, the identification of the basis for the problems will depend upon corroborative data from other tests and analysis of error patterns.

Normative data are available for the age range from two years four months to ten years eleven months when a ceiling effect is observed in the average normal child. The subtest performances are of good consistency over time with five-month stability coefficients ranging from .83 to .93. The internal consistency of the subtest is adequate with split-half correlations ranging from .74 to .85. Performances have been reported to correlate positively with Stanford-Binet MA with correlation coefficients ranging from .34 to .58.

Learning disabled youngsters will frequently produce incorrect responses to the test items which suggest problems in target word identification and retrieval. They may produce an unacceptable synonym for a target word, or an associated word that belongs to the same semantic and grammatical category. Wiig and Semel (1975) have reported that LD adolescents may experience deficits in perceiving and formulating verbal analogies. Performances on the *Auditory Association* subtest have been observed to correlate positively with measures of receptive vocabulary (PVVT), comprehension of syntactic structures (NSST), and controlled associations for foods, animals, and toys (Wiig, Lapointe, & Semel, 1975). These findings support the observation that identification of the basis of performance reductions depends upon corroborative test results. They also suggest that reductions in the divergent production of semantic classes observed in a controlled association task may be indicative of deficits in accurate recall and retrieval from long-term memory store.

Assessing Divergent Language Production Abilities

The ability to identify, retrieve, and recall a variety of words or concepts in response to a specific object, picture, word, or word sequence reflects divergent language production (Guilford, 1967). Learning disabled children and adolescents have been reported to demonstrate reductions in verbal fluency, that is, the accuracy and speed with which they can retrieve a variety of words and concepts (Bannatyne, 1971; Johnson & Myklebust, 1967; Wiig & Semel, 1975). The findings suggest that they may not have developed adequate strategies to facilitate recall and retrieval from long-term memory store.

The rationale for assessing the free and controlled association abilities is that the long-term memory system is characterized by relationships between everything stored within it (Lindsay & Norman, 1972). Furthermore, the organization or structure of the output is directly related to the organization within the memory system.

Within a well organized long-term memory system we can therefore expect to observe associative or logical groupings or links between words. The associative grouping strategies are also known to facilitate retrieval (Bousfield, Cohen, & Whitmarsh, 1958; Gerjoy & Spitz, 1966). In a disorganized long-term memory system, the responses may be unrelated or the structure may be irrational and reflect bizarre associations (Rockeach, 1964). Learning disabled youngsters would not be expected to produce bizarre associations. They may show a lack of associatively and logically related groupings in both free and controlled association or show a pattern of shifting from one potential group to another (Wiig & Semel, 1975).

The divergent semantic production abilities of language disabled children and adolescents may be evaluated using one or more of the following tests and tasks: (1) the *Verbal Expression* subtest of the *Illinois Test of Psycholinguistic Ability* (Kirk, McCarthy, & Kirk, 1968); (2) the *Stanford-Binet Intelligence Scale: Word Naming* subtest (Terman & Merrill, 1960); (3) the *Free Association* subtest of the *Detroit Tests of Learning Aptitude* (Baker & Leland, 1959); and the (4) *Controlled Association* subtest of the *Boston Diagnostic Asphasia Examination* (Goodglass & Kaplan, 1972)

ITPA: Verbal Expression

The *Verbal Expression* subtest of the *Illinois Test of Psycholinguistic Ability* (ITPA) (Kirk, McCarthy, & Kirk, 1968) assesses the ability to abstract and formulate a diversity of the attributes of four common objects: a ball, a block, an envelope, and a button. The examiner initially presents the demonstration items, a nail and a hammer, to the child and elicits responses to a series of questions requiring labeling of various characteristics. The test items are presented with the instruction "Tell me all about this." The child's responses are scored to reflect verbal references to the following categories: (1) label and class, (2) color, (3) shape, (4) composition, (5) function of action, (6) major parts, (7) quantity, (8) other physical characteristics, (9) comparison, and (10) person, place, or thing.

Normative data are available for the age range from two years to ten years eleven months. The inter-scorer reliabilities reported for experienced examiners range from .98 to 1.00. Internal consistency coefficients range from .51 to .79, suggesting inadequacies in this measure of consistency.

Performances on the *Verbal Expression* subtest reflect the ability to abstract and formulate characteristics and attributes of objects, an area in which language disabled children may experience difficulties. The responses also reflect flexibility, fluency, and originality in abstracting and formulating alternative responses, a divergent semantic production ability (Guilford, 1967). The responses do not, however, reflect syntactic formulation abilities. Interpretation of the responses on this subtest may be corroborated by responses to other tests that require abstraction and formulation of attributes (DTLA: Likenesses and Differences subtest; WISC Similarities subtest, etc.) and responses to tests of divergent language production (DTLA: Free Association; Boston Diagnostic Aphasia Examination: Controlled Associations). The responses may also be analyzed to identify the attributes which are consistently described or which are never mentioned. This analysis may provide an estimate of the relative saliency of various attributes to the child.

Stanford-Binet: Word Naming

The *Stanford-Binet Intelligence Scale* (Terman & Merrill, 1960) contains a *Word Naming* subtest (year X) which may be used to assess the divergent production of semantic units. The youngster is required to name as many different words as he can within a one-minute period. The subtest is passed successfully if twenty-eight words are produced in one minute, exclusive of repetitions. Use of up to three numbers in counting is allowed. The youngster cannot give sentences, but credit is given for the portion of the sentence produced before the examiner becomes aware that a sentence is being formed and stops the subject. Automatic series such as months of the year or days of the week and proper names are credited. Learning disabled youngsters ten years of age or above may pass this subtest successfully. They may, however, exhibit reductions in the speed of word retrieval when the time period is extended as it is on the *Free Association* subtest of the *Detroit Tests of Learning Aptitude*.

DTLA: Free Association

The *Free Association* subtest of the *Detroit Tests of Learning Aptitude* (Baker & Leland, 1959) evaluates the flexibility and speed of retrieval of associated verbal labels (words), a divergent semantic production skill (Guilford, 1967). The subtest requires that the youngster retrieve and formulate a series of associated words within a given time period. The directions given by the examiner include an associated word sample, for example, "Say any words you think of like tree, sky, train, boy—any words at all'' (Baker & Leland, 1958, p. 56).

The time period allotted for responding increases from one minute for ages three to seven to five minutes for ages fourteen and older. The responses are scored to reflect the number of words produced during each one-minute period; the total number of words produced during the time period is used to evaluate age-equivalent performances. Words which appear in logical sequences such as one, two, three or a, b, c (automatic series) are not credited. Normative data are available for the age range from five years three months to nineteen years.

Learning disabled youngsters frequently run out of words after the first one-minute period. Subsequent responses may suggest a random search pattern for words with few apparent associative ties or groupings between words. Analysis of the response patterns can therefore suggest whether associative organization or grouping strategies are available to facilitate word retrieval.

Boston Diagnostic: Fluency of Controlled Association

Controlled association tasks may be used to assess the divergent production abilities for semantic classes (Guilford, 1967). The *Boston Diagnostic Aphasia Examination* (Goodglass & Kaplan, 1972) features a *Fluency of Controlled Association* subtest which requires rapid retrieval and naming of animals. The total time allowed for the task is ninety seconds. Raw scores are assigned according to the total number of animals named in the most productive sixty–second period. The raw scores may be converted to z-scores to allow comparison between the performances on various subtests and charting of a profile of aphasia subscores.

Wiig and Semel (1975) adapted this task to include naming of foods, animals, and toys during a sixty-second period. Learning disabled adolescents from twelve years five months to sixteen years four months were observed to produce significantly fewer food names than their academically achieving controls.

The data obtained from the thirty-two academic achievers for food and animal naming may be used to compare the individual performances by learning disabled adolescents. The academic achievers named an average of 23.16 food items per minute (Range 14 to 30; SD = 4.6) and an average of 18.75 animals (Range 13 to 28; SD = 3.43). Learning disabled adolescents in the appropriate age range who score below the range or two standard deviations below the mean of the academic achievers may be considered to experience reductions in verbal fluency for semantic classes.

Assessing the Productive Control of Linguistic Structure

Learning disabled children and adolescents have been reported to demonstrate delays in the acquisition of productive control of linguistic rules and structure. They may not have acquired control of morphological and syntactic rules in elicited or spontaneous language production (Rosenthal, 1970; Se-

mel & Wiig, 1975; Vogel, 1974; Wiig & Semel, 1975). Johnson and Myklebust (1967) have suggested that learning disabled children are not able to
retain the linguistic structure of sentences they hear; as a result, they do not
adequately control the linguistic patterns necessary to generate appropriately
structured sentences.

The development of expressive language and the control of syntactic structures and transformations in language production may be evaluated using
one or more of the following tests and measures: (1) *Measures of length and
complexity* (McCarthy, 1930; Davis, 1937; Templin, 1957; Johnson, Darley,
& Spriestersbach, 1963); (2) *Developmental Sentence Scoring* (Lee & Canter, 1971; Koenigsknecht & Lee, 1971; Lee, 1974); (3) the *Word Association
Test* (Brown & Berko, 1960); (4) the *Grammatic Closure* subtest of the *Illinois Test of Psycholinguistic Ability* (Kirk, McCarthy, & Kirk, 1968); (5) the
Michigan Picture Language Inventory (Lerea, 1958; Wolski, 1962); (6) the
Expressive subtest of the *Northwestern Syntax Screening Test* (Lee, 1969,
1971); and (7) *Sentence Repetition Tests* (Menyuk, 1963; Carrow, 1974;
Newcombe & Marshall, 1967).

Measures of Length and Complexity

The development of expressive language has been assessed extensively by
measures obtained from spontaneous language samples (Johnson, Darley, &
Spriestersbach, 1963). Among these measures are

1. Mean length of response (MLR)
2. Mean of the five longest responses (M5L)
3. Standard deviation of response length (SD−RL)
4. Number of one-word responses (N1W)
5. Number of different words (NDW)
6. Structural complexity score (SCS)

The spontaneous language sample providing the data for further analysis is
to be elicited and recorded verbatim or on audio tape. It should contain fifty
consecutive utterances, a sample size originally specified by McCarthy
(1930). It has later been observed to be the smallest sample size that results in
adequate reliability of the measures (Darley & Moll, 1960). The spontaneous
language samples have generally been elicited by using picture books or toys
(Davis, 1937; McCarthy, 1930; Templin, 1957). The procedure has been
slightly modified to include responses to interjected remarks or questions
from the examiner (Minifie, Darley, & Sherman, 1963; Shriner & Sherman,
1967).

Mean Length of Response (MLR) was introduced by Nice (1925) and has
later been used in extensive studies of language development by McCarthy
(1930) and Templin (1957). It is a relatively easy measure to obtain since it
requires only counting of the number of words in each utterance, totaling the
numbers, and dividing by fifty. It has been found to be the best single measure for assessing language development since it correlates positively (.80)
with psychological scale values of degree of language development (Shriner
& Sherman, 1967). Normative data for MLR have been reported for the age

range from one year nine months to nine years five months based on the results of nine studies (Johnson, Darley, & Spriestersbach, 1963, p. 188).

Shriner (1969) has reviewed the MLR as a measure of expressive language development. The MLR has been shown to vary as a function of manipulations and situational factors, indicating that it is sensitive to experimenter and stimulus bias; furthermore, it provides little information about changes in the control over morphology and syntax as a function of age. Cazden (1972) has also pointed to the fact that with development there is a greater density of ideas in a single sentence and embedding increases. In a similar vein, Hass and Wepman (1974) have also reported that the major syntactic change with age reflected increases in embeddedness.

The *Mean of the Five Longest Responses* (M5L) was suggested by Davis (1937) as an indicator of the child's maximum linguistic skills. It is obtained by counting the total number of words in the five longest utterances and dividing by five. This measure also correlates positively with psychological scale values of degree of language development (.77) (Shriner & Sherman, 1967). Normative data for the increase in M5L as a function of development have been presented by Templin (1957, p. 79).

The *Standard Deviation of Response Length* (Shriner & Sherman, 1967) provides a measure of the relative variability in sentence length. The SD−RL does not correlate with psychological scale values of degree of language development (.00) (Shriner & Sherman, 1967), suggesting limited value in diagnosis.

The *Number of One Word Responses* (N1W) has been used by Davis (1937) and Templin (1957) to assess relative language maturity. Templin (1957, p. 174) has presented normative data for this measure for the range from three to eight years. They indicate that the number of one-word responses decreases with age. N1W has been reported to correlate at -.59 with psychological scale values of degree of language development (Shriner & Sherman, 1967); this relatively low negative correlation suggests that this measure does not adequately predict the status of language development.

The *Number of Different Words* (NDW) was introduced as a measure of "use vocabulary" (Templin, 1957). Normative data have been presented for the range from three to eight years indicating that the number of different words in spontaneous language increases with age (Templin, 1957, p. 116). Shriner and Sherman (1967) have reported a positive correlation between this measure and psychological scale values of degree of language development (.78).

The *Structural Complexity Score* (SCS) has been used by Davis (1937), McCarthy (1930), and Templin (1957) as a quantitative measure of completeness and complexity. The SCS is obtained by classifying utterances and assigning weighted scores according to the following criteria (Johnson, Darley, & Spriestersbach, 1963, pp. 170-72):

1. Incomplete responses are assigned a score of zero.
2. Simple sentences (subject-predicate-object) or sentences with a compound subject, object, or predicate receive a score of one.
3. Simple sentences with two or more phrases are given a score of two.

4. Compound sentences are given a score of three.

5. Complex and elaborated sentences recieve a score of four.

Normative data for the Mean SCS have been reported for the range from three to eight years by Templin (1957, p. 191).

The reliability of the weighting procedure has been questioned by Darley and Moll (1960) and Minifie, Darley, & Sherman, (1963). Shriner and Sherman (1967) report a correlation coefficient of .76 between SCS and psychological-scale value of degree of language development. They suggest that the use of the structural complexity score could be improved by applying the results of linguistic analyses.

Developmental Sentence Scoring

This method of scoring (Lee & Canter, 1971; Koenigsknecht & Lee, 1971; Lee, 1974) was developed to provide a quantitative measure of children's syntactic development in spontaneous speech. It emphasizes eight grammatical-form categories which have been shown to have the most significant developmental progression in children's language: (1) indefinite pronoun or noun modifier, (2) personal pronoun, (3) main verb, (4) secondary verb, (5) negative, (6) conjunction, (7) interrogative reversal in questions, and (8) wh- question. The method of analysis is based on transformational generative grammar (Chomsky, 1957, 1965) and case grammar (Brown, 1973; Fillmore, 1968).

The *Developmental Sentence Scores* (DSS) are obtained from analysis of a spontaneous speech sample containing fifty complete sentences. Fragmentary and incomplete sentences are discarded from the sample. Sentences are considered complete when they express a subject-predicate relationship. Lee (1974) discusses methods for obtaining a representative spontaneous speech sample in a clinical setting. The following stimulus materials are suggested to stimulate the child's verbalizations: toys, pictures, or illustrations for a familiar story. The stimulus pictures suggested are from a preprimer series by Robinson, Monroe, and Artley (1962a, 1962b). The suggested illustrations for a familiar story, "The Three Bears," are from *What's its name?* (Utley, 1950).

All spontaneous speech samples are to be recorded on audio-tape for accurate transcription. Lee (1974) provides comprehensive guidelines for making allowances for articulatory errors, nonfluencies, grammatical reformulations, and word finding. The sample to be analyzed and scored must consist of a block of consecutive utterances. The procedure allows for exclusion of stereotyped repetitions, and unintelligible and echoed utterances.

Lee (1974) has suggested a separate analysis for *Developmental Sentence Types* (DST) to be used for presentence utterances, that is, fragmentary and incomplete sentences. This analysis is appropriate for preschoolers with significant language delays. The *Developmental Sentence Scoring* (DSS) procedure is suggested for the analysis of syntactic structures which involve elaboration of the basic subject-predicate construction or transformation.

In the DSS procedure, each grammatical form is scored independently using a weighted scoring system. The weighted scores reflect a progressive sequence of grammatical growth for each category, and scores range from one to eight points for the majority of the grammatical categories. In addition, a score of one is added for each sentence that meets adult English standards. This score is withheld for semantic irregularities, omissions, or confusions of syntactic rules and structures, and word-order changes.

Lee (1974) presents a Reweighted DSS scoring system (chart 8) and samples of analyzed speech samples (charts 10, 12, 14, 15). In addition, the scoring of each grammatical category is described in detail (pp. 138–63). The Developmental Sentence Score (DSS) reflects the mean value, that is, the sum of the individual sentence scores divided by the number of sentences.

Normative data are presented in the form of selected percentiles for the DSS scores of 160 children, from three years to six years eleven months old, by one-year intervals (Lee, 1974, p. 167). The DSS performance of an individual child may also be judged against the mean of a lower age group to obtain an estimate of the language delay (Lee, 1974, p. 169). Successive DSS scores may be further used to evaluate the rate of progress in response to language training (Lee, 1974, pp. 173–74). The author stresses that the method measures the degree of delay in the acquisition of syntax in spontaneous speech. It does not purport to provide a differential diagnosis of etiology or handicapping condition. An adaptation of the Developmental Sentence Analysis method has been developed for Spanish-speaking children (Toronto, 1972).

Koenigsknecht (1974) reported the results of extensive statistical analysis of the performances by the standardization group. The results indicated significant increases in syntax usage (DSS) as a function of age. The most discriminating DSS categories were main verbs, conjunctions, and indefinite pronouns-noun modifiers. The rank order of the remaining DSS categories from the most to the least discriminating was personal pronouns, secondary verbs, negatives, sentence points, wh- questions, and interrogative reversals. Measures of length of utterances and DSS increased progressively as a function of age. This finding suggests that length-maturity measures (McCarthy, 1930; Davis, 1937; Templin, 1957) and the present measures of the acquisition of syntax were related.

Analysis of the internal consistency of the DSS indicated increasing consistency between components of the test and the total test as a function of age with an overall reliability coefficient of .71. The split-half reliability coefficient for the DSS was .73, indicating good internal consistency. The DSS score was not found to vary significantly as a result of changes in the use of stimulus materials. There were, however, significant differences in the scores for four of the grammatical categories: indefinite pronouns, personal pronouns, secondary verbs, and interrogative reversals. When the DSS scores for four repeated applications within a two-week period were compared, there was a significant-trial effect, suggesting that the method should be limited to the assessment of longitudinal changes.

Developmental Sentence Scoring (DSS) has been reported to differentiate learning disabled (dyslexic) and achieving children (Vogel, 1974). Similarly, Slegman (1974) observed significant delays in the acquisition of syntax by four learning disabled ranging in age between ten years eight months and twelve years four months. Based on DSS scores within the various grammatical categories, their spontaneous speech was devoid of interrogative reversals and wh- questions. Negations were infrequent as were secondary verbs. These findings suggest that the DSS method may be used to identify deficits in the spontaneous control and production of specific grammatical categories in learning disabled children in the elementary grades. It seems of clinical-educational importance that the two grammatical categories, wh- questions and interrogative reversals, proved deficient. These categories were observed to be the least discriminating measures for the various age levels compared by Koenigsknecht (1974).

Word Association Test

Word association tasks such as the *Word Association Test* designed by Brown and Berko (1960) may be used to indirectly assess developmental delays in the acquisition of grammar. In this test, the immediate associative responses to count nouns, mass nouns, adjectives, transitive and intransitive verbs, and adverbs are recorded and scored based on the relationship to the stimulus words. Responses are scored as homogenous when they belong to the same part of speech as the stimulus word and as heterogeneous when they do not. Normal children in the first three grades exhibited an obvious increase in the number of homogeneous responses as a function of age, and the development of count nouns and adjectives preceded other parts of speech. Adults produced significantly more homogeneous responses than children.

The *Word Association Test* may provide information regarding the acquisition of grammar by some LD children in the early and middle grades. It appears able to complement or substantiate the results of other tests that tap linguistic rule learning. Bartel, Grill, & Bartel (1973) have, however, observed that learning disabled and normal children do not differ significantly in the shift from syntactic (across grammatical class) to paradigmatic (within grammatical class) word association. This observation suggests that the *Word Association Test* may not be sensitive enough to the language production deficits that may be associated with learning disabilities.

ITPA: Grammatic Closure

The *Grammatic Closure* subtest of the *Illinois Test of Psycholinguistic Ability* (Kirk, McCarthy, & Kirk, 1968) assesses the ability to formulate and complete sentences by applying the appropriate morphological and syntactic rules. The subtest contains thirty-three items requiring application of the rules for forming regular and irregular noun plurals, noun possessive singulars, noun derivations, regular and irregular past tenses, past participles, the adjective *any* and comparative and superlatives, adverbs, prepositions, and pronouns.

The subtest has been standardized for the range from two years two months to ten years four months, when a ceiling effect is evident in the average normal child. The consistency of the test results over time ranges from inadequate to good depending upon age with five-month stability coefficients ranging from .46 to .87. The reported internal reliability coefficients range from .60 to .74.

Learning disabled children have been observed to experience problems in applying rules for and formulating irregular noun plurals, noun possessives, irregular past tenses, past participles, comparative and superlative of adjectives, and pronouns. These problems may also be observed in spontaneous speech. The *Grammatic Closure* subtest may be used as a screening device to identify language disabled children with delays in the acquisition of productive control of syntactic rules. It does not provide in-depth analysis of problem areas.

Michigan Picture Language Inventory

This inventory (Lerea, 1958) assesses the expressive use of vocabulary and language structure. The language structure section of the test evaluates the formulation of the following grammatical categories: (1) singular and plural nouns, (2) personal pronouns, (3) possessives, (4) adjectives, (5) demonstratives, (6) articles, (7) adverbs, (8) prepositions, and (9) verbs and auxiliaries. The representation of items within these categories has been discussed in chapter 5 (pp. 120−21). The reliability coefficient for language structure expression (.95) indicates a high degree of consistency of the test results.

Normative data have been presented for four-, five-, and six-year-olds (Wolski, 1962). The data indicate that a ceiling effect was not established in six-year-olds, suggesting that the test may be used for children in the early grades. The advantages of the test are considered to relate to the diversity of the structures that are included and to the relative ease of administration. Guidelines have not been presented for the interpretation of error responses. The structure of the test lends itself to easy identifcation of areas of expressive deficits, and the format of the items may be duplicated in remedial intervention.

Northwestern Syntax Screening Test: Expressive

The *Expressive* portion of the *Northwestern Syntax Screening Test* (Lee, 1971) contains twenty items, each consisting of a sentence pair. They are presented in a progression that reflects the order of difficulty. Each sentence pair is represented pictorially on a page of the test manual. The examiner presents the sentence pair orally without identifying which picture is associated with each of the sentences. Subsequently, the examiner points to each of the pictures to elicit the test sentences while asking "What's this one?" and "What's that one?" Only verbatim repetitions of the original sentences are scored as correct. Responses that are not grammatically identical are not acceptable even though the intended grammatical distinction between the sentence pair may be retained. This procedure is justified on the basis that the grammatical structure being tested "may have introduced enough complexity to cause the specific structure to be dropped" (Lee, 1970, p. 109).

The test was designed to compare the receptive and expressive use of grammatical features and structures such as prepositions, personal pronouns, negatives, plurals, reflexive pronouns, verb tenses, subject-object identification, possessives, wh- and yes/no questions, passives, and indirect object transformation (Lee, 1970). It was standardized on 242 children between the ages of three years and seven years eleven months from middle and upper income communities. Data are presented for the nintieth, seventy-fifth, fiftieth, twenty-fifth, and tenth percentiles. Critical cut-off points (tenth percentile) are presented at one-year intervals. Toronto (1973) has recently developed a Spanish version of the test.

The test is considered a screening test only and was not designed to provide a detailed evaluation of syntactic skills in language production. This point has been emphasized in research by Prutting, Gallagher, and Mulac (1975). They compared responses to the items of the *Expressive* subtest of the NSST with the results of analysis of spontaneous language samples. The results indicated that, on the average, 30% of the children who missed a particular item on the NSST produced the grammatical feature correctly in spontaneous speech. The findings were considered to support the recommendation by Slobin and Welsh (1971, 1973) that information obtained from sentence repetition tasks should be supplemented by analysis of spontaneous language.

The NSST has been reported to differentiate between learning disabled and academically achieving children (Semel & Wiig, 1975). Performances on the *Expressive* and *Receptive* portions of the test correlated significantly and both correlated with measures of achievement on the *Peabody Individual Achievement Test* (PIAT) (Dunn & Markwardt, 1970). These findings suggest that the NSST may assist in identifying LD youngsters with delays in the acquisition of control of syntactic structures in expressive language. Because the test requires delayed recall of sentences, it may also tap aspects of the ability to retain the items in short-term memory through rehearsal and possibly the resistance to interference (Atkinson & Shiffrin, 1971; Murdock, 1962).

Sentence Repetition Tests

The knowledge and control of grammatical structure may be assessed using sentence repetition tasks. In this procedure, the need to obtain a sample of the child's or adolescent's spontaneous speech for comprehensive linguistic analysis is avoided. Sentence repetition tasks have been widely used to assess the linguistic competence of children, adolescents, and adults (Brown & Bellugi, 1964; Ervin, 1964; Fraser, Bellugi, & Brown, 1963; Luterman & Bar, 1971; Menyuk, 1964, 1969; Menyuk & Looney, 1972; Newcombe & Marshall, 1967; Wiig & Roach, 1975).

Ervin (1964) observed that the child's grammar was the same in spontaneous speech as in imitating the speech of adults. Furthermore, linguistic structures that cannot be related to deep structure tend to be omitted in the imitation of surface structure (McNeill, 1970). Experimental evidence consistently indicates interactions among grammatical structure and semantic aspects and memory for sentences (Blumenthal, 1967; Blumenthal & Boakes, 1967; Miller & Isard, 1964; Rohrman, 1968; Savin & Perchonock, 1965). This finding suggests a need for evaluating short-term auditory memory capacities using verbal stimuli without linguistic structure (digits, syllables, words) in association with sentence-imitation tasks.

Sentence repetition has been reported to differentiate among language disordered, learning disabled, and normal children, learning disabled and academically achieving adolescents, and brain-damaged aphasic and normal adults (Menyuk, 1964; Menyuk & Looney, 1972; Newcombe & Marshall, 1967; Rosenthal, 1970; Wiig & Roach, 1975).

Newcombe and Marshall (1967) extended the analytic possibilities of a sentence-repetition task by varying both the syntactic and semantic constraints. Their research indicated that deficits in the recall of syntactically and semantically varied sentences distinguished left-hemisphere-damaged (aphasic) from right-hemisphere-damaged and nonbrain-damaged adults. In a related study, Wiig and Roach (1975) reported that recall of these sentences also distinguished between learning disabled and academically achieving adolescents.

Among sentence-repetition tests that may be used for the differential diagnosis of deficits in the production of linguistic structures are (1) the *Model Elicited Imitation Sentences* (Menyuk, 1963); (2) the *Carrow Elicited Language Inventory* (Carrow, 1974); and (3) the *Newcombe-Marshall Experimental Sentences* (Newcombe & Marshall, 1967).

The *Model Elicited Imitation Sentences* (Menyuk, 1963) may be used to assess the child's control of sentence transformations in immediate recall. The experimental test contains twenty-seven sentences, ranging in length from three to nine words, designed to reflect the transformational rules used by nursery-school and kindergarten children to generate sentences. These rules were abstracted from responses to a projective test (Blum, 1950) and conversations with adults and age peers. The sentences reflect the following transformations: passive, negative, question, contraction, inversion, relative question, imperative, pronominalization, separation, *got*, auxiliary placement (be and have), *do*, possessive, reflexive, conjunction (deletion, *if, so, because*, pronouns), adjective, relative clause, complement, iteration, nominalization, and nominal compound.

The results of comparison between the nonrepetitions (omissions or modifications) by nursery-school and kindergarten children indicated significant growth in the imitative control of the transformations. Nursery-school children were able to repeat all items except (1) the question, "Are you nice," (2) *got*, I've got a lollipop," (3) auxiliary *have*, "I've already been there," (4) conjunction with *so*, "He saw him so he hit him," (5) conjunction with *because*, "He'll eat the ice cream because he wants to," and (6) nominalization, "She does the shopping and cooking and baking." Kindergarten children repeated all transformations except *got* and the auxiliary *have*. There was no correlation between nonrepetition of sentences and sentence length. The results also indicated that more children were able to control the transformations in repetition than in spontaneous language use.

These findings suggest that the *Model Elicited Imitation Sentences* may be used as a screening test in kindergarten and in the first grade to identify children with reductions in the imitative control of transformations. It may also be used to identify delays in the acquisition of imitative control of transformations by high-risk or LD children in the early grades.

The *Carrow Elicited Language Inventory* (Carrow, 1974) was designed to assess the child's productive control of grammar, using a sentence imitation procedure. It is based on the observation that "analysis of the imitations of systematically-varied model sentences can determine the child's knowledge of transformational rules and the syntactic and semantic markers borne by lexical items" (Slobin & Welsh, 1973, p. 2). The procedure is described to allow analysis of grammatic forms and syntactic structures that the child may be capable of producing in imitation but may not produce in a spontaneous language sample.

The inventory contains fifty-two stimuli, fifty-one sentences and one phrase. The verbal stimuli range in length from two to ten words (mean six words). The stimuli were developed to contain basic sentence types and specific grammatical morphemes and transformations. The stimuli have been classified as follows: (1) forty-seven are active and four are passive, (2) thirty-seven are affirmative, fourteen negative, (3) thirty-seven are declarative, twelve interrogative, and two imperative. The grammatical categories and features have been classified and include: nouns (59), noun plurals (8), verbs (103), adjectives (9), adverbs (12), pronouns (41); articles (41), negatives (13), prepositions (14), demonstratives (2), conjunctions (7), and contractions (12). Examples of stimuli are the first item, *Big girl* (phrase) and the last, "If it rains, we won't go to the beach."

The stimulus phrase and sentences are read by the examiner. The child's imitations are recorded on audio-tape to permit analysis of responses and of error patterns. Total error scores and subscores for each grammatical category and error types may be obtained. The test manual provides directions for scoring error types (substitutions, omissions, additions, transpositions, reversals). Normative data were developed on the 475 children who were also used for the standardization procedures. The raw scores for the total test are converted to derived scores. Normative data for mean total error scores and mean subcategory error scores are provided at one-year intervals for the age range from three years to seven years eleven months. Percentile rank scores and stanine scores (normalized standard scores) are also provided to determine an individual child's relative performance in relation to the standardization sample.

The author describes the inventory as a diagnostic tool that may be used to (1) identify children with language problems, (2) determine which linguistic structures contribute to inadequate linguistic performance, and (3) quantify language status. She cautions that performance reductions may reflect auditory memory deficits, suggesting that other tests need to be used in conjunction with the inventory for appropriate diagnosis.

The scoring and analysis forms accompanying the inventory provide a detailed scoring section and verb protocol which prove of value in determining areas for educational or clinical intervention. The verb protocol classifies each verb as modal, auxiliary, copula, verb, infinitive, or gerund. The structure of the sentence in which the verb occurs is also specified as declarative, interrogative, negative, or affirmative. Finally, the error type may be specified to reflect incorrectly formulated tense, person, or number.

The *Newcombe-Marshall Experimental Sentences* (Newcombe & Marshall, 1967) may be used to assess the effects of varying linguistic and semantic constraints on immediate recall. The twenty sentences contain between five and nine words and were constructed to include the following sentence types:

1. Fully grammatical and meaningful sentences, varying in length and complexity, for example, "The boy hit the girl" and "Wasn't the stone wall built by the kind husband?"
2. Grammatically well-formed sentences that were semantically deviant and violated selectional rules of the grammar, for example, "Colorless green ideas sleep furiously."
3. Well-formed sentences (semantically and syntactically) for which the possibility of semantic confusion between subject and object nouns exists (reversible sentences), for example, "Didn't the lion chase the tiger?"
4. Sentences containing modifier strings in correct and incorrect order, for example, "She has bought five large brown leather cases" and "She has washed plastic red small eight cups."
5. Random word strings, for example, "Walk some by hard of clearly table very."

The twenty experimental sentences have been presented in Chapter 4, Table 7.

In experimental use, the sentences are read individually, in random order, and subjects are required to repeat each sentence immediately after hearing it. For diagnostic purposes, the sequence of presentation may be adapted to avoid two sentences of similar type or similar transformations being presented consecutively. Normative data are not available for comparison with age expectations. The sentences may be used with LD, language-disordered adolescents and young adults for the differentiation of linguistic coding difficulties. The research by Wiig and Roach (1975) indicated that learning disabled adolescents exhibited significant reductions in the recall of sentences that violated semantic (selectional) rules, contained correctly and incorrectly sequenced modifier strings, contained a random word string, or were syntactically complex with embedding. Similar observations in the diagnostic use of the test would suggest heavy dependence on semantic aspects for language processing, deficits in linguistic processing, and short-term memory and sequencing problems for modifier strings.

References

Aten, J., & Davis, J. Disturbances in the perception of auditory sequence in children with minimal brain dysfunction. *Journal of Speech and Hearing Research*, 1968, **11**, 236-45.

Atkinson, R. C., & Shiffrin, R. M. The control of short-term memory. *Scientific American*, 1971, **225** (2), 82-90.

Baker, H. J., & Leland, B. *Detroit tests of learning aptitude*. Indianapolis: Test Division of Bobbs-Merrill, 1959.

Bannatyne, A. *Language, reading, and learning disabilities*. Springfield, Ill.: Charles C Thomas, 1971.

Bartel, N. R., Grill, J. J., & Bartel, H. W. The syntactic-paradigmatic shift in learning disabled and normal children. *Journal of Learning Disabilities*, 1973, **6**, 59-64.

Blum, G. S. *The Blacky pictures*. New York: Psychological Corp., 1950.

Blumenthal, A. L. Prompted recall of sentences. *Journal of Verbal Learning and Verbal Behavior*, 1967, **6**, 203-6.

Blumenthal, A. L., & Boakes, R. Prompted recall of sentences. *Journal of Verbal Learning and Verbal Behavior*, 1967, **6**, 674-76.

Bousfield, W., Cohen, B., & Whitmarsh, G. Associative clustering of words of different taxonomic frequencies of occurrence. *Psychological Reports*, 1958, **4**, 39-44.

Brown, R. *A first language: the early stages*. Cambridge: Harvard University Press, 1973.

Brown, R., & Bellugi, U. Three processes in the child's acquisition of syntax. *Harvard Educational Review*, 1964, **34**, 133-50.

Brown, R., & Berko, J. Word association and the acquisition of grammar. *Child Development*, 1960, **31**, 1-14.

Carrow, E. *Carrow elicited language inventory*. Austin, Tex.: Learning Concepts, 1974.

Cazden, C. B. *Child language and education*. New York: Holt, Rinehart & Winston, 1972.

Chomsky, N. *Syntactic structures*. The Hague: Mouton, 1957.

Chomsky, N. *Aspects of the theory of syntax*. Cambridge: M.I.T. Press, 1965.

Cohen, J. The factorial structure of the WISC at ages 7½, 10½, and 13½. *Journal of Consulting Psychology*, 1959, **23**, 285-99.

Cronbach, L. J. *Essentials of psychological testing*. (3rd ed.) New York: Harper & Row, 1970.

Darley, F. L., & Moll, K. L. Reliability of language measures and size of language sample. *Journal of Speech and Hearing Disorders*, 1960, **3**, 166-73.

Davis, E. *The development of linguistic skills in twins, singletons with siblings, and only children from age five to ten years*. Minneapolis: University of Minnesota Press, 1937.

Denckla, M. B. Naming of pictured objects by dyslexic and non-dyslexic "MBD" children. Paper presented at the Academy of Aphasia, 1974.

Dunn, L. M., & Markwardt, F. C. *Peabody individual achievement test*. Circle Pines, Minn.: American Guidance Service, 1970.

Ervin, S. M. Imitation and structural change in children's language. In E. H. Lenneberg (Ed.), *New directions in the study of language*. Cambridge: M.I.T. Press, 1964. Pp. 163-89.

Fillmore, C. J. The case for case. In E. Bach & R. T. Harms (Eds.), *Universals in linguistic theory*. New York: Holt, Rinehart & Winston, 1968.

Fraser, C., Bellugi, U., & Brown, R. Control of grammar in imitation, comprehension, and production. *Journal of Verbal Learning and Verbal Behavior*, 1963, **2**, 121-35.

Gerjoy, I., & Spitz, H. Associative clustering in free recall: intellectual and developmental variables. *American Journal of Mental Deficiency*, 1966, **70**, 918-27.

Glasser, A. J., & Zimmerman, I. L. *Clinical interpretation of the Wechsler intelligence scale for children*. New York: Grune & Stratton, 1967.

Goodglass, H., & Kaplan, E. *Boston diagnostic aphasia examination*. Philadelphia: Lea & Febiger, 1972.

Guilford, J. P. *The nature of human intelligence*. New York: McGraw-Hill, 1967.

Hainsworth, P. K., & Siqueland, M. L. *Early identification of children with learning disabilities: the Meeting Street School screening test*. Providence, R. I.: Crippled Children and Adults of Rhode Island, 1969.

Hass, W. A., & Wepman, J. M. Dimensions of individual difference in the spoken syntax of school children. *Journal of Speech and Hearing Research*, 1974, **17**, 455-69.

Johnson, W., Darley, F. L., & Spriestersbach, D. C. *Diagnostic methods in speech pathology*. New York: Harper & Row, 1963.

Johnson, D. J., & Myklebust, H. R. *Learning disabilities: educational principles and practices*. New York: Grune & Stratton, 1967.

Kirk, S. A., McCarthy, J. J., & Kirk, W. D. *Illinois test of psycholinguistic ability*: (Rev. ed.) Urbana: University of Illinois Press, 1968.

Koenigsknecht, R. A. Statistical information on developmental sentence analysis. In L. L. Lee (Ed.), *Developmental sentence analysis*. Evanston, Ill.: Northwestern University Press, 1974. Pp. 222-68.

Koenigsknecht, R. A., & Lee, L. L. Validity and reliability of developmental sentence scoring: a method for measuring syntactic development in children's spontaneous speech. Paper presented at the American Speech and Hearing Association Convention, Chicago, 1971.

Lee, L. *Northwestern syntax screening test*. Evanston, Ill.: Northwestern University Press, 1969, 1971.

Lee, L.A. screening test for syntax development. *Journal of Speech and Hearing Disorders*, 1970, **35**, 103-12.

Lee, L. *Developmental sentence analysis*. Evanston, Ill.: Northwestern University Press, 1974.

Lee, L. L., & Canter, S. M. Developmental sentence scoring: a clinical procedure for estimating syntactic development in children's spontaneous speech. *Journal of Speech and Hearing Disorders*, 1971, **36**, 315-40.

Lerea, L. Assessing language development. *Journal of Hearing Research*, 1958, **1**, 75-85.

Lerner, J. *Children with learning disabilities*. Boston: Houghton Mifflin Co., 1971.

Lindsay, P. H., & Norman, D. A. *Human information processing: an introduction to psychology*. New York: Academic Press, 1972.

Luterman, L. B., & Bar, A. The diagnostic significance of sentence repetition for language impaired children. *Journal of Speech and Hearing Disorders*, 1971, **36**, 29-39.

McCarthy, D. *The language development of the preschool child*. Minneapolis: University of Minnesota Press, 1930.

McCarthy, D. *McCarthy scales of children's abilities*. New York: Pscyhological Corp., 1970.

McCarthy, J. J., & McCarthy, J. F. *Learning disabilities*. Boston: Allyn & Bacon, 1969.

McNeill, D. *The acquisition of language: the study of developmental psycholinguistics*. New York: Harper & Row, 1970.

Menyuk, P. A preliminary evaluation of grammatical capacity in children. *Journal of Verbal Learning and Verbal Behavior*, 1963, **2**, 429-39.

Menyuk, P. Comparison of grammar of children with functionally deviant and normal speech. *Journal of Speech and Hearing Research*, 1964, **7**, 109-21.

Menyuk, P. *Sentences children use*. Cambridge: M.I.T. Press, 1969.

Menyuk, P., & Looney, P. A problem of language disorder: length versus structure. *Journal of Speech and Hearing Research*, 1972, **15**, 264-79.

Miller, G. A., & Isard, S. Free recall of self-embedded English sentences. *Information and Control*, 1964, **7**, 292-303.

Minifie, F. D., Darley, F. L., & Sherman, D. Temporal reliability of seven language measures. *Journal of Speech and Hearing Research*, 1963, **6**, 139-49.

Murdock, B. B., Jr. The serial effect of free recall. *Journal of Experimental Psychology*, 1962, **64**, 482-88.

Newcombe, F., & Marshall, J. C. Immediate recall of sentences by subjects with unilateral cerebral lesions. *Neuropsychologia*, 1967, **5**, 329-34.

Nice, M. M. Length of sentences as a criterion of a child's progress in speech. *Journal of Educational Psychology*, 1925, **16**, 370-79.

Prutting, C. A., Gallagher, T. M., & Mulac, A. The expressive portion of the NSST compared to a spontaneous language sample. *Journal of Speech and Hearing Disorders*, 1975, **40**, 40-48.

Robinson, H. M., Monroe, M., & Artley, A. S. *Before we read*. Chicago: Scott Foresman & Co., 1962. (a)

Robinson, H. M., Monroe, M., & Artley, A. S. *We read pictures*. Chicago: Scott Foresman & Co., 1962. (b)

Rockeach, M. *The three Christs of Ypsilanti*. New York: Alfred A. Knopf, 1964.

Rohrman, N. The role of syntactic structure in the recall of English nominalizations. *Journal of Verbal Learning and Verbal Behavior*, 1968, **7**, 904-12.

Rosenthal, J. H. A preliminary psycholinguistic study of children with learning disabilities. *Journal of Learning Disabilities*, 1970, **3**, 391-95.

Savin, H., & Perchonock, E. Grammatical structure and the immediate recall of English sentences. *Journal of Verbal Learning and Verbal Behavior*, 1965, **4**, 348-53.

Semel, E. M., & Wiig, E. H. Comprehension of syntactic structures and critical verbal elements by children with learning disabilities. *Journal of Learning Disabilities*, 1975, **8**, 53-58.

Shriner, T. H., A review of mean length of response as a measure of expressive language development in children. *Journal of Speech and Hearing Disorders*, 1969, **14**, 61-67.

Shriner, T. H., & Sherman, D. An equation for assessing language development. *Journal of Speech and Hearing Research*, 1967, **10**, 41-48.

Slegman, D. Sentence formulation deficits of learning-disabled children. Unpublished clinical paper, Boston University, 1974.

Slobin, D., & Welsh, C. A. Elicited imitation as a research tool in developmental psycholinguistics. In C. Lavatelli (Ed.), *Language training in early childhood education*. Urbana: University of Illinois Press, 1971. Pp. 170-85.

Slobin, D. I., & Welsh, C. A. Elicited imitation as a research tool in developmental psycholinguistics. In C. Ferguson & D. Slobin (Eds.), *Studies of child language development*. New York: Holt, Rinehart & Winston, 1973. Pp. 485-97.

Templin, M. C. *Certain language skills in children*. Minneapolis: University of Minnesota Press, 1957.

Terman, L. M., & Merrill, M. A. *Stanford-Binet intelligence scale*. Boston: Houghton Mifflin Co., 1960.

Toronto, A. S. A developmental Spanish language analysis procedure for Spanish-speaking children. Doctoral dissertation, Northwestern University, 1972.

Toronto, A. S. *Spanish syntax screening test*. Evanston, Ill.: Northwestern University Press, 1973.

Utley, J. *What's its name*. Urbana: University of Illinois Press, 1950.

Vogel, S. A. Syntactic abilities in normal and dyslexic children. *Journal of Learning Disabilities*, 1974, **7**, 47-53.

Wechsler, D. *Manual for the WISC*. New York: Psychological Corp., 1949.

Whimby, A. E., & Fischhof, V. Memory span: a forgotten capacity. *Journal of Educational Psychology*, 1969, **60**, 56-58.

Whimby, A. E., & Ryan, S. F. Role of short-term memory and training in solving reasoning problems mentally. *Journal of Educational Psychology*, 1969, **60**, 361-64.

Wiig, E. H., Lapointe, C., & Semel, E. M. Relationships among language processing and production abilities of learning-disabled adolescents. Paper presented at the Annual Convention of the American Speech and Hearing Association, Washington, D.C., 1975.

Wiig, E. H., & Roach, M. A. Immediate recall of semantically and syntactically varied "sentences" by learning-disabled adolescents. *Perceptual and Motor Skills*, 1975, **40**, 119-25.

Wiig, E. H., & Semel, E. M. Productive language abilities in learning disabled adolescents. *Journal of Learning Disabilities*, 1975, **8**, 578-86.

Wolski, W., Language development of normal children four, five, and six years of age as measured by the Michigan picture language inventory. Unpublished doctoral dissertation, University of Michigan, 1962.

Zigmond, N. K. Auditory processes in children with learning disabilities. In L. Tarnapol (Ed.), *Learning disabilities: introduction to educational and medical management*. Springfield, Ill.: Charles C Thomas, 1969. Pp. 196-216.

10 Remediation of Language Production Deficits

Overview

The present chapter introduces principles and methods for remedial intervention with children and adolescents with language production deficits. Remedial strategies are discussed which focus on improving (1) auditory memory for words, phrases, and sentences, (2) convergent and divergent production of language, and (3) productive control of syntax. The rationales for selecting areas for remedial intervention, deciding the purpose of intervention, and developing remedial procedures and methods are discussed against a background of available research.

The principles and methods introduced for improving auditory memory are based on knowledge of (a) the organization of memory based on models introduced by, among others, Bartlett (1932), Cofer (1941, 1967, 1973), Guilford (1967), Miller (1956), and Simon and Chase (1973); (b) factors that influence immediate recall and retrieval from long-term memory store; and (c) order of difficulty of contents based on psycholinguistic research. Principles and methods for improving immediate recall of verbal materials are discussed separately from the principles and methods introduced for improving delayed recall.

Variables that have been observed to facilitate retrieval from long-term memory are introduced and cueing techniques based on formal data (Tulving, 1974) and clinical observations are suggested. A variety of methods and procedures are discussed for improving convergent and divergent semantic production. Among these are conceptual grouping, sentence completion, verbal analogies, and cloze procedures. Among methods and techniques introduced for improving the productive control of syntax are *Interactive Language Development Teaching* (Lee, Koenigsknecht, & Mulhern, 1975), rearranging scrambled sentences, sentence completion, cloze procedures, and sentence formulation which incorporates key words. Sources for additional methods or programmed materials are suggested.

Improving Auditory Memory for
Words, Phrases, and Sentences

Language production deficits associated with learning disabilities have been reported to reflect, among others:

1. Reductions in the speed and accuracy with which words, phrases, and sentences can be recalled and retrieved (Bannatyne, 1971; Denckla, 1974; Johnson & Myklebust, 1967; Wiig & Semel, 1975).
2. Deficits in the convergent production of semantic units, classes, and relations (Wiig & Semel, 1975).
3. Deficits in the divergent production of semantic units (Wiig & Semel, 1975).
4. Delays in the acquistion of control of syntactic structures and transformations in language production (Semel & Wiig, 1975; Vogel, 1974; Wiig & Roach, 1975; Wiig & Semel, 1975).

Ahmann and Glock (1971) have suggested that language production is facilitated by cognitive storage and retrieval in association with affective domain behaviors such as internalization of ideas, practices, standards, or values and psychomotor behaviors such as sensory perception and mental, physical, and emotional set. In a similar vein, Winitz (1973) has emphasized that language processing and comprehension is based primarily on recognition but language production involves retrieval and recall. On this basis, the remediation of language production deficits should not be emphasized before adequate cognitive and linguistic processing skills have been established.

Remediation procedures designed to improve the language production abilities of learning disabled children and adolescents must focus on each of the observed deficit areas. It is also recognized that auditory memory factors may affect both language processing and production.

Accordingly, the auditory memory and verbal retention deficits which may be associated with learning disabilities should receive attention in designing a program of remediation (Aten & Davis, 1968; Grossman, 1972; Johnson & Myklebust, 1967; Semel & Wiig, 1975; Wiig & Roach, 1975). On this basis, remediation procedures for deficits in the retention and immediate recall of words, phrases, and sentences will be dealt with as part of the discussion of improving language production abilities.

Definitions and Organization of Memory

In its widest sense, memory can be defined as the conservation of acquired reactions. Piaget and Inhelder (1973) modify this definition by referring to (1) "memory in the wider sense" and (2) "memory in the strict sense." Memory in the wider sense refers to the type of memory involving the "conservation of schemata," that is, the ability to reproduce whatever can be generalized in a system of actions or operations (habitual, sensori-motor, conceptual operational, and other schemata) (p. 4). Memory in the strict sense refers to reactions associated with recognition or recall (p. 4).

The development of memory with age is considered to be closely related to the structuring activities of intelligence. In the developmental sequence, recognition memory develops before recollection memory which is considered dependent upon the semiotic functions, that is, use of figurative symbols, and upon conceptual representation or representative images. The following quote describes the relationship between memory and cognition:

> once we realize that, in order to discover an organization, we must either construct it at least reconstruct it, things begin to look quite different, and once we consider the memory adequate to this construction or reconstruction, we must also grant that it has an inner capacity for organization or reorganization, isomorphous with that of intelligence. But, in that case, there is no reason for separating the two, rather must we consider the memory as part of intelligence, though differentiated and specialized to perform a precise task, namely, the structuring of the past. . . . [Piaget & Inhelder, 1973, pp. 400-401]

The view that verbal memory is a constructive, generative, and productive process is shared by Bartlett (1932) and Cofer (1941, 1967, 1973), among others. It has received support from several investigations of verbal memory (Bransford & Franks, 1971; Jarvella, 1971; Sachs, 1967). These studies have indicated that (1) the exact (verbatim) memory for verbal material is not long-lasting, (2) memory for meaning is preserved over time while memory for wording and linguistic structure is discarded. Tzeng (1972) has also established that sentence recognition reflects established schemata that govern a person's judgments whether or not sentences are old or new.

The organization of memory is described differently by authorities. Piaget and Inhelder (1973) differentiate three major hierarchic types of memory, each of which contains several subclasses. These are (1) *recognitive memory*, involving the assimilation of data into schemata, (2) *mnemonic reconstruction*, involving intentional reproduction of an action or its results, and (3) *mnemonic recall*, involving internalized reconstruction based on the "memory image."

Guilford (1967) distinguishes between short- and long-term memory and between various memory factors. In relationship to language, memory factors have been reported for (1) semantic units, (2) semantic classes, (3) semantic relations (associative-memory), (4) semantic systems, (5) semantic transformations, and (6) semantic implications. The perceived relationship between memory and cognition is expressed in the statement: "There is memory if, and only if, there has been cognition" (p. 211). The relationship between memory and language production is expressed as follows: "The distinction between memory abilities and production abilities means that retention and retrieval of information are distinctly different operations. Of course, if there has been no retention, there cannot be retrieval" (p. 136).

Miller (1956) supports a dual-stage memory process consisting of short-and long-term memory. He observed invariances in memory-span experiments which indicated that the short-term memory capacity is about seven, plus or minus two familiar units or chunks of any kind. The existence of chunks, that is, coherent memory or perceptual units, in language processing and recall has since been supported by research (Fodor and Bever, 1965; McLean & Gregg, 1967). Fodor and Bever (1965) observed that the major syntactic break in sentences influenced the subjective location of noise (clicks) perceived during speech. These findings suggested that segments of sentences marked by constituent structure analysis, such as the noun or verb phrase, function as perceptual units (chunks).

McLean and Gregg (1967) observed that stimulus grouping facilitated serial verbal learning. The effect of stimulus grouping (induced chunking) was also evident in the backward recall of verbal series. The chunks were furthermore observed to be stable, especially for stimulus groupings of three and four. When the stimuli were presented one at a time, stable chunks were also produced but they varied in size, that is, in the number of units contained in a chunk. Other studies have supported that chunks (memory or perceptual units) can be induced. Bollinger and Gerstman (1957) demonstrated that in the absence of other cues and isolated from sentences, acoustic pauses can induce structural organization (chunks).

Simon and Chase (1973) have reviewed investigations of relative efficiency in chess-playing tasks. The mechanisms involved have suggested a memory system with (1) a limited-capacity short-term memory, (2) a vast repertory of familiar patterns stored as chunks in long-term memory and a recognition mechanism for retrieval, and (3) a related chunking process. They have presented data which support that a limited-capacity short-term visual memory can be bypassed by perceptual knowledge, acquired through experience based on chunking, and stored in long-term memory. They propose that "the length of time required for a learning task will be proportional to the number of new chunks that have to be familiarized in order to perform the task" (p. 399).

These findings have direct bearing upon remedial strategies and procedures. In combination with observations that in long-term memory the act of recall increases the strength of the memory trace (Horowitz, Norman, & Day, 1966; Tulving, 1967), they suggest that remedial procedures emphasizing immediate recall may result in improved performances on tasks requiring recall from long-term memory.

Factors Influencing Short-Term Auditory Memory

In designing remediation strategies to improve auditory-verbal memory, procedures emphasizing short-term auditory memory processes must be delimited from those emphasizing long-term auditory memory. Short-term auditory memory, measured by the immediate recall of auditory-verbal input, may be facilitated by several variables. Among those that must be considered in planning remediation are (1) word frequency, (2) associative strength, (3) linguistic structure, (4) logical relationship, (5) length, (6) suprasegmental features, (7) salience, that is, immediate relevance to the individual, and (8) serial position.

Word Frequency

Word frequency may affect the immediate recall of verbal materials, in that a series of high-frequency words such as *man, woman, dog* is more easily recalled than a series of lower-frequency words such as *rose, tulip, uncle*. In order to account for word frequency in planning remediation, the educator may consult reference works that provide word counts and indices of relative frequency in English (Rinsland, 1945; Thorndike & Lorge, 1944).

Associative Strength

The associative strength between words in sequences may affect the immediate recall, in that word sequences with a high degree of association such as *knife-fork-spoon* are easier to recall than unrelated word sequences such as *dog-car-apple*. There are several reference works that may be used to establish the associative relationships between words when planning remediation. Among these are the free association norms reported by Palermo and Jenkins (1964) and the restricted association norms reported by Riegel (1965).

Linguistic Structure

The linguistic structure of sentences is known to influence the immediate recall. Savin and Perchonock (1965) have reported the mean number of words recalled in a variety of sentences and sentence transformations. Based on these means, the order of difficulty in the immediate recall of sentences progresses from the easiest to the hardest as follows: (1) active declarative, (2) wh- question, (3) question (yes/no), (4) passive, (5) negative, (6) negative question, (7) emphatic, (8) passive question, (9) negative passive question, (10) emphatic passive, and (11) negative passive.

Menyuk and Looney (1972) investigated the accuracy of sentence repetitions by language-disordered and normally speaking children, ranging in age from four years five months to seven years nine months. They observed that normally speaking children were able to repeat imperative, active—declarative, negative, and question sentences with little difficulty. They experienced only slightly greater difficulty with a negative subject and a passive sentence. The language-disordered children demonstrated that some sentence types (imperative and active-declarative) were less difficult than negative, question, negative subject, and passive sentences. Within the group of more difficult sentences the order of difficulty progressed as follows: (1) negative, (2) question, (3) negative subject, and (4) passive.

Wiig and Roach (1975) observed a similar order of difficulty in the immediate recall of sentences by LD adolescents. It progressed from the easiest to the most difficult as follows: (1) active-declarative without adjective sequences, (2) question (yes/no), (3) negative question, (4) relative clause transformation (embedding), and (5) active-declarative sentences with extended adjective sequences.

Sachs (1967) has reported data which support that "Form which is not relevant to the meaning is normally not retained." The data indicated that subjects were able to recognize semantic and syntactic changes in sentences with no intervening delays. When sentences were presented with about twenty-seven seconds delay, syntactic changes were not recognized consistently; in contrast, semantic changes were consistently recognized with delays of about forty-six seconds.

The combined findings suggest that the educator must consider the order of presentation of various sentence types in planning remediation. Furthermore, recall of sentence structure must be required immediately and recall of semantic aspects may be delayed.

Logical Relationship

The logical relationship between words may also influence immediate recall. Word sequences which are logically related such as "Put the car in the garage" appear easier to retain and recall than sequences with a less logical or illogical relationship; for example, "Put the car on top of the roof."

Zivian (1966) investigated word identification as a function of the semantic (logical) relationship and restricted association strength of verbal cues using college students as subjects. The cues for the word identification task were related to the target word at either high or low restricted association strength and with either a logical (class membership or class relationship) or infralogical (temporal or spatial) relationship based on the Michigan Restricted Association Norms (Riegel, 1965). An example of a logical cue for the target word *car* would be: similar . . . *auto,* while an infralogical cue would be: location . . . *garage.*

The results indicated that more correct target words were given to clues with high restricted association strength than to clues with low restricted association strength. More target words were also identified from logical than from infralogical cues.

Wiig and Globus (1971) observed similar patterns of facilitation of target word identification for aphasic and non-brain-damaged adults. The results indicated:

1. The most facilitating cues combined high restricted association strength and logical (class membership) relationship.
2. The second most efficient cues combined high restricted association strength and infralogical (spatial and temporal) relationship.
3. The third most facilitating cues combined low restricted association strength and infralogical relationship.
4. The least efficient cues combined low restricted association strength and logical relationship.

The educator may use the work by Riegel (1965) as a reference in considering logical relationships between the words used in remediation.

Length of Sequences

The length of word sequences will influence immediate recall differently depending upon the structural aspects of the sequence. Length is a critical variable in digit recall and in the recall of unrelated words (Baker & Leland, 1959; Terman & Merrill, 1960; Wechsler, 1949). Sentence recall, however, appears much less sensitive to length than to structure (Menyuk & Looney, 1972; Savin & Perchonock, 1965; Wiig & Roach, 1975). As a result, the educator should consider structural aspects as well as length in using verbal materials for remediation. When structure is absent and recall is minimally facilitated by associative and logical relationships, the consideration of length becomes critical. The number of units (length) incorporated in the verbal materials should be determined by (1) the maximum number of units that can be retained by the individual youngster and (2) the number of units that can be retained by the child's age peers based on normative data.

Normative data from the Stanford-Binet (Terman & Merrill, 1960) indicate the following relationships between chronological age and the mean number of digits that can be recalled:

Age	Number of digits (forward) recalled
2 1/2 years	2
3 years	3
4 1/2 years	4
7 years	5
10 years	6
Adulthood	7

Johnson and Myklebust (1967) have reported that dyslexic children may demonstrate better immediate recall for unrelated words than for sentences, though they may perform below age level. This observation is interpreted to indicate that syntactical deficits may interfere with the immediate recall of both the structure and meaning of sentences.

Suprasegmental Features

Suprasegmental features such as intonation contours (phrasing) and stress patterns may facilitate word and sentence recall (Blasdell & Jensen, 1970; Sitko & Semmel, 1967). It is easier to recall a set of seven digits when they are divided into two chunks (perceptual units) by intonation contours, stress, and juncture. Telephone numbers are more easily recalled when the seven digits are divided into two groups, and the digits in each group are held together by a common intonation contour. Sentences said in a monotonous voice are harder to recall than sentences with normal intonation patterns.

Sitko and Semmel (1967) have studied the effects of phrasal cueing on free recall by EMR and nonretarded children. They observed that recall was facilitated by suprasegmental cueing in the following order from most to least effective:

a. Phrasal cueing with correct syntactic structure. (The baby/who ate the food/drank the milk.)

b. Linear cueing with correct syntax. (The/baby/who/ate/ the/food/drank/the/milk.)

    c. Distorted phrasal cueing with correct syntax. (The boy who/got the horse saw/the fish)

    d. Phrasal cueing with distorted syntax. (Dog the/man the bit who/cat the chased.)

    e. Linear cueing with distorted syntax. (Bird/the/worm/the/dropped/who/bath/the/took.)

    f. Distorted phrasal cueing with distorted syntax. (Dog the man/the bit who cat/the chased.)

Salience

Word salience, that is, the relevance or value of a word to an individual, has been observed to influence the grouping of kinship terms. Romney and D'Andrade (1964) observed that the terms *mother* and *father* were of high salience to high school youngsters while *daughter* and *son* were of low salience. Similarly, words and sentences with high salience seem easier to recall than their low salience counterparts. Since salience is a subjective variable, the relative salience for words must be established with the individual youngster. To some youngsters cars and mechanical items may be of high salience; to others food items may be of greater personal value. The youngster may be asked to indicate hobbies and favorite activities before the content and vocabulary to be used in remediation is established.

Serial Position

The serial position of words or elements of a stimulus series affects recall in that final elements are easier to recall than initial elements, and middle elements are hardest to recall (Jarvella, 1971; Murdock, 1962). Children with deviant language development have been reported to recall only final elements and less frequently to retain only initial elements (Menyuk, 1969). In contrast, LD adolescents recalled the initial words in sentences better than the final elements but the middle elements were least well recalled (Wiig & Roach, 1975). The combined findings suggest that expansion of sentences to improve chunking should occur first in the final phrase, next in the initial phrase, and finally in the middle portion.

    Among other factors observed to affect memory are (1) intensity of attention, (2) interest in subject, and (3) amount of drill and overlearning (Marsh, 1973). The educator should attempt to control as many as possible of the variables that may influence short-term auditory memory and immediate recall. Some variables may be controlled when intervention materials are selected or designed. Others, such as attention, interest in subject, and amount of drill and overlearning must be considered during each session and may vary from youngster to youngster.

Improving Short-Term Memory

The purpose of intervention for short-term auditory memory deficits may not be to increase the number of units (digits, syllables, words, etc.) which can be retained by the language disabled child. Observations suggest that the educator may have little success in expanding short-term memory capacities by emphasizing the number of units that are retained. This observation is supported by results indicating that *Interactive Language Development Teaching* (Lee, Koenigsknecht, & Mulhern, 1975) has resulted in significant gains in a variety of receptive and expressive language abilities with the exception that *Auditory Sequential Memory* (ITPA) measures were not improved. The emphasis in remediation must instead be on increasing the size of the perceptual-conceptual units (chunks) that can be retained.

Efficient chunking in processing auditory language appears to depend upon establishing adequate perceptual, cognitive-semantic, and linguistic processing strategies. This observation suggests that remediation procedures designed to improve language processing should precede procedures designed to improve short-term auditory memory abilities. Winitz (1973) has emphasized a similar sequence in foreign language learning, stating that language processing involves primarily recognition but language production depends upon recall and retrieval. Chunking of digit and word series may be induced by association, meaning, pairing syllables, ease of pronunciation, familiarity, or phrasing (Blasdell & Jensen, 1970; Kausler, 1974).

Recall of Word Sequences

Procedures designed to improve the recall of word sequences should progress using sequences with increasingly weaker associative-logical relationships:

1. Related:
    Apple - pear
    Apple - pear - orange - banana
    Apple - orange - pear - banana
    Pear - banana - orange - apple
2. Unrelated:
    Clock - jet
    Turtle - shoe
    Clock - jet - turtle
    Clock - jet - turtle - shoe
    Clock - turtle - jet - shoe
    Turtle - clock - shoe - jet

Recall of Sentences

Materials designed to improve the immediate recall of sentences may initially use *sentence patterning* in which a simple subject-predicate relationship is expanded to a subject-predicate-object one. Subsequent expansions of the basic sentence should occur first within the last phrase, the NP (object) of the verb phrase, following the "recency" principle (Murdock, 1962). Secondly, the noun phrase (subject) of the sentence may be expanded. The middle section, the verb of the verb phrase, should be expanded last. Chunking may be facilitated by phrasing (Blasdell & Jensen, 1970; Sitko & Semmel, 1967):

1. The boy/hit.
   The boy/hit/the ball.
   The boy/hit/the big ball.
   The little boy/hit/the big ball.
   The little boy/is hitting/the big ball.
   The little boy/has been hitting/the big ball.

2. The man/drove.
   The man/drove/the car.
   The man/drove/the new car.
   The man/drove/the big new car.
   The tall man/drove/the big new car.
   The tall man/was driving/the big new car.
   The tall man/has been driving/the big new car.

Next, to improve short-term auditory memory, *transformations* may be introduced according to the experimentally established order of difficulty (Menyuk & Looney, 1972; Savin & Perchonock, 1965; Wiig & Roach, 1975):

1. Interrogative, passive, negative, emphatic (Savin and Perchonock, 1965, p. 351):
   The boy hit the ball.
   What did the boy hit?
   Did the boy hit the ball?
   The ball was hit by the boy.
   The boy did not hit the ball.
   Didn't the boy hit the ball?
   The boy *hit* the ball.
   Wasn't the ball hit by the boy?
   The ball *was hit* by the boy.
   The ball was not hit by the boy.
2. Embedding:
   The girl/lives/next door.
   The girl/has/a dog.
   The girl/who has a dog/lives next door.
   The girl/who lives next door/has a dog.

Songs, poems and *jingles* may also be used in designing remedial procedures. "Backward chaining" may be selected as a format for the drills. In this procedure, the last items (word, phrase, sentence, or line) are omitted consecutively to establish recall of the complete sequence:

Roses are red, violets are blue, sugar is sweet and so are you.
Roses are red, violets are blue, sugar is sweet and_____
Roses are red, violets are blue,_____.
Roses are red, _____
_____.
Roses_____
_____.

Improving Delayed Recall

Oral Commands

Oral commands may be used in procedures to improve delayed auditory recall of sentences. The oral commands may require gross or fine motor actions. Learning disabled youngsters often find it easier to follow verbal directions requiring gross motor actions such as walking or jumping than to follow directions requiring fine motor actions such as manipulating objects, coloring, or drawing on command. In responding to both gross and fine motor commands, they may find it difficult to retain and recall the directions if they require left-right discrimination or contain prepositional phrases, number facts, adjective sequences, or linguistic concepts.

Simple oral commands such as "Raise your hand" may be executed on the basis of short-term auditory memory abilities by immediate interpretation. Complex, lengthy verbal directions may be retained indefinitely in short-term auditory memory by conscious effort through rehearsal of the items involved. The main purpose of using oral commands in remediation therefore seems to be to develop the ability to consciously rehearse verbal sequences in short-term memory. This rehearsal of auditory-verbal information requires reauditorization, an ability that may be deficient in learning disabled youngsters (Johnson & Myklebust, 1967).

Silent, internal rehearsal by reauditorization (inner speech) has a second function. It allows material in short-term memory to be retained and transferred to permanent storage in long-term memory (Horowitz, Norman, & Day, 1966; Tulving, 1967). The rate of presentation has also been reported to influence transfer to long-term memory store. Glanzer and Cunitz (1966) have shown that a decrease in presentation rate improves recall from long-term memory store but not from short-term memory.

Learning disabled youngsters often find it easier to follow verbal directions when the items involved are separated by *and* as in the command "Go to the table and pick up the book and bring it to me." This observation suggests that chunking of the words into the obvious word groups facilitates reauditorization and recall. Chunks may also be induced by introducing pauses between the individual word groups.

Sequencing Oral Commands

The remedial procedures should be designed to control (1) level of difficulty, (2) induced chunking, (3) rate of presentation, and (4) vocabulary and syntax. They should be sequenced to progress from one to two or more level commands. They should also be sequenced to introduce *and* between the components of the commands initially, followed by introducing pauses between the components and finally by using normal phrasing. The rate of presentation should also be controlled. Initially, the rate of presentation may be slower than the ordinary conversational rate to facilitate retention and recall from long-term memory store. Later, the rate of presentation should gradually approximate usual speech rates. Finally, left-right directions, difficult prepositional phrases, number facts, adjective sequences, and linguistic concepts should be introduced. Based on these principles, the activities may progress to require:

1. Following patterned oral commands of increasing length that require gross motor actions in which the components are separated by *and*:
   Go to the blackboard.
   Go to the blackboard and pick up a piece of chalk.
   Go to the blackboard and pick up a piece of chalk and write your name.
   Go to the blackboard and pick up a piece of chalk and write your name and then go to your desk.

2. Following unpatterned oral commands of increasing length that require gross motor actions in which the components are separated by *and*:
Go to the door.
Walk to the desk and pick up the book.
Run to the closet and get your coat and put it on.
Skip to the blackboard and take a piece of chalk and carry it to your desk and put it down.

3. Following patterned or unpatterned oral commands of increasing length that require gross motor actions in which the components are separated by pauses:
Go to the door. (pause.) Open it.
Go to the door. (pause) Open it. (pause) Close the door. (pause) Run to your desk.
Go to the door. (pause) Open it. (pause) Close the door. (pause) Run to your desk. (pause) Sit down.

4. Following oral commands of increasing length that require fine motor actions in which the components are separated by *and*:
Materials: Paper dolls and clothes
Put on the dress.
Put on the shirt and the blouse.
Put on the hat and the shoes and the coat.
Put on the shirt and the blouse and the scarf and the shoes.

5. Following oral commands of increasing length that require fine motor actions in which the components are separated by pauses:
Materials: Paper and crayons
Draw a red circle.
Draw a yellow flower. (pause) Write your name.
Draw a blue square. (pause) Take the green crayon. (pause) Draw a tree.
Draw a black triangle. (pause) Take the yellow crayon. (pause) Draw a yellow circle. (pause) Take the red crayon. (pause) Draw a red flower.

6. Following oral commands that contain adjective sequences:
Materials: Colored tokens (big, little; circle, square, triangle; red, blue, yellow, etc.)
Touch the blue circle.
Touch the small yellow square.
Touch the big blue circle and the small yellow square.
Touch the blue circle, (pause) the yellow square and the green triangle.
Touch the small blue circle, (pause) the big yellow square and the big green triangle.

7. Following oral commands that contain a variety of prepositional phrases and left-right directions:
Pick up the book. Put it on top of my desk.
Hold a pencil in the air in your left hand.
Stand on your chair, turn around, and jump down.
With your ruler, point to the window to the right of the door.

8. Following oral commands that contain number facts:
   Materials: A deck of cards
   Find an ace. Find a king.
   Find a heart. Find a two. Find a spade.
   Find two aces. Find the queen of hearts. Find a seven of spades.
   Find the jack, queen, and king of spades, the ace of hearts, and the ten of diamonds.
9. Following oral commands that contain linguistic concepts:
   Pick up *all* your books.
   Take *any* of your crayons and *some* of your paper.
   If today is Monday, draw a line on your paper.
   Take the *longest* pencil, place it next to the *smallest* crayon, and pick up the *biggest* piece of chalk.
   Point to the pencil that is *shorter than* this line.

Improving Long-Term Memory and Delayed Recall

Learning disabled youngsters may demonstrate strengths as well as limitations in long-term memory. They may have exceptionally good long-term memory for telephone numbers, car names, or unessential details; however, they may have poor long-term memory for proper names, for details in conversation or stories, or for numbers or monetary terms.

Procedures designed to improve long-term memory and delayed recall of verbal materials must emphasize the recall of semantic details rather than of linguistic structure. Research has indicated that within a period of thirty seconds after the presentation of verbal material it can be recalled almost perfectly. This observation suggests that there is no decay in memory as a function of time within that period. After a delay of thirty seconds, memory is fragile and highly susceptible to interference (Atkinson & Shiffrin, 1971). The implications for therapy are that the responses required to lengthy verbal materials must reflect deep-structure and semantic interpretation and tap semantic details. According to Miller, Chomsky (1963), Slobin (1971), deep structure and semantic interpretation are represented in long-term memory.

Facilitating Variables

Among materials that may be used to strengthen the delayed recall of semantic details are (1) oral directions, (2) paragraphs, and (3) stories. The variables that may facilitate delayed recall are essentially the same as those that facilitate immediate auditory recall. Among them are

1. Word frequency.
2. Associative strength between elements.
3. Logical relationship between elements.
4. Length of the materials, that is, the number of sentences included.
5. Suprasegmental features, such as stress, applied to significant details.
6. Salience of the content to the individual.
7. Serial position of the semantic details.

Space, Time, and Quantity in Oral Commands

Learning disabled youngsters may demonstrate significant problems in recalling details pertaining to space, time, and quantity (number facts). As a result, these details should be emphasized in designing materials for remediation. The materials may require:

1. Listening to oral directions and answering questions about them.
   a. Go down to the corner and take a right turn.
       Where do you take the right turn?
   b. Go half a mile up Highland Park and bear left at the park.
       How far up Highland Park do you go?
       Which way do you go at the Park?
   c. Drive 25 miles till you get to Exit 9. Take that exit and follow Route
       17 for about 10 miles.
       How far away is Exit 9?
       Which route do you follow when you get off at Exit 9?
       How far do you go on Route 17?
2. Listening to paragraphs of increasing length (newscasts, weather reports, newspaper clippings, etc.) and answering questions about them:
   a. Today temperatures will be in the upper fifties, with rain probable
       this morning, clearing in the early afternoon.
       What will the temperature be today?
       When will it rain?
       When will the rain stop?
   b. A one-hundred-thousand-ton oil tanker broke up off the coast of Mi-
       ami this evening, spreading a slick that extends for twenty-eight
       miles. Cleanup operations have begun on the slick which has not yet
       reached shore.
       Where did the tanker break up?
       How large was the oil slick?
       Where was the slick when cleanup was started?

Among sources for programmed materials designed to improve auditory
memory and listening for details are *Perceptual Communication Skills* (Herr,
1969), and the *Sound-Order-Sense* and the *SAPP* programs (Semel, 1970, in
press). Methods and procedures have also been discussed and presented by
Battin and Haug (1968), Bush and Giles (1969), Johnson and Myklebust
(1967), Kranyik (1970), Lerner (1971), and Wiseman (1965). Elementary and
junior-high school reading books may also provide a variety of materials
which can be adapted for remediation.

Improving Convergent Language Production

The ease with which a person can identify and retrieve a specific word or
concept that satisfies the semantic constraints imposed by a context reflects
convergent semantic production abilities (Guilford, 1967). Convergent language production is reflected in tasks such as naming an object or a picture,
naming a verbal opposite, and completing a verbal analogy or a sentence or
paragraph from which one or more words have been deleted.

Learning disabled youngsters may experience difficulties on verbal tasks requiring convergent semantic production. They may be slow and inaccurate in naming objects and pictures (Denckla, 1974; Johnson & Myklebust, 1967; Wiig & Semel, 1975). They may also be slow and inaccurate in naming verbal opposites and in completing verbal analogies (Wiig & Semel, 1975). Observations further suggest that they may experience problems in completing sentences which express cause-effect, comparative, temporal—sequential, or familial relationships or contain linguistic concepts of inclusion-exclusion, such as *all, none, some, any, all except, all but, not, neither . . . nor.* In a similar vein, they may demonstrate difficulties in completing sentences or paragraphs with deleted words (cloze passages) in which word selection is determined by semantic and linguistic constraints.

The errors made by learning disabled youngsters on tasks requiring convergent language production indicate that

1. Word substitutions (verbal paraphasias) are common even on relatively easy tasks such as naming the verbal opposite of *brother* (Wiig & Semel, 1975).
2. Word substitutions generally belong to the same semantic and grammatic class as the intended word; that is, the name of a fruit such as *orange* may be substituted by *banana,* and nouns are generally substituted by nouns, verbs by verbs, etc. (Denckla, 1974; Wiig & Semel, 1975).
3. Perseverative responses, that is, repetition of a previously produced word, may occur in naming objects or pictures, naming antonyms, or completing verbal analogies (Wiig & Semel, 1975).

These observations suggest that the word-finding difficulties associated with learning disabilities are similar to the verbal paraphasias characteristic of adult aphasics with left temporal, parieto-temporal, or parieto-occipital-temporal lesions (Goldstein, 1948; Goodglass & Kaplan, 1972; Luria, 1966, 1973). Goldstein (1948) has suggested that verbal paraphasias reflect figure-ground problems; Luria (1973), on the other hand, proposes that word substitutions result from inability to discover a required dominant word from within a set of related words of equal probability. The latter suggestion seems to describe the problems experienced by LD youngsters. Accordingly, the purposes of remediation become to (1) facilitate the identification and accurate retrieval of a target word within a set of related words and (2) inhibit retrieval of related words from a set with similar probabilities. Increasing the speed with which target words can be identified in long-term memory store and retrieved should also be emphasized in remediation.

Variables Facilitating Retrieval

Investigations of variables influencing the accuracy and speed with which specific words may be retrieved from long-term memory store provide suggestions relevant to designing remedial procedures. Dixon and Horton (1968) and Tulving (1974) have pointed out that the accessibility to relevant information depends upon the contents of storage as well as on the retrieval cues. Tulving (1974) further suggests that "forgetting is a cue-dependent phenomenon, reflecting the failure of retrieval of perfectly intact trace information"

(p. 74). Retrieval from memory store is viewed as cue-dependent, and this view is supported by the results of several verbal memory experiments. These experiments have provided relevant information for the use of cues in remediation. They indicate that

1. The presentation of specific retrieval cues following noncued recall of verbal materials has a significant effect upon the accuracy of recall (Tulving & Pearlstone, 1966).
2. Associative cues are more effective in facilitating the recall of target words than rhyming word cues (Tulving, 1974).
3. The proportion of accurately recalled target words increases with increases in the number of the inital letters, that is, the size of the word fragment, given in the cue word (Tulving, 1974).
4. Target words presented either in isolation or as part of a sentence are better recalled using synonyms as cue words than without cues. Homonyms are more effective as cues than synonyms, and cue words identical to the target words are most effective (Light, 1972).
5. Names of conceptual categories, for example, types of buildings, metals, insects, carpenter's tools, etc., may serve as cues to restore recall to levels similar to the original learning (Tulving & Psotka, 1971).
6. Retrieval is considerably better in the presence of cues that appeared with the target words during learning than in the presence of target words in a subject-generated recognition list (Tulving & Thomson, 1973).

Cueing for Retrieval

The implications for cueing during remediation seem evident. The findings suggest that

1. Retrieval cues should be used during intervention when the youngster fails to produce a response or has produced an inaccurate response.
2. Retrieval cues naming the conceptual category (semantic class) of a target word, or words highly associated with the target words may be most effective in facilitating accurate recall.
3. Although homonyms and synonyms are not the most effective retrieval cues, they may facilitate specific word recall. Furthermore, homonyms may be more effective in facilitating recall than synonyms.
4. Parts of words may be used as retrieval cues to facilitate accurate word recall. Larger word fragments such as syllables may facilitate accurate recall better than small word fragments such as the initial sound.

The recall of target words in convergent semantic production tasks may also be facilitated using gestural cues, motor cues depicting an activity, or nonsymbolic sound cues. Gestural cues may be used most appropriately to facilitate recall of the names of common objects such as toys, utensils, furniture, and so forth. Motor cues may be used to facilitate the recall of specific action verbs. Nonsymbolic sound cues may be used to facilitate the recall of names of objects associated with specific sounds such as trains, telephones, doorbells, and so forth.

The relationships between target word indentification, stimulus situation, and associative strength or logical relationship of verbal cues have also been explored. Wyke (1962) has provided experimental evidence that correct verbal responses by adult aphasics were facilitated when the possible choice of response words was restricted by the stimulus situation as it is in a sentence completion task. Zivian (1966) has reported that more correct target words were given to verbal cues with high restricted association strength than to cues with low restricted association strength when association strength was based on the *Michigan restricted association norms* (Riegel, 1965). More correct target words were identified from logical cues, that is, cues related to target words by class membership and class relationship (Flavell, 1963), than from infralogical cues implying a temporal or spatial relationship. An example of a logical cue for the target word *car* would be: similar . . . *auto* while an infralogical cue would be: location . . . *garage*. Wiig and Globus (1971) have reported a similar pattern of facilitation for word identification by adult aphasics.

Inhelder and Piaget (1958) have reported that logical (class) and infralogical (temporal or spatial) relationships are equally well formulated by adulthood but logical relationships are most efficiently translated. Zivian (1966) also pointed to the fact that sets of words delineated by logical relations (class membership) are better defined. On the other hand, Zivian (1966) observed longer latencies in responding when logical cues or multiple cues were presented, suggesting that the reductions in the size of the word set from which a target word was to be selected required more complex identification processes. The implications for remediation of the combined findings suggest that

1. Cues with high associative strength and/or logical relationship to a target word should be used to increase the probability of a correct response.
2. Responses may be delayed relatively longer when logical or multiple cues are used which restrict the size of the appropriate word set.
3. Speed of retrieval may be improved by increasing the set from which a target word may be selected.
4. Sentence completion procedures may be used effectively in intervention to improve the accuracy of word retrieval. These procedures may also be used to improve the speed of retrieval when the word set from which a target word must be selected is sufficiently large.

Convergent Production of Semantic Units

The convergent production of semantic units may be improved using visual confrontation naming or sentence completion tasks. Visual confrontation naming tasks may progress from naming objects for which tactile information or motor activities may facilitate recall to naming pictures as follows:

1. Naming a series of grouped objects that are common in the youngsters' everyday environment:
   a. Toys (ball, boat, car, plane, train, etc.)

       b. Fruits (apple, pear, banana, orange, grape, etc.)
       c. Dollhouse furniture (chair, table, refrigerator, sink, bed, etc.)
       d. Clothes items (pants, shirt, socks, coat, skirt, etc.)
2. Naming pictures of grouped objects such as toys, furniture, foods, clothes, etc.
3. Naming pictures of a series of grouped actions related to:
       a. Getting up in the morning (brushing teeth, combing hair, getting dressed, eating breakfast, etc.)
       b. Sports or gym sessions (running, jumping, catching, throwing, walking, swimming, etc.)
       c. Hobbies (sewing, baking, knitting, hammering, sawing, weaving, etc.)
       d. School activities (reading, writing, knitting, swimming).
4. Naming colors progressing from the primary colors to others within the color spectrum.
5. Naming pictorial representations of ungrouped objects, actions, colors, etc.

Rapid Naming Drills

Rapid naming drills may also be introduced for youngsters who are slow in responding. Johnson and Myklebust (1967) suggest that the educator and/or the youngster time these rapid naming drills. They indicate that a rate of word naming of one word per second is a desirable goal.

It may be necessary to sacrifice accuracy for speed in word retrieval during the initial sessions. The educator may indicate that errors are acceptable to begin with and accept up to 15% errors in return for an increase in the speed of retrieval and word naming. As the rate of responding stabilizes, the criteria for accuracy of the responses may be gradually raised from 85% to close to 100%.

The effectiveness of word naming drills with adult aphasics has recently been investigated by Wiegel Crump and Koenigsknecht (1973). They provided four adult aphasics with a total of eighteen sessions given two or three times a week. The patients were drilled on the recall of twenty words (household items, clothes, foods, action verbs, and living things), all words which the aphasics failed to retrieve before therapy. To facilitate naming, the patients were cued with visual and auditory cues (gestures, associated words, synonyms, carrier phrases, or word fragments). A measure of word naming was obtained after every six therapy sessions. The interesting finding was that the aphasics made similar gains in retrieving both drilled (twenty items) and nondrilled words (twenty additional items) within the same superordinate category, suggesting transfer of retrieval skills within conceptual groups. Similar findings should be obtained for language disabled youngsters with word finding and naming difficulties.

Keenan (1966) has described a programmed approach for eliciting naming behavior from aphasic patients. The program was designed for use with a Language Master using Language Master cards. The total program contained a noun, a verb, and a number program. One set of Language Master cards (Set I) was prepared to present pictures of two referents for either nouns, action verbs, or numbers. The name of each referent was recorded on the magnetic tape strip of each card, and each card contained the printed name of one of the referents centered above the two pictures. The reverse side of each card repeated the printed word and the associated referent. An alternate set (Set II) of cards presented a printed word, the picture of the referent, and the recorded name. The program progressed in the following steps:

1. Identification of referent followed by imitation of the spoken and printed words (Set I).
2. Identification of referent based on printed word only followed by imitation of spoken and printed words (Set I).
3. Identification of referent based on spoken word only followed by imitation of spoken and printed words (Set I).
4. Recall of printed word based on referent and spoken word (Set II).
5. Recall of spoken word based on referent and printed word (Set II).
6. Recall of printed word based on spoken word only (Set II).
7. Recall of spoken word based on printed word only (Set II).
8. Recall of printed word based on referent only (Set II).
9. Recall of spoken word based on referent only (Set II).

This program may be adapted for use with language disabled youngsters with limited reading skills by leaving out steps which require recall of printed words. Steps 1, 3, 5, and 9 would seem appropriate for improving word naming by learning disabled youngsters.

Sentence Completion

Procedures designed to improve the accuracy and speed of word retrieval may also incorporate sentence completion tasks. The sentence to be completed may initially introduce limited constraints on the possible words that may satisfy the context. Since a large word set would satisfy the context, the speed of retrieval should be at maximum. Later, sentences may be introduced that increase the semantic constraints and limit the set of possible words. Initially, the speed of retrieval may decrease. The remedial procedures may require:

1. Sentence completion with word selection from a large set of possible words:
   a. Cars are _____.
      Jets are _____.
   b. Tigers are _____.
      Elephants are _____.
   c. Children like _____.
      Monkeys like _____.
   d. You can eat _____.
      You can drink _____.
      You can wear _____.

2. Sentence completion with word selection from a more restricted word set:
   a. You can row _____.
      You can drive _____.
      You can fly _____.
   b. I live in _____.
      I drive in _____.
   c. I brush my teeth with _____.
      I comb my hair with _____.
3. Sentence completion with word selection based on association by simultaneous occurrence.
   a. I like bread and _____.
   b. I drink coffee from a _____.
   c. I fry bacon and _____.
   d. I fix my hair with a brush and _____.

Procedures designed to improve the convergent production of semantic classes may require recall of:

1. Contrasting words (antonyms):
   a. man-woman
      boy-girl
   b. walk-run
   c. big-little
   d. up-down
      in-out
   e. happy-sad
2. Similar words (synonyms) by presenting the least frequent word first to elicit the most frequent term:
   a. swift-fast
   b. blossom-flower
   c. giggle-laugh
3. Subordinates based on logical relationship:
   a. fruit-banana
   b. animal-dog
   c. furniture-chair
4. Superordinates based on logical relationship:
   a. tiger-animal
   b. apple-fruit
   c. table-furniture
5. Spatially related words (infralogical relationship):
   a. garage-car/*bus*
   b. airport-plane/*helicopter*
   c. zoo-animal/*tiger*
6. Temporally related words (infralogical relationship):
   a. winter-snow
   b. summer-hot
   c. morning-breakfast

7. Verbs for predication:
   a. dog-bark
   b. lion-growl
   c. plane-fly

Associated and logically related words may also be recalled in sentence completion tasks such as:

1. Antonym: Some cars are big; some cars are (little).
2. Synonym: When you giggle you (laugh).
3. Subordinate: My favorite fruit is _____.
4. Superordinate: A tiger is one of many (animals).
5. Spatially related words: I park my car in (a garage).
6. Temporally related words: In the winter we have (snow).
7. Predication: Dogs bark and tigers (growl).

Convergent Production of Semantic Relations

The convergent production of semantic relations may be improved using (a) verbal analogy tasks, (b) sentence completion tasks requiring completion of comparative sentences, temporal-sequential events, and familial relationships, or (c) sentence completion tasks using sentences containing linguistic concepts of inclusion-exclusion (some, any, all, etc.) or cause-effect relationships (If . . . then, because). *Verbal analogies* should be introduced in a sequence reflecting their relative levels of difficulty. The various types and the order of difficulty of verbal analogies have been discussed in Chapter 7. Procedures designed to improve the convergent production of semantic relations may require completion of verbal analogies expressing:

1. Whole-part relationshps: A dog has hair; a bird has (feathers).
2. Part-whole relationships: A roof belongs on a house; a feather belongs on a (bird).
3. Opposite relationships (antonyms): A father is big; a baby is (little).
4. Similar relationships (synonyms): When I am happy I laugh or smile; when I am sad I cry or (weep).
5. Spatial (infralogical) relationships: A car is parked in a garage; a plane is parked in a (hangar).
6. Temporal-sequential (infralogical) relationships: Summer comes before winter; Halloween comes before (Thanksgiving).
7. Familial relationships: A boy can be a brother; a girl can be (a sister).
8. Purpose (instrumental) relationships: You play tennis with a racket; you play baseball with (a bat).
9. Predication: A cat meows; a dog (barks).
10. Action-object or object-action relationships: (a) You drive a car; you fly a (plane); (b) Planes are for flying; horses are for (riding).

Sentences requiring logical operations (comparative, spatial, temporal, and familial relationships) may also be used in sentence completion tasks to improve the convergent production of semantic relations. The order of difficulty of these sentences has been discussed in Chapter 3 (pp. 67-70). Comparative sentences and spatial relationships may be completed with one of a relatively large set of words and should therefore be relatively easy and fast to complete. Sentences expressing temporal-sequential relationships require completion from a much smaller set of words and may require more time for responding. Comparative sentences expressing logical relationships should be easier to complete than sentences with spatial or temporal (infralogical) relationships (Inhelder & Piaget, 1958; Wiig & Globus, 1971; Zivian, 1966). Accordingly, the activities may require completion of:

1. Comparative sentences with positive comparisons: Elephants are bigger than (tigers).
2. Comparative sentences with negative comparisons. Apples are smaller than (watermelons).
3. Spatial (infralogical) relationships: Mother put the flowers on (the table).
4. Temporal-sequential (infralogical) relationships: a. Breakfast comes before (lunch). b. Summer comes after (spring).
5. Familial relationships: My mother's sister is my (aunt).

Linguistic concepts of inclusion-exclusion or cause-effect may also be used in sentence completion tasks to faciilitate convergent production of semantic relations. Generally, linguistic concepts of inclusion-exclusion (some, any, all, none, etc.) may be completed from a large set of possible words while cause-effect relationships (If . . . then, because) must be completed from a limited set. The procedures may require completion of:

1. Sentences contain linguistic concepts of inclusion:
   a. I like all _____.
   b. I like some _____.
   c. I like all kinds of ice cream but/except _____.
2. Sentences containing linguistic concepts of exclusion:
   a. I do not like _____.
   b. I like neither cats nor _____.
3. "Fanny Doodles" (*ZOOM*, Public Broadcasting System, Station WGBH, Boston) reflecting the principles of inclusion-exclusion:
   a. Fanny Doodle loves sweets but hates (candy).
   b. Fanny Doodle loves apples but hates (fruit).
4. Sentences expressing cause-effect relationships:
   a. I wore a raincoat because it (rained).
   b. If there is smoke there is (fire).

Convergent Production of Semantic Systems

The convergent production of semantic systems may be improved by using oral cloze paragraphs and passages. The cloze procedure was introduced by Taylor (1953) based on the concept of *gestalt closure*. Cloze passages are narrative material in which various words are deleted. Written cloze passages have been used effectively to test and teach reading comprehension, language arts skills, and other subjects (Blackwell, Thompson, & Dzuiban, 1972; Bormuth, 1962; Culhane, 1970; Jenkinson, 1957; Schneyer, 1965). Hafner (1965) proposes that the cloze procedure taps cognitive retrieval.

Cloze passages may be constructed according to a variety of principles. The word deletions may occur at regular intervals by deleting every nth word. Culhane (1970) suggests deletion of every fifth word. Weaver and Bickly (1967) have studied deletion of every seventh word while Bormuth (1962) suggests deletion of every tenth word.

Studies have also utilized cloze passages with deletion of specific words and phrase-marked cloze passages and compared specific and random word deletions (Blackwell, 1975; Bloomer, 1966; Rankin, 1957; Rankin & Dale, 1969). Bloomer (1966) deleted nouns, verbs, modifiers (adjectives and adverbs), function words (prepositions, conjunctions, and noun determiners), auxiliaries, and pronoun substantives. He observed that noun deletion produced better prediction results than all other deletion types. Rankin (1957) suggested that cloze responses may be based on cognition rather than perception. He concluded that noun and verb deletions measure factual information while random deletions tap the comprehension of structural relationships. Rankin and Dale (1969) observed that both lexical and structural cloze passages provide valid measures of reading comprehension.

Weaver (1965) introduced the oral cloze procedure. He reported that about forty words may be encoded for each cloze item, suggesting that the responses reflect divergent as well as convergent production abilities. This aspect led to the suggestion that any word would be acceptable in completing a cloze passage as long as the word made sense in the context.

Oral cloze passages may be constructed by the educator according to the principles described above. They may reflect:

1. Random word deletion of the fifth, seventh, or tenth word
2. Specific lexical word deletion (noun, verb, etc.)
3. Phrase-marker deletion, that is, deletion of the first or last word of a phrase or of a single word acting as a phrase (noun, verb, adjectival, or adverbial phrase)

The following cloze passage designed according to the principle of phrase-marker deletion by Blackwell (1975) illustrates the format of a cloze passage. The procedures and processes involved in completing the passage may be discerned by personal experience in completing this passage.

The Lion and the Mouse

Long ago in the forest there lived a lion and some mice. One day the _____ wanted to play. The _____ up and down some hills and _____ jumped on piles of leaves. They ate some seeds and they _____ some sweet flowers. _____ was a happy day.

"_____ is fun," said the little gray _____.

But one _____ named Fuzzy did not _____.

"Look!" he said. "_____ is the lion. He is _____!"

The little _____ ran away. They hid _____ the forest. Only one mouse was _____.

"Don't be afraid," _____ said. "Come on! We can play _____ the soft fur."

"No, no!" _____ the other little _____. "He will wake up and _____ us!"

"Well, I am _____ to play in the soft _____
even if you _____!" Then he ran up _____ lion's
back. "Eek! Eek!" he said. "This is lots of _____!"

The big lion _____. "Roar!" said the _____.

"Eek! Eek!" said Fuzzy.

"I am _____ to eat you," said the lion. "You woke me up!"

"Oh, no!" _____ Fuzzy. "Do not eat _____! I
will not _____ in your soft _____ again!"

"I _____ let you go this time," said the _____.
"But do not bother me _____."

Quickly _____ poor little mouse ran away. _____
did not see the lion _____ a long time. _____ day
he heard the lion roar. Fuzzy felt sorry _____ the lion. The
_____ knew what he had to _____. He chewed
and _____ the net. Soon the _____ was free!
_____ lion had saved _____ mouse. The mouse had
saved the lion.

[Blackwell, 1975, pp. 115–16]

Improving Divergent Language Production

The ease with which a person can produce a variety of verbal responses (words, phrases, or sentences) to describe objects, events, or ideas reflects the divergent semantic production abilities (Guilford, 1967). Several abilities can be identified which contribute to facility in divergent language production. Among them are (1) *verbal fluency,* reflected by ready availability of verbal responses (words, phrases, or sentences), (2) *flexibility,* reflected by willingness to shift from one set to another in terms of word classes or sentence types (spontaneous flexibility) and to change strategies (adaptive flexibility), (3) *originality,* reflected by unusual responses, and (4) *elaboration,* reflected by attention and description of details and embellishment of verbal responses.

Learning disabled children have been reported to lack verbal fluency when required to produce divergent verbal responses (Bannatyne, 1971; Johnson & Myklebust, 1967; Lerner, 1971). These reductions appear to persist into adolescence (Wiig and Semel, 1975). The responses to divergent semantic production tasks by learning disabled adolescents further showed that they may shift from one set (class) to another in their search for words and fail to employ efficient strategies for retrieval. These observations suggest a high level of spontaneous but limited adaptive flexibility.

Clinical observations of verbal descriptions of objects, events and ideas further suggest that learning disabled youngsters may show limited abilities for elaboration. They may neglect details in their descriptions and provide terse, stereotyped, concrete responses. As examples, they may fail to describe (a) attributes of objects such as form, size, or composition, (b) possessive relationships (ownership, etc.), or (c) object-action or action-agent relationships.

There is evidence in the literature that divergent production abilities can be developed using general as well as specific training procedures. Torrance (1965) described five general training principles that resulted in significant gains in divergent production abilities (originality, elaboration, fluency, and flexibility). The principles were (1) treating student questions with respect, (2) treating imaginative ideas with respect, (3) supporting the value of student ideas, (4) permitting practice without evaluation, and (5) associating evaluations with causes and consequences. These training principles can be translated directly to language training sessions designed to improve divergent semantic production skills.

Specific training procedures have been reported to be effective at first grade and college levels, among others. Cartledge and Krauser (1963) provided twenty-five-minute daily sessions for first graders during which they were directed to think about how they could improve toys. They showed significant gains in fluency, flexibility, and originality. College students have been trained to produce remote and uncommon word-associations by Maltzman, Bogartz, and Berger (1958) and Maltzman et al. (1960). As a result of training, there was an observable transfer of effects from one divergent semantic production task to another (Maltzman, Bogartz, & Berger, 1958). The results also indicated that practice in giving uncommon word-associations with reinforcement may be effective in developing divergent semantic production abilities. The implications for remediation suggest that procedures designed to improve verbal fluency, flexibility, and originality may incorporate: (1) specific directions to produce uncommon responses, (2) word—association tasks, and (3) immediate reinforcement of responses reflecting fluency, flexibility, originality, and elaboration.

Divergent Production of Semantic Units

Activities designed to increase the attention to details of objects and events and improve the production of semantic units may progress from requiring immediate descriptions of objects or pictures to requiring descriptions of past events. Since divergent semantic production is dependent upon previous experiences and amount of information stored in long-term memory, it may be necessary to describe the stimulus objects or events verbally before any verbal descriptions are requested by the youngsters. The procedures and activities may require:

1. Description of familiar objects in response to questions about details, followed by immediate verbal reinforcement:
   Presentation of a toy car or a picture of a car followed by specific questions such as:
   a. What is it?
   b. What color is it?
   c. What kind of car is it?
   d. What is it made of?
   e. What size is it?
   f. Where (what places) can you find cars?
   g. What can it be used for?
   h. Who has a car in your family?
   i. What would you need to buy a car?

2. Spontaneous verbal description of familiar objects using pictorial presentations followed by general questions and by immediate verbal reinforcement of descriptions of attributes and relationships:
   Presentation of a pictured object, such as a telephone, followed by general questions such as:
   a. What can you tell me about this thing?
   b. What else can you tell me about it?
   c. What more can you think of to tell me about it?
3. Description of pictures of familiar events, for example, washing the car, playing baseball, baking a cake, a Thanksgiving dinner, etc., in response to specific questions, emphasizing details, temporal and spatial aspects of the event and cause-effect relationships:
   Presentation of a picture of a family breakfast followed by specific questions such as:
   a. What is happening?
   b. What time of the day is it?
   c. Where is the family?
   d. What are they eating?
   e. How many people are there?
   f. Who are the people?
4. Spontaneous verbal description of a pictured event followed by open-ended questions and immediate verbal reinforcement of descriptions of temporal, spatial, and cause-effect relationships:
   Presentation of a picture of a current sports event (ball game, tennis match, etc.) followed by general questions such as:
   a. Can you tell me about this picture?
   b. What else can you tell me about it?
   c. What else can you think of to tell me about it?
5. Description of a sequence of events pictured in slides or film followed by specific questions, emphasizing details of the events (people present, objects present, attributes of people and objects, etc.) and temporal-spatial and cause-effect relationships:
   Slide or film presentation of a familiar event such as a shopping trip followed by specific questions such as:
   a. What happened?
   b. Who were the people?
   c. What did they do before leaving home?
   d. How did they get to the store?
   e. What type of store did they go to?
   f. What did they buy at the store?
   g. What happened after they left the store?
6. Spontaneous description of a sequence of events pictured in slides or film followed by general question such as:
   a. What was this all about?
   b. What else can you tell me about?
   c. What else happened?

Divergent Production of Semantic Classes, Systems, and Implications

The remedial procedures may also emphasize word associations in either free- or controlled-association tasks. Procedures designed to improve the production of semantic classes may require:

1. Free word-association during a ninety-second period in a response to an object or a pictured object or event. The number of responses given during the most fluent sixty seconds may be used to chart progress in verbal fluency.
2. Controlled word-association during a sixty- or ninety-second period in response to superordinate (class) names or function categorization such as foods, fruits, clothes, furniture, things to build with, etc. The number of responses produced in repeated drills in response to a specific superordinate (class) or functional description may be used to chart improvements in verbal fluency.

The *divergent production of semantic systems* may be improved in tasks requiring formulation of a variety of sentences incorporating a key word in appropriate semantic contexts. The emphasis in these procedures is on varying the semantic contexts in which the key words appear, not necessarily on the formulation of a variety of sentence types or transformations, responses that reflect syntactic production skills. The remedial procedure may require formulation of a variety of sentences incorporating:

1. Nouns such as *boy, cat, car, telephone*, etc.
2. Verbs such as *walk, run, drive, have, want, like*, etc.
3. Adjectives such as *young, old, new, big, little, slow, fast*, etc.

Procedures designed to improve the *divergent production of semantic implications* may emphasize the formulation of a variety of cause-effect relationships. They may require:

1. Completion of sentences by formulating a variety of plausible causes for an action:
   a. John went to the store because . . .
   b. Jane went home because . . .
   c. George went to New York because . . .
2. Completion of sentences describing a cause by formulating a variety of plausible effects:
   a. Yesterday in the storm . . .
   b. When the car broke down, Mr. Jones . . .
   c. Paul was hungry so he . . .
3. Completion of stories (paragraphs) with a variety of appropriate and probable endings (causes-effects):
   a. Last summer Joan went to the beach every day. She always brought her lunch and a snack. One day . . .

   b. Yesterday I went to New York on the bus. I sat right behind the
      driver. On the way I saw . . .
   c. Al bought a marvelous gadget last week. It looked like a wrench. He
      wanted to use it . . .
4. Formulation of a serial story by a group of youngsters in which only the
   immediately preceding sentence of the story is known to each youngster. The story may be started with a sentence such as: "Last week when
   I was walking along the road, I saw a boy . . ."

Among sources that discuss strategies and methods for improving divergent semantic production are *The structure of intellect: its interpretation and
uses* (Meeker, 1969) and *New directions in creativity* (Renzulli, 1973). Meeker (1969) provides suggestions for testing and training a variety of cognitive,
convergent, and divergent production abilities and relates training to curriculum design. Renzulli (1973) emphasizes divergent semantic production in a
language arts curriculum for the fifth through the eighth grade.

Improving Syntax in Language Production

Learning disabled children and adolescents have demonstrated deficits in the
ability to formulate syntactic structures and transformations in language production (Vogel, 1974; Wiig & Semel, 1975). They may also exhibit reductions in the imitative control of syntactic structures and transformations
(Rosenthal, 1970; Semel & Wiig, 1975; Wiig & Roach, 1975).

Procedures designed to improve the productive control of syntax and sentence transformation should be introduced when adequate linguistic processing skills have been established (Asher, 1972; Brown, Cazden, & Bellugi,
1968; Fraser, Bellugi, & Brown, 1963; Winitz, 1973). The specific remedial
strategies and procedures may be selected on the basis of age appropriate-
ness. They should also be selected to reflect increases in the level of difficulty
of recall and retrieval of the various syntactic structures and transformations.
The order of presentation may be based on either clinical observation, research findings, linguistic theories, or psycholinguistic principles.

Interactive Language Development Teaching

Lee, Koenigsknecht, and Mulhern (1975) have introduced a language development teaching method based on psycholinguistic findings and principles.
It introduces syntactic structures and sentence transformations according to
their relative levels of difficulty. The teaching program is appropriate for
high-risk and LD children with language delays in nursery school, kindergarten, and the early elementary grades.

The *Interactive Language Development Teaching* method (Lee, Koenigsknecht, & Mulhern, 1975) was designed to utilize a conversational setting
closely resembling the setting for normal language development. In order to
capitalize on the developmental features, a setting is created "where language can be spontaneous, nominative, and meaningful and where both receptive and expressive skills can be practiced" (p. 7).

The format chosen centers around storytelling in which the child responds to specific questions or prompts relating to the plot line of the story. This format emphasizes the semantic-cognitive aspects of language while facilitating the abstraction and recall of syntactic and transformational rules.

The narrative material presented in the lessons is selected to reflect the experiences and background of the young child. It is concrete and describes everyday activities involving typical families. Each story functions as an independent unit with a plot that comes to a logical conclusion. In addition, lessons and stories were selected and sequenced to:

1. Provide sufficient narrative to keep the child's attention. [p. 11]
2. Provide adequate build-up of semantic content for the target structures. [p. 12]
3. Introduce new structures as receptive tasks before eliciting them as targets. [p. 14]
4. Provide frequent review to stabilize structures previously introduced as target responses. [p. 14]
5. Clarify the concepts underlying the contentive vocabulary. [p. 14]
6. Include questions which elicit creative thinking. [p. 16]

Each new lesson is preceded by an overview of (a) the concepts and vocabulary to be introduced, (b) the materials needed for the lesson, and (c) a list of the elicited grammatical structures which receive primary or secondary emphasis in the lesson. The format of each lesson is similar. The narrative is presented in one column, the target responses are listed adjacently, and the total *Developmental Sentence Score* (DSS) (Lee, 1974) obtainable for a complete, grammatical response is provided. This format reflects the fact that the goals for the lessons were derived from *Developmental Sentence Analysis* of children's spontaneous language samples (Lee, 1974).

The *Interactive Language Development Teaching* program also provides guidelines for the verbal interactions between the educator-clinician and the child (pp. 18-23), a feature which is uncommon and educationally relevant. The first step suggested in eliciting complete target responses requires sentence repetition of the complete model. The second step provides opportunities for repetition of parts of the desired target response which were omitted by the child, that is, a reduced model is presented by the educator for imitation. The third step introduces expansion requests which require that the child must expand an incomplete response without a model to imitate. The fourth step suggests that the child repeat and correct an incorrect target response. In the fifth step, the educator repeats the child's response to elicit self-correction. The sixth step introduces a self-correction request to the child to stimulate spontaneous self-correction. In the seventh step the original question may be rephrased to elicit the correct target response.

The language program is divided into two levels. Level I emphasizes the acquisition and productive control over basic sentence structures, coordination, and simple transformations. Level II emphasizes grammatical structures which develop later and stresses elaboration of the verb phrase, secondary verbs, conjunction, and complex transformations. The program may be used with small groups of children or in remedial sessions with a single child.

The *Interactive Language Development Teaching* program has been assessed experimentally (Lee, Koenigsknecht, & Mulhern, 1975). After a treatment period of 8.3 months, twenty-five children with language delays, ranging in age from three years two months to five years nine months, showed gains in both receptive and expressive language abilities. Clinically significant gains in the control of syntax in language production were observed on several measures. *Developmental Sentence Scores* (DDS) (Lee, 1974) indicated a mean gain of 10.8 months. Performances on the *Grammatic Closure* subtest of the ITPA (Kirk, McCarthy, & Kirk, 1968) indicated a mean gain of 15.0 months. The mean gain on the *Expressive* section of the *Northwestern Syntax Screening Test* (Lee, 1971) was 6.8 months. These findings suggest that LD children in the early grades with language delays or language disorders may experience similar gains in the productive control of syntax.

Rearranging Scrambled Word Sequences

Among methods and procedures which may be considered in planning intervention for the language production deficits of older language disabled children are (1) rearranging scrambled word sequences, (2) sentence completion, (3) oral cloze tasks, (4) sentence transformation, and (5) formulation of sentences that incorporate key words or phrases.

Johnson and Myklebust (1967) have suggested that tasks requiring that scrambled sentences be rearranged should be incorporated to improve word sequencing skills. They suggest that the youngster should be given three or four flash cards containing single, printed words to be arranged into a sentence (pp. 140-41). The exercises suggested emphasize rearrangement of words such as *run can I* into simple active-declarative sentences.

An alternative strategy may be used which introduces three or four flash cards, most containing phrases rather than single words for forming sentences such as "The boy ate the ice cream." In this procedure, the noun phrase (the boy) is introduced as a unit, the verb of the verb phrase (ate) constitutes one unit and the noun phrase of the verb phrase (the ice cream) a separate unit. This format appears to be easier for some LD youngsters than a format presenting single words. When segments of sentences marked by constituent structure analysis are presented, they may act as perceptual units (memory units) and may therefore facilitate recall of syntactic structures and transformations from long-term memory store (Fodor & Bever, 1965; McLean & Gregg, 1967). This procedure may also be used for the introduction of complex sentence transformations. The remedial procedures may require:

1. Rearrangement of scrambled phrases into active-declarative sentences of increasing length.
   a. kicked—the boy—the ball
   b. the boy—the ball—kicked—into the yard
   c. the big boy—into the yard—kicked—the blue ball—next door

2. Rearrangement of scrambled phrases into interrogative, passive, and negative sentence transformations according to order of difficulty (Savin & Perchonock, 1965):
   a. the boy—*What*—kick—did (wh- question)
   b. the boy—the ball—*Did*—kick (question)
   c. by the boy—was kicked—the ball (passive)
   d. did not kick—the boy—the ball (negative)
3. Rearrangement of scrambled phrases into contrasting active-declarative and interrogative, and passive and negative sentence pairs:
   a. Rearranging *The book—the girl—gave—to the boy—was given—the book—the boy—by the girl* into an active-declarative sentence (The girl gave the boy the book) and a contrasting passive sentence (The book was given to the boy by the girl). A model sentence pair such as "The boy hit the ball" (active) and "The ball was hit by the boy" (passive) may be provided initially for a guide.
   b. Rearranging *The book—the boy—did the boy give—the girl—the girl—gave—the book—the boy* into an active sentence (The boy gave the girl the book) / (The girl gave the boy the book) and an interrogative sentence (Did the boy give the girl the book?). A sentence pair such as "The boy hit the ball" (active) and "Did the boy hit the ball?" (interrogative) may be provided initially as a model.
   c. Rearranging *The bike—gave—the mother—the boy—did not give—the boy—the bike—the mother* into an active sentence (The mother gave the boy the bike)/(The boy gave the mother the bike) and a negative sentence (The mother did not give the boy the bike)/(The boy did not give the mother the bike). A model sentence pair such as "The boy hit the ball" (active) and 'The boy did not hit the ball" (negative) may be provided initially.
4. Rearrangement of scrambled phrases into sentences with various *and* conjunctions:
   a. the boy—the father—the ball—kicked—and
   b. ate—and—the hotdog—the boy—the ice cream
   c. the boy—the milkshake—the bone—ate—the dog—drank—and
5. Rearrangement of scrambled phrases into sentences with various conjunctions using *but, because, so,* etc., introduced according to order of difficulty (Lee, 1974, p. 40):
   a. the book—remembered—the bag—the boy—but—forgot
   b. because—the sun—it—was shining—hot—was
   c. the boy—so—the bike—walked—was gone
6. Rearrangement of scrambled phrases and words into sentences with relative clauses or embedding:
   a. the boy—took—the bike—who—saw—John
   b. the girl—ate—the apple—who—ran

Sentence Completion and Cloze Procedures

Sentence tasks may also be introduced to develop control of syntactic structures in language production. Johnson and Myklebust (1967) suggest this type of sentence completion task for developing subject-verb agreement in language production. In their examples, the noun phrases of sentences are provided, for example, "The boy _____." The youngsters are requested to use the words *is* or *are* and to finish the sentences. Sentence completion procedures may also be used to establish the use of verb tense, indirect object, prepositional and adverbial phrases, and interrogatives. The procedures may require completion of:

1. Sentences requiring a specified tense:
   a. Yesterday the boy . . .
   b. Tomorrow the man . . .
   c. Today the girl . . .
   d. Right now the dog . . .
   e. Sometimes our cat . . .
2. Sentences with transitive verbs that require direct-indirect object sequences or a direct object and a prepositional phrase:
   a. The boy gave . . .
   b. The boy handed . . .
   c. The girl sent . . .
3. Sentences requiring prepositional or adverbial phrases:
   a. The girl put the flowers . . .
   b. The boy kicked the ball . . .
   c. The man went . . .
   d. The woman drove . . .
4. Wh- questions and interrogatives introduced in order of difficulty:
   a. What . . .
   b. Who . . .
   c. Where . . .
   d. When . . .
   e. How . . .
   f. Why . . .
   g. Is/are . . .
   h. Does/did . . .
   i. Can/could . . .
   j. Has/have . . .
5. Sentences beginning with various linguistic concepts:
   a. If . . .
   b. When . . .
   c. After . . .
   d. Before . . .
   e. Because . . .

Cloze procedures have been reported to be effective in testing and teaching reading comprehension, language arts skills, and other subjects (Blackwell, Thompson, & Dzuiban, 1972; Bormuth, 1962; Culhane, 1970; Jenkinson, 1957; Schneyer, 1965). The characteristics and design of cloze passages have been discussed (pp. 280-82). Oral cloze passages may be designed to establish lexical and structural formulation in language production using fifth or seventh word random deletions (Rankin, 1957). Johnson and Myklebust (1967) have suggested the use of cloze sentences and passages to establish the correct use of, among others, prepositions, adjectives, and noun plurals in language production.

Sentence Formulation .

Wiig and Semel (1975) have reported that learning disabled adolescents may experience difficulties in sentence formulation when they are required to incorporate key words. Learning disabled adolescents produced significantly more incorrect and incomplete sentences than academically achieving adolescents when they were given a key word with an inflectional ending such as *belongs* or a key word such as *After* . . . which requires a conjunction. These findings suggest that sentence formulation tasks requiring incorporation of key words that impose semantic and linguistic constraints should be introduced in intervention. The procedures may require:

1. Sentence formulation with incorporation of key words marked by inflectional or derivational suffixes. Examples of key words are (a) *boys* (noun plural), (b) *painter* (derived noun), (c) *running* (present progressive), (d) *went* (irregular past tense), (e) *bigger* (comparative), (f) *fastest* (superlative), (g) *quickly* (derived adverb), etc.
2. Sentence formulation with incorporation of key words requiring sentence transformations. Examples of key words are (a) conjunctions such as *and, or, but,* etc., (b) *not* (negation), (c) wh- forms such as *who, when, where* (interrogatives), (d) *didn't* (negative interrogative), etc.

Among sources providing procedures and activities for improving the control of linguistic structures in language production are *The world of language books* (Bennett, Mysliviec, & Beckman, 1972), *A student-centered language arts curriculum,* Grade K-6 and K-13 (Moffett, 1973a, 1973b), *Teaching the universe of discourse* (Moffett, 1968), and the *Sound-Order-Sense* and *SAPP* (Semel, 1970, in press).

References

Ahmann, J. S., & Glock, M. D. *Evaluating pupil growth*. Boston: Allyn & Bacon, 1971.

Asher, J. J. Children's first language as a model for second language learning. *Modern Language Journal*, 1972, **56**, 133-318.

Aten, J., & Davis, J. Disturbances in the perception of auditory sequence in children with minimal cerebral dysfunction. *Journal of Speech and Hearing Research*, 1968, **11**, 236-45.

Atkinson, R. C., & Shiffrin, R. M. The control of short-term memory. *Scientific American*, 1971, **225**, 82-90.

Baker, H., & Leland, B. *Detroit tests of learning aptitude*. Indianapolis: Test Division of Bobbs-Merrill, 1959.

Bannatyne, A. *Language, reading and learning disabilities*. Springfield, Ill.: Charles C Thomas, 1971.

Bartlett, F. C. *Remembering: a study in experimental and social psychology*. Cambridge: Cambridge University Press, 1932.

Battin, R. R., & Haug, C. O. *Speech and language delay*. Springfield, Ill.: Charles C Thomas, 1968.

Bennett, R. A., Mysliviec, N., & Beckman, B. *The world of language books*. (Teacher's ed.) Chicago: Follett Publishing Co., 1972.

Blackwell, J. M. An investigation into phrase-marked and non-phrase-marked cloze scores. Doctoral dissertation, Boston University, 1975.

Blackwell, J. M., Thompson, R. A., & Dzuiban, C. D. An investigation into the effectiveness of the cloze procedure as a vocabulary teaching tool. *Journal of Reading Behavior*, 1972, **4**, 53-54.

Blasdell, R., & Jensen, P. Stress and word position as determinants of imitation in first-language learners. *Journal of Speech and Hearing Research*, 1970, **13**, 193-202.

Bloomer, R. H. Non-overt reinforced cloze procedure. Microfiche: ED010-270, Florida Technological University Library, 1966.

Bollinger, D., & Gerstman, L. J. Disjuncture as cue to constructs. *Word*, 1957, **13**, 246-55.

Bormuth, J. R. Cloze tests as measures of readability and comprehension ability. Doctoral dissertation, Indiana University, 1962.

Bransford, J. D., & Franks, J. J' The abstraction of linguistic ideas. *Cognitive Psychology*, 1971, **2**, 331-50.

Brown, R., Cazden, C., & Bellugi, U. The child's grammar from I to III. In J. P. Hill (Ed.), *The 1973 Minnesota symposium on child psychology*. Minneapolis: University of Minnesota Press, 1968.

Bush, W. J., & Giles, M. T. Aids to psycholinguistic teaching. Columbus, Ohio: Charles E. Merrill, 1969.

Cartledge, C. J., & Krauser, E. L. Training first-grade children in creative thinking under quantitative and qualitative motivation. *Journal of Educational Psychology*, 1963, **54**, 295-99.

Cofer, C. N. A comparison of logical and verbatim learning of prose passages of different lengths. *American Journal of Psychology*, 1941, **54**, 1-20.

Cofer, C. N. Does conceptual organization influence the amount retained in free recall. In B. Kleinmuntz (Ed.), *Concepts and the structure of memory*. New York: John Wiley & Sons, 1967.

Cofer, C. N. Constructive processes in memory. *American Scientist*, 1973, **61**, 537-43.

Culhane, J. W. Cloze procedures and comprehension. *Reading Teacher*, 1970, **23**, 410-13.

Denckla, M. B. Naming of pictured objects by dyslexic and non-dyslexic "MBD" children. Paper presented at the Academy of Aphasia, 1974.

Dixon, T., & Horton, D. (Eds.) *Verbal behavior and general behavior theory*. Englewood Cliffs, N.J.: Prentice-Hall, 1968.

Flavell, J. H. *The developmental psychology of Jean Piaget*. New York: Van Nostrand Reinhold Co., 1963.

Fodor, J. A., & Bever, T. G. The psychological reality of linguistic segments. *Journal of Verbal Learning and Verbal Behavior*, 1965, **4**, 414-20.

Fraser, C., Bellugi, U., & Brown, R. Control of grammar in imitation, comprehension, and production. *Journal of Verbal Learning and Verbal Behavior*, 1963, **2**, 121-35.

Glanzer, M., & Cunitz, A. R. Two storage mechanisms in free recall. *Journal of Verbal Learning and Verbal Behavior*, 1966, **5**, 351-60.

Goldstein, K. *Language and language disorders*. New York: Grune & Stratton, 1948.

Goodglass, H., & Kaplan, E. *The assessment of aphasia and related disorders*. Philadelphia: Lea & Febiger, 1972.

Grossman, R. Auditory and visual sequencing ability in dyslexic children. Master's thesis, University of Denver, 1972.

Guilford, J. P. *The nature of human intelligence*. New York: McGraw-Hill, 1967.

Hafner, L. E. Implications of cloze. In E. L. Thurston & L. E. Hafner (Eds.), *The philosophical and sociological bases of reading*. Milwaukee, Wis.: National Reading Conference, 1965. Pp. 188-202.

Herr, S. E. *Perceptual communication skills: developing auditory awareness and insight*. (Teacher's handbook). Los Angeles: Imed, 1969.

Horowitz, L. M., Norman, S. A., & Day, R. S. Availability and associative symmetry. *Psychological Review*, 1966, **73**, 1-15.

Inhelder, B., & Piaget, J. *The growth of logical thinking from childhood to adolescence*. New York: Basic Books, 1958.

Jarvella, R. J. Syntactic processing of connected speech. *Journal of Verbal Learning and Verbal Behavior*, 1971, **10**, 409-16.

Jenkinson, M. E. Selected processes and difficulties in reading comprehension. Doctoral dissertation, University of Chicago, 1957.

Johnson, D. J., & Myklebust, H. R. *Learning disabilities: educational principles and practices*. New York: Grune & Stratton, 1967.

Kausler, D. H. *Psychology of verbal learning and memory*. New York: Academic Press, 1974.

Keenan, J. S. A method for eliciting naming behavior from aphasic patients. *Journal of Speech and Hearing Disorders*, 1966, **31**, 261-66.

Kirk, S. A., McCarthy, J. J., & Kirk, W. D. *Illinois test of psycholinguistic ability:* (Rev. ed.) Urbana: University of Illinois Press, 1968.

Kranyik, M. A. Music can help. *Grade Teacher*, 1970, **87**, 60-64.

Lee, L. L. *Northwestern syntax screening test*. Evanston, Ill.: Northwestern University Press, 1971.

Lee, L. L. *Developmental sentence analysis*. Evanston, Ill.: Northwestern University Press, 1974.

Lee, L., Koenigsknecht, R. A., & Mulhern, S. T. *Interactive language development teaching*. Evanston, Ill.: Northwestern University Press, 1975.

Lerner, J. W. *Children with learning disabilities*. Boston: Houghton Mifflin Co., 1971.

Light, L. L. Homonyms and synonyms as retrieval cues. *Journal of Experimental Psychology*, 1972, **96**, 255-62.

Luria, A. R. *Higher cortical functions in man*. New York: Basic Books, 1966.

Luria, A. R. *The working brain*. New York: Basic Books, 1973.

McLean, R. S., & Gregg, L. W. Effects of induced chunking on temporal aspects of serial recitation. *Journal of Experimental Psychology*, 1967, **74**, 455-59.

Maltzman, I., Bogartz, W., & Berger, L. A procedure for increasing word association originality and its transfer-effects. *Journal of Experimental Psychology*, 1958, **56**, 392-98.

Maltzman, I., Simon, S., Raskin, D., & Licht, L. Experimental studies in the training of originality. *Psychological Monographs*, 1960, **74**, No. 6 (Whole No. 493).

Marsh, D. H. Auditory figure-ground ability in children. *American Journal of Occupational Therapy*, 1973, **27**, 218-25.

Meeker, M. N. *The structure of intellect: its interpretation and uses*. Columbus, Ohio: Charles E. Merrill, 1969.

Menyuk, P. *Sentences children use*. Cambridge: M.I.T. Press, 1969.

Menyuk, P., & Looney, P. L. A problem of language disorder: length versus structure. *Journal of Speech and Hearing Research*, 1972, **15**, 264-79.

Miller, G. A. The magical number seven, plus or minus two. *Psychological Review*, 1956, **63**, 81-97.

Miller, G. A., & Chomsky, N. Finitary models of language users. In R. D. Luce, R. R. Bush, & E. Galanter (Eds.), *Handbook of mathematical psychology*. Vol. 2. New York: John Wiley & Sons, 1963. Pp. 419-91.

Moffett, J. *Teaching the universe of discourse*. Boston: Houghton Mifflin Co., 1968.

Moffett, J. *A student-centered language arts curriculum, grade K-6: a handbook for teachers*. Boston: Houghton Mifflin Co., 1973. (a)

Moffett, J. *A student-centered language arts curriculum, grade K-13: a handbook for teachers*. Boston: Houghton Mifflin Co., 1973. (b)

Murdock, B. B., Jr. The serial effect of free recall. *Journal of Experimental Psychology*, 1962, **64**, 482-88.

Palermo, D. S., & Jenkins, J. J. *Word association norms: grade school through college*. Minneapolis: University of Minnesota Press, 1964.

Piaget, J., & Inhelder, B. *Memory and intelligence*. New York: Basic Books, 1973.

Rankin, E. F. An evaluation of the cloze procedure as a technique for measuring reading comprehension. Doctoral dissertation, University of Michigan, 1957.

Rankin, E. F., & Dale, L. H. Cloze residual gain: a technique for measuring learning through reading. In G. B. Schick & M. M. May (Eds.), *The psychology of reading behavior*. Milwaukee, Wis.: The National Reading Conference, 1969. Pp. 17-25.

Renzulli, J. S. *New directions in creativity*. New York: Harper & Row, 1973.

Riegel, K. F. *The Michigan restricted association norms*. University of Michigan, Department of Psychology, Report No. 3, 1965.

Rinsland, H. D. *A basic vocabulary of elementary school children*. New York: Macmillan, 1945.

Romney, A. K., & D'Andrade, R. G. Cognitive aspects of English kin terms. In A. K. Romney & R. G. D'Andrade (Eds.), *Transcultural studies in cognition. American Anthropologist*, 1964, **66**, 3:2, 146-70.

Rosenthal, J. H. A preliminary psycholinguistic study of children with learning disabilities. *Journal of Learning Disabilities*, 1970, **3**, 391-95.

Sachs, J. S. Recognition memory for syntactic and semantic aspects of connected discourse. *Perception and Psychophysics*, 1967, **2**, 437-42.

Savin, H. B., & Perchonock, E. Grammatical structure and the immediate recall of English sentences. *Journal of Verbal Learning and Verbal Behavior*, 1965, **4**, 348-53.

Schneyer, J. W. Use of the cloze procedure for improving reading comprehension. *Reading Teacher*, 1965, **19**, 1978.

Semel, E. M. *Sound-Order-Sense: a developmental program in auditory perception*. Chicago: Follett Educational Corp., 1970.

Semel, E. M. *Semel auditory processing program*. Chicago: Follett Publishing Corp., in press.

Semel, E. M., & Wiig, E. H. Comprehension of syntactic structures and critical verbal elements by children with learning disabilities. *Journal of Learning Disabilities*, 1975, **8**, 53-58.

Simon, H. A., & Chase, W. G. Skill in chess. *American Scientist*, 1973, **61**, 394-403.

Sitko, M. C., & Semmel, M. I. The effect of phrasal cueing on free recall of EMR and non-retarded children. *American Educational Research*, 1967, **10**, 348-53.

Slobin, D. I. *Psycholinguistics*. Glenview, Ill.: Scott Foresman & Co., 1971.

Taylor, W. L. Cloze procedure: a new tool for measuring readability. *Journalism Quarterly*, 1953, **30**, 415.

Terman, L., & Merrill, M. *Stanford-Binet intelligence scale*. Boston: Houghton Mifflin Co., 1960.

Thorndike, E. L., & Lorge, F. *The teacher's word book of 30,000 words*. New York: Columbia University, 1944.

Torrance, E. P. *Rewarding creative behavior*. Englewood Cliffs, N.J.: Prentice-Hall, 1965.

Tulving, E. The effects of presentation and recall of material in free-recall learning. *Journal of Verbal Learning and Verbal Behavior*, 1967, **6**, 175-84.

Tulving, E. Cue-dependent forgetting. *American Scientist*, 1974, **62**, 74-82.

Tulving, E., & Pearlstone, Z. Availability versus accessibility of information in memory for words. *Journal of Verbal Learning and Verbal Behavior*, 1966, **5**, 381-91.

Tulving, E., & Psotka, J. Retroactive inhibition in free recall: inaccessibility of information available in the memory store. *Journal of Experimental Psychology*, 1971, **87**, 1-8.

Tulving, E., & Thomson, D. M. Encoding specificity and retrieval processes in episodic memory. *Psychological Review*, 1973, **80**, 352-73.

Tzeng, O. J-L. An empirical study of the difference between components of a dual-memory system. Unpublished doctoral dissertation, Pennsylvania State University, 1972.

Vogel, S. A. Syntactic abilities in normal and dyslexic children. *Journal of Learning Disabilities*, 1974, **7**, 47-53.

Weaver, W. W. Theoretical aspects of the cloze procedure. In E. L. Thurston & L. E. Hafner (Eds.), *The philosophical and sociological bases of reading*. Milwaukee, Wis.: National Reading Conference, 1965, Pp. 115-32.

Wechsler, D. *Wechsler intelligence scale for children*. New York: Psychological Corp., 1949.

Wiegel Crump, C., & Koenigsknecht, R. Tapping the lexical store of the adult aphasic: analysis of the improvement made in word retrieval skills. *Cortex,* 1973, **9**, 411-18.

Wiig, E. H., & Globus, D. Aphasic word identification as a function of logical relationship and association strength. *Journal of Speech and Hearing Research,* 1971, **14**, 195-204.

Wiig, E. H., & Roach, M. A. Immediate recall of semantically varied "sentences" by learning disabled adolescents. *Perceptual and Motor Skills,* 1975, **40**, 119-25.

Wiig, E. H., & Semel, E. M. Productive language abilities in learning disabled adolescents. *Journal of Learning Disabilities,* 1975, **8**, 578-86.

Winitz, H. Problem solving and the delaying of speech as strategies in the teaching of language. *American Speech & Hearing Assn.,* 1973, **15**, 583-86.

Wiseman, D. E. A classroom procedure for identifying and remediating language problems. *Mental Retardation,* 1965, **3**, 20-24.

Wyke, M. An experimental study of verbal association in aphasia. *Brain,* 1962, **85**, 679-86.

Zivian, M. T. Word identification as a function of semantic clues and association strength. University of Michigan, Department of Psychology, Report No. 12, 1966.

11 Social Perception: A Component Language Skill

Overview

The final chapter emphasizes the need to consider deficits in social perception in the educational and clinical management of children and adolescents with language and learning disabilities. The characteristics and possible bases for reduced social perception are presented. The relationship between social perception and personality development is discussed with reference to Cooley (1956), Mead (1934), and Sullivan (1953, 1954, 1964). Parameters of nonverbal communication are introduced with emphasis on studies of the significance of kinesics and proxemics by, among others, Birdwhistell (1952, 1970) and Hall (1959, 1966).

Observations of social imperception in learning disabled children and adolescents are presented. The discussions emphasize observations of classroom behaviors reflecting social imperception and its implications during adolescence. Counseling experiences are introduced that focus on the relationships between social imperception and social-sexual development. Tests are suggested that may assist in the diagnosis of deficits in the perception and interpretation of nonverbal communication cues. Several approaches for intervention are discussed. Specific methods are suggested for improving the interpretation of body language, and the need for counseling is emphasized.

Characteristics and Implications

Children and adolescents with learning disabilities have been reported to exhibit deficiencies in social perception, that is, reduced ability to acquire the significance of the nonverbal aspects of communication that indicate the attitudes, feelings, and intentions of others (Giffen, 1968; Johnson & Myklebust, 1967; Lerner, 1971; Wiig & Harris, 1974).

Learning disabled children may demonstrate difficulties and confusions in interpreting everyday expressions of affect and attitudes through facial expressions, gestures, caresses, or touches. They may respond inappropriately and therefore risk rejection and ridicule by their peers. They may become indifferent, aggressive, and hostile if they continually receive the impression that they are not accepted or loved. Because they may not be able to recognize a smile or a touch as an expression of love, affection, or approval they may lack the basic security provided by the knowledge of being loved. This deprivation may in turn result in deviant personality development (Sullivan, 1953, 1954, 1964).

The problems encountered by the LD youngster as a result of reductions in affective sensitivity may be further compounded by problems in acquiring unspoken social rules and amenities. Among the adaptive social skills the learning disabled youngster may fail to acquire are the rules relating to who enters a room first, who enters last, who is in line for the next turn, how to win or lose gracefully, and how and where to assert one's self in a social situation and how and when to enter into or withdraw from it. These social skills are important in adapting to a variety of educational, social, and competitive situations. The learning disabled child or adolescent with poor social abilities may suffer rejection and frustration, which may lead to nonadaptive or unacceptable social behaviors such as withdrawal, aggression, anger, or open hostility.

The quality of interpersonal interactions depends as much on nonverbal as on verbal communication ability (Allport, 1961; Argyle, 1967, 1972; Birdwhistell, 1952, 1970; Cook, 1971). Sensitivity to the affective, nonverbal aspects of interpersonal communication is also recognized to contribute to adaptive patterns of social behavior (Johnson & Myklebust, 1967; Sullivan, 1953; Swensen, 1973). Reductions in social perception appear to constitute significant communication deficits and result in poorer interpersonal relations and social adjustment for some children and adolescents with learning disabilities (Bryan, 1974; Cowgill, Friedland, & Shapiro, 1973; Wiig and Harris, 1974).

Bases for Reductions in Social Perception

Reduced ability to recognize affective cues may have various bases and reflect either cognitive, conceptual, visual-perceptual, or symbolic deficits. Johnson and Myklebust (1967) attribute deficiencies in the social behavior of LD children to a neurological basis. In adults with aphasia, reductions in the ability to recognize faces and interpret emotions have been attributed to a general cognitive deficit or to impaired concept formation (Bay, 1962; De Renzi, Faglioni, & Spinnler, 1966; Faglioni, Spinnler, & Vignolo, 1969; Horenstein, 1970; Milgram, 1960). Similarly, reduced ability to recognize affective cues may relate to conceptual deficits commonly reported in children with learning disabilities (Lerner, 1971).

In a different vein, deficiencies in the recognition of affective cues associated with learning disabilities may reflect specific visual processing deficits (Johnson & Myklebust, 1967). The interpretation of nonverbal aspects of expressed emotions has generally been considered to involve at least a two-stage process. Kagan and Krathwohl (1967) consider affective sensitivity to depend upon a sensory and a labeling stage. Warrington and James (1967) concluded that recognition and interpretation of facial expression are two distinct cerebral processes based on their finding that patients with lesions in the left hemisphere made errors in naming while patients with lesions in the right hemisphere made errors in recognition. Fridja (1969) describes the two stages in interpreting facial expressions to involve (1) assessment of the pattern of changes in facial expression and (2) subsequent specification of this pattern on the basis of situational and other contextual cues. Based on these models, reduced affective sensitivity associated with learning disabilities may reflect visual processing deficits interfering with the assessment or recognition of kinesic patterns or symbolic deficits interfering with the specification, interpretation, or labeling of the perceived kinestic patterns.

Bruner (1951) offers a model for social perception that comprises a three-step cycle. The first step of the cycle asserts that the act of perceiving begins with an expectancy hypothesis, suggesting that we not only perceive social cues but also that we anticipate them. The second step in the model relates to the processing of the input data. The third step is viewed as the confirmation or checking process. At this level, the perceiver judges whether the information is congruent with the expectancy hypothesis. If the initial hypothesis is not confirmed, it shifts in a direction determined by personal experience and cognitive factors as well as by the feedback from the immediately preceding, unsuccessful information-checking cycle. The expectancy hypothesis—confirmation model suggested by Bruner for social perception has very similar features to the model proposed here for auditory language processing. This suggests that the same analytic framework may apply to processing visual, nonverbal communication cues and auditory verbal information. The implications of this similarity suggest that the remedial strategies may be based on the same principles. It is not surprising, in this context, that Davitz (1964) observed that people who were sensitive to nonverbal communication cues expressing the emotions of others are also sensitive to emotional expression by voice through prosody (pitch, loudness, duration, and timbre). They were also observed to be high in verbal intelligence and abstract symbolic abilities, linking the nonverbal and verbal communication abilities to each other.

Social Perception and Personality Development

The role of interpersonal relations in personality development and in the development of the self has been discussed by, among others, Cooley (1956), Mead (1934), and Sullivan (1953). They agree that the self develops out of interaction with other people but disagree about the origin of the person's feelings about the reactions of others to him.

Mead (1934) postulated a cognitive basis for the self and felt the self developed as a result of internalized conversation between the *I* and the *me*. In this conversation the *me* was thought to represent what the person thinks others think about him. The *I* represented how the person himself thought, felt, or acted based on the reactions of the *me*. The internal, interactive dialogue is considered to develop and constitute the self, and this self can only be developed through interactions with others.

Mead takes the process a step further and asserts that "selves can only exist in definite relationships to other selves. No hard-and-fast line can be drawn between our own selves and the selves of others, since our own selves exist and enter as such into our experience only insofar as the selves of others exist and enter as such into our experience" (p. 164). Although this statement may seem extreme to some, the implications are awesome when we consider the disadvantages and deficits with which the learning disabled child and adolescent enter into interpersonal relationships.

Cooley (1956) considers the self to originate from our perceptions of the reactions (verbal and nonverbal) of others to us. He states that "the kind of self-feeling one has is determined by the attitude toward this attributed to the other mind. A social self of this sort might be called the reflected or looking glass self" (pp. 183-84). Swensen (1973) discusses that this self is composed of (1) our conception of how we appear to others, (2) our conception of how this appearance is judged by others, and (3) our reactions to and feelings about the appearance and judgment. He concludes that "anyone's social situation is of crucial importance to his existence. A person with disturbed or unsatisfying relationships with others will unquestionably be a disturbed person" (pp. 4-5).

Sullivan (1953, 1954, 1964) applied the concepts of Mead and Cooley to his psychiatric work and developed a theory of interpersonal relations and personality development. The development of personality and self is described by Sullivan (1953) within the developmental stages of *infancy, childhood, the juvenile era, preadolescence*, and *late adolescence*. The discussion of significant variables in the various stages of personality development and the implications of atypical developmental factors may provide insight into the personality development of the LD child and adolescent.

During *childhood*, socialization unfolds and self-system develops and changes, based on experiences gained in interactions with significant adults. In the *juvenile era*, socialization widens to include significant people outside the home. The increased communication and interaction with others provide opportunities for consensual validation so that public facts will be discriminated from personal fantasies. It is also during this period that the child with limited communication (verbal and nonverbal) abilities may be rejected and ridiculed by others because he does not "make sense." The *preadolescent* period provides new opportunities for consensual validation of the self-concept, which occurs through interactions with one or more good friends of the same sex. Sullivan asserts that youngsters who have been deprived of positive experiences with a "chum" during this period may never be able to relate to peers in adulthood or feel secure among strangers.

During early adolescence and adolescence, the development of sexual identity and patterns of sexual behavior assume primary importance. It should lead to the establishment of an intimate relationship with a person of the opposite sex during *late adolescence* and the development of a sexual role. Sullivan stresses the importance of positive interpersonal relationships during adolescence and discusses the contributions of verbal and nonverbal communication modes to the adequate development of the self. He further states that "unfortunate experience at any developmental phase may do great damage to one's possibilities of future interpersonal relations and . . . very fortunate experience at any developmental stage may do much to remedy the limitations already introduced by previous developmental misfortunes" (1964, p. 266).

The complexities of the development of personality and the self and the grave implications of communication deficits for adequate social development are relevant to the total management of the youngster with a learning disability. Recent reports of relationships between juvenile delinquency and learning disabilities (Berman & Siegal, 1975; Tarnopol, 1970) underscore this point.

Parameters of Nonverbal Communication

The parameters of nonverbal communication have been studied in considerable detail (Birdwhistell, 1952, 1970; Davitz, 1964; Ekman & Friesen, 1968; Hall, 1959, 1966; Mahl, 1968; Scheflen, 1967). The observations reveal a complex nonverbal system of communication involving kinesics (body language), proxemics (distance and space) and "paralanguage" (vocal characteristics) which may function independently of or in relationship with verbal communication.

Scheflen (1967) categorizes the modalities involved in interpersonal, face-to-face communication as (1) verbal language (includes linguistics and paralanguage), and (2) nonverbal language (includes kinesic, tactile, odorous, territorial, and artifactual (dress) cues). The relationships between the verbal and nonverbal language modalities are viewed differently by authorities.

Birdwhistell (1970) considers interpersonal communication to be "a system which makes use of the channels of all the modalities" (p. 70). The nonverbal channels are considered to be of equal importance in communicating as the verbal channels. Ekman and Friesen (1968), on the other hand, emphasize the relationships between verbal and nonverbal communication modes. These relationships have been outlined as follows by Swensen (1973, p. 85-86):

1. The nonverbal act expresses the same meaning as the verbal act.
2. The nonverbal act anticipates future amplification of concurrent verbal content.
3. The nonverbal act can convey a meaning which contradicts the meaning of the verbal act.
4. The nonverbal act can emphasize global aspects of an interaction, rather than specific aspects of the verbal act.
5. The nonverbal act can accent a specific part of the verbal act.
6. The nonverbal act can fill or explain silences.
7. The nonverbal act can maintain or regulate the verbal interaction.
8. The nonverbal act can substitute for a word or phrase in the verbal act.
9. The nonverbal act can provide a delayed registration of meaning which has already been expressed verbally.

The complexity of expressing and interpreting nonverbal communication cues is further increased by the parameters of kinesics (body language) and proxemics (space language). The kinesic cues that are an essential part of interpersonal communication are generally referred to as nonverbal communication cues. They are the primary conveyors of attitudes and emotions which may be expressed consciously or unconsciously. Proxemics, communication through personal and social distance and space, conveys information which reflects intimacy and status in interpersonal relations.

Kinesics (body language) has been viewed to express personality as well as to convey information during interpersonal interaction (Allport, 1961; Birdwhistell, 1952, 1970; Davitz, 1964). Birdwhistell (1952) describes two levels of nonverbal communication (1) the macrokinesic level which relates to body movements carrying meaning or conveying information, and (2) the parakinesic level which relates to body movements accenting or qualifying the verbal communication. At the macrokinesic level, Birdwhistell identifies the *kineme,* the smallest unit of body movement that can change the meaning of a body movement, and the *kinemorph,* the smallest unit that can carry meaning in body language. The analogy to the phoneme and morpheme in linguistics should be evident.

Aspects of Body Language

Ekman and Friesen (1968) have attempted to delineate the kinds of information that can be conveyed by body language. They consider body language primarily a relationship language, indicating that the message could have been conveyed verbally but that the verbal statement may be difficult or embarrassing. Nonverbal behavior is also considered to have a special symbolic language to express emotions and attitudes towards the self. It may accent and qualify verbal behavior and is less subject to censorship than verbal language.

There seems to be general agreement that facial expressions are the main conveyors of emotions but that they differ among cultures (Birdwhistell, 1952; Davitz, 1964; Ekman & Friesen, 1968). Although each facial expression must be interpreted within a context, gross categories of emotion (positive-negative and active-passive) can be identified (Davitz, 1964). Slow-motion movies have also revealed "micromomentary expressions" lasting about one-fifth of a second. These expressions may be incongruent with both the verbal and nonverbal behavior context in which they occurred (Haggard and Isaacs, 1966). The micromomentary expressions (MME) have been interpreted to serve as "a safety valve to permit at least the very brief expression of unacceptable impulses and affects" (p. 165). Eye contact appears to reflect variables such as like-dislike, content, and listening-speaking, and to serve as a signal in conversation (Duncan, 1969; Ekman & Friesen, 1968; Exline, Gray, & Schuette, 1965; Mehrabian, 1969, 1970; Sommer, 1967).

Body posture generally does not communicate the same effect as facial expression (Ekman & Friesen, 1968). It seems to reflect attitude towards the other person or persons involved in the interaction and to indicate relative tension and relaxation. Body orientation seems to reflect liking and esteem. The level of body movement seems to indicate responsiveness, and an isolated high rate of leg movement when seated seems to reflect a negative attitude.

Egolf and Chester (1973) have advocated that the professional concerned with disorders of language and communication needs to be aware of the characteristics and implications of nonverbal communication cues and deficits. In an effort to bring about heightened awareness, they have discussed parameters affecting nonverbal communication such as physical attributes, costuming and cosmetics, eye movements, and use of space, time, touch, body movement and vocal quality and related these to quantitative and qualitative aspects of therapeutic interactions. Their observations of the implications of nonverbal communication cues for speech and language therapy apply equally to interactions between the educator-clinician and language and learning disabled children and adolescents.

Nonverbal Communication Deficits in Learning Disabilities

Johnson and Myklebust (1967) state that the LD child "does not comprehend his social word to the extent that he can do so" (p. 295). They further stress that although LD children may be deficient in social perception, they do not demonstrate severely abnormal behaviors as do autistic children (Goldfarb, 1961; Kanner, 1957; Myklebust, 1964) and do not show fundamental differences in personality.

Their observations indicate that learning disabled children may not perceive and interpret nonverbal behaviors correctly unless they are taught and unless the relationships among nonverbal experiences are verbalized. He has problems in perceiving and interpreting facial expressions, gestures, and other nonverbal behaviors and may be judged to be "tactless" and "stupid." Furthermore, social imperception in learning disabled children was observed to be associated with low performances on the *Picture Arrangement* subtest of the WISC (Johnson & Myklebust, 1967).

Lerner (1971) describes the nonverbal communication problems of learning disabled children as being based on deficits in interpreting stimuli in the social environment and in relating the interpretations appropriately to the social situation. As a result, they have difficulty in making appropriate social judgments and in adapting to social situations. Both Johnson and Myklebust (1967) and Lerner (1971) infer a right hemispheric impairment in these children and point to associated deficits in body image, directionality in space, and left-right orientation. They indicate that the LD child with problems in social perception may demonstrate evidence of a confused perceptual field, inaccurate estimations of space, and difficulties in adhering to the territorial boundaries in social interactions. As a result, he may move inappropriately in space, misinterpret directional gestures, bump into objects and people, stand too close to other people, talk before it is appropriate, and break into closed groups.

Classroom Behaviors Reflecting Social Imperception

These observations of social imperception in youngsters with learning disabilities have been corroborated by investigations of the predictors of learning disabilities, of teacher's perceptions of educationally high-risk children, and of classroom behaviors (Bryan, 1974; Cowgill, Friedland, & Shapiro, 1973; Keogh, Tchir, & Windeguth-Behn, 1974). Cowgill, Friedland, and Shapiro (1973) report that the best predictors of learning disabilities from kindergarten reports were immaturity, poor social and emotional adjustment, poor speech and language, and impulsivity.

In a similar vein, Keogh, Tchir, and Windeguth-Behn (1974) report that the most frequent descriptors of the learning disabled child given for kindergarten and primary-grade children described behavioral personality problems. Among the characteristics attributed to the learning disabled child were aggression, hyperactivity, short attention span, no responsibility, poor interpersonal relationships, disruptive, disinterested, angry, and hostile.

Bryan (1974) further observed that learning disabled children spent significantly less time in attending behavior for a variety of school subjects than did academically achieving children. They also demonstrated differences in their interpersonal relationships with teachers and with peers: learning disabled children spent as much time interacting with others, but were more likely to be ignored by regular classroom teachers and by age peers when they initiated interactions.

Social Imperception in Adolescence

The problems experienced by learning disabled youngsters in social interaction appear to be augmented in puberty when sexual identities and roles develop, and physical and sexual changes require adjustments of previously established body images and self-concepts. During this period, affective sensitivity, that is, the ability to adequately perceive and interpret the attitudes and affects of others, may constitute an important means of receiving external evaluations for consensual validation to assist in the development of an appropriate body image, a realistic self-concept, and a sexual identity. At the same time, the complexity of relevant affective cues increases and therefore places greater demands on affective sensitivity.

There is evidence that the difficulties in social perception experienced by the learning disabled child persist into adolescence (Wiig & Harris, 1974). They administered a videotape of a young female's nonverbal expressions (pantomimes) of anger, embarrassment, fear, frustration, joy, and love to seventeen learning disabled and seventeen academically achieving adolescents (Mean age = sixteen years one month) matched for sex, age, full-scale WISC or WAIS IQ, ethnic and socioeconomic background. The results indicated that the LD adolescents made significantly more substitutions in the labeling of the nonverbally expressed emotions than achieving controls, indicating quantitative reductions in the recognition of affective cues.

Qualitative differences were also observed when the substitution patterns were compared in the two groups. Achieving adolescents most frequently substituted love for embarrassment. This substitution is considered to reflect the common teen-age expression of love as an embarrassing emotion (Table 28).

TABLE 28
Comparison of Most Frequent Substitutions in Interpretation of Emotions by
17 Adolescents With Learning Disabilities and 17 Controls

Misinterpretations		Total substitutions	
Stimulus	Substitution	Learning Disabled	Controls
Love	Joy	16	4
Embarrassment	Joy	15	0
Embarrassment	Love	10	23
Joy	Embarrassment	8	2
Joy	Love	6	0
Frustration	Love	5	0
Anger	Frustration	4	11
Frustration	Anger	4	4
Fear	Frustration	4	0
Frustration	Joy	3	0
Joy	Frustration	2	0
Embarrassment	Frustration	2	0
Frustration	Fear	2	0
Anger	Joy	2	0

SOURCE: Reprinted with permission of publishers from: Wiig, E. H., and Harris, S. P. Perception and interpretation of nonverbally expressed emotions by adolescents with learning disabilities. *Perceptual and Motor Skills*, 1974, **38**, 239-45.

In contrast, substitutions of love for embarrassment were low in frequency by the thirty college students of the pilot study and by young adult stutterers and their controls (Litz, 1973), suggesting an age-related difference in the recognition of love and embarrassment in normal subjects. The remaining substitutions involved emotions that were either ranked adjacently or received a wide range of ranks in a pilot evaluation of the emotions by achieving adolescents (Wiig & Harris, 1974), a finding agreeing with early studies of errors in the interpretation of emotions (Woodworth, 1938).

The substitutions made by the adolescents with learning disabilities were not limited to emotions that were ranked adjacently or received variable ranks in the evaluation by achieving adolescents. They frequently substituted emotions judged as relatively positive for ones judged as relatively negative. Their responses also lacked the "teen-age quality" observed in academically achieving adolescents. The substitutions suggest a high proportion of undifferentiated responses to both the positive and negative feeling tone of the expressed emotions.

The number of correct interpretations of emotions correlated positively with scaled scores on the *Block Design* (r = .53, p< .05) and *Object Assembly* (r = .67, p< .01) subtests of the WISC or WAIS and the *Design* subtest of the Detroit tests (r = .71, p< .01) for the learning disabled adolescents, indicating that the present measure of affective sensitivity related to measures of visual-motor organization (Wechsler, 1958). This finding contrasts with previous reports that social imperception in learning disabilities is generally associated with low performance on the *Picture Arrangement* subtest of the WISC (Johnson & Myklebust, 1967). The positive correlations suggest that reductions in affective sensitivity in learning disabled adolescents relate to reduced visual-motor organization (Wechsler, 1958) and to the assessment or recognition of kinesic patterns (Fridja, 1969; Kagan & Krathwohl, 1967; Warrington & James, 1967).

The educational and social significance of the observed reductions in affective sensitivity was further stressed by the reports from the special education teacher. Learning disabled adolescents scoring in the lower half on the experimental test were generally poor in adaptive social behaviors and exhibited inadequate social perceptions in the classroom. Their development of social perception relative to cultural expectations for roles as men and women also seemed uneven, supporting a need to consider nonverbal communication in the clinical management of learning disabled children and youth.

Problems in Social-Sexual Interactions

Clinical observations suggest that the problems experienced by the learning disabled youngster in social perception, interpersonal relations, and adaptive social behaviors are intensified during adolescence. The critical contributing factor seems to relate to the increased desire as well as to the increased expectations for social and personal interactions with persons of the opposite sex.

Learning disabled adolescents may enter into these interactions with conflicts relating to their self-concepts. The concept of self, and the concepts of the ideal and the public selves, may be in conflict as a result of previous frustrations and rejections. They may not have developed appropriate body images, acquired adaptive social behaviors, or gained insight into the cultural expectations for behaviors during the period when sexual identity and sexual roles are developed. As a result, they may demonstrate a blatant naivete in their social-sexual interactions, misinterpret friendly gestures as sexual overtures, show aggressiveness in initiating social-sexual contacts, and be very naive in discerning the implications of sexual advances by others.

The nature of the problems experienced by some LD adolescents and young adults in developing sexual identities and sexual roles may be illustrated by observations from counseling. Learning disabled adolescents frequently express puzzlement over rejections experienced when they touch others during social interactions. They often express a need to touch others to indicate their approval and like for them. Denied the approval by society and by others to indicate their emotions by touch, they may feel deprived because of perceived limitations in expressing themselves effectively, either verbally or nonverbally.

Some LD adolescents and young adults express a need to be touched by others in order to establish and maintain an image of their bodies. They may indicate that they feel deprived and sense a loss of security without the validation of their bodies provided by the tactile input from the touch of others.

Some young adults with learning disabilities express a sense of wonder when they achieve a body image which has previously eluded them in positive sexual interactions.

Some adults with learning disability backgrounds have expressed a need to maintain or reestablish their body images through the caress and touch by another person in intimate sexual interactions. These reflections are often offered by learning disabled persons with visual-perceptual and visual-motor deficits and with revisualization problems. They suggest that problems in establishing a body image may be reflected in excessive touching in social interactions and a need for establishing body awareness and image.

Learning disabled adolescents frequently describe problems in interpreting a gaze and they themselves may not follow the cultural expectations for the duration of a gaze. Typically, they describe a need to visually survey other people to form a total impression of the person or of the person's non-verbal reactions during the interaction. The duration and direction of their gazes may cause others embarrassment and result in rejection or withdrawal. The culture dictates that visual surveys of the characteristics and reactions of others occur surreptitiously, and a sustained gaze is inappropriate unless the situation is intimate. The learning disabled female who depends on sustained visual survey to analyze and synthesize kinesic cues may be perceived as forward and often expresses surprise that this behavior is interpreted as a sexual advance.

Social imperception and lack of affective sensitivity is often associated with problems in appropriately expressing emotion. In some learning disabled adolescents, this may reflect itself as a lack of emotional tone and expression; in others, the nonverbal communication cues may be overexaggerated, or inappropriate, failing to convey the intended emotion. They may perceive the inappropriateness and withdraw from social-sexual interactions during adolescence, and they may compensate with blatant, aggressive, socially inappropriate verbal overtures. Each of these reactions may result in further rejection and lead to problems in the development of a sexual identity and role. Social imperception and reduced affective sensitivity also interfere with the process of consensual validation considered important in the *juvenile era* for adequate personality development (Sullivan, 1953).

Assessment of Nonverbal Communication Deficits

The diagnosis of deficits in the perception of nonverbal communication cues is hampered by the fact that there are presently no standardized tests available. Clinical observations and research findings suggest relationships among deficits in social perception and affective sensitivity and depressed scores on standardized tests (Johnson & Myklebust, 1967; Lerner, 1971; Wiig & Harris, 1974). These standardized tests may therefore be used to obtain indirect evidence of difficulties in perceiving and interpreting nonverbal communication cues: (1) the *Bender Gestalt Test for Young Children*, (2) the *Picture Arrangement*, *Block Design* and *Object Assembly* subtests of the *WISC*, (3) the *Memory for Design* subtest of the *Detroit Tests of Learning Aptitude*, and (4) the *Vineland Social Maturity Scale*.

Bender Gestalt Test for Young Children

This (Koppitz norms) (Koppitz, 1964) is a copy-drawing test designed to assess visual-motor perception. The test contains nine designs that serve as models for the child's copy-drawing. The copy-drawings are done using a pencil on plain white paper. The model designs are presented in a sequence progressing from simple to complex. The resulting drawings are scored using a checklist that considers direction, integration, rotation, and perseveration. Normative data are available for the age range between five and ten.

The test manual provides information regarding administration and scoring. Test-retest and scorer reliability correlations have been reported to be high, ranging from .88 to .96. The validity of the test has been determined by including only items that differentiated academically achieving first- and second-graders from poor achievers. Lerner (1971) suggests that social imperception in LD children is associated with reduced performances on the *Bender Gestalt* test, suggesting that it has predictive value.

WISC: Picture Arrangement

The *Picture Arrangement* subtest of the WISC (Wechsler, 1949a,b) contains eleven items requiring cut up comic strip pictures to be assembled in a logical sequence. The picture sequences depict sequential and causal events presented in order of difficulty. Performances reflect visual perception, comprehension, and synthesis abilities; reductions may indicate social or interpersonal imperception (Johnson & Myklebust, 1967). In a factor analysis, Cohen (1959) observed no specific factors for this subtest. Glasser and Zimmerman (1967) provide interpretations of qualitative performance differences which appear relevant to the diagnostic use of the subtest with learning disabled children who demonstrate problems in social perception and interpersonal relations.

WISC: Block Design

The *Block Design* subtest of the WISC (Wechsler, 1949a, b) assesses the ability to perceive, analyze, synthesize, and reproduce abstract, two—dimensional geometrical patterns. The subtest contains ten items generally of increasing difficulty. The subject is required to reproduce designs with a set of multi-colored blocks within a given time limit. The subtest has been found to reveal a specific factor of perceptual organization (Cohen, 1959). It can therefore be used independently to assess perceptual organization and spatial visualization ability.

Glasser and Zimmerman (1967) provide an excellent discussion of the interpretation of error patterns and qualitative performance differences. Their interpretations may assist in identifying the nature of specific perceptual organization deficits contributing to social imperception in learning disabilities. The significant, positive correlations (53 and .67) reported by Wiig and Harris (1974), between measures of ability to perceive and interpret nonverbally expressed emotions and performances on the *Block Design* and *Object Assembly* subtests of the WISC and WAIS suggest predictive relationships.

WISC: Object Assembly

The *Object Assembly* subtest of the WISC (Wechsler, 1949a,b) assesses the ability to synthesize parts of familiar objects into complete, integrated figures. The subtest consists of four items, using cut up (jigsaw) picture puzzles of a man, a horse, a face, and a car, to be assembled within a time limit. It taps visual perception, anticipation of part-whole relationships, and visual synthesis abilities. Cohen (1959) indicates that performances on the subtest reflect perceptual organization ability, a skill also tapped by the *Block Design* subtest of the WISC. The *Object Assembly* subtest is, however, considered to be of inadequate reliability, suggesting that interpretation of performances on this subtest in isolation may have low validity. Wechsler (1949, 1955) reports high inter-correlations between subtest performances on the *Object Assembly* and *Block Design* subtests of the WISC for 13½-year-olds (r = .63) and for 18- to 19-year-olds (r = .69). This correlation plus the shared perceptual organization factor in the two subtests suggest that they should be used in combination to evaluate the bases for social imperception in learning disabilities.

DTLA: Memory for Designs

The *Memory for Designs* subtest of the *Detroit Tests for Learning Aptitude* (Baker & Leland, 1959) contains three groups of geometrical figures. Of these, eight figures (Group A) are to be copied with the model present; eight additional figures are to be reproduced after five-seconds exposure, assessing memory for the designs. Each copy drawing or reproduction is scored using a point scoring scale presented in the test manual. The maximum score obtainable is forty-four points.

Norms are available for the age range from three years to fifteen years nine months. No test-retest reliability data are provided for this subtest. A test-retest coefficient over a five-month period has been reported at .68. The significant, positive correlation (r = .71) reported by Wiig and Harris (1974) between a measure of affective sensitivity and learning quotients on the *Memory for Designs* subtest by LD adolescents suggests predictive value.

Vineland Social Maturity Scale

This scale (Doll, 1936, 1947a, 1947b) utilizes a format in which either the parent or the child is interviewed to obtain a measure of social maturity in terms of self-help, self-direction, occupation, communication, locomotion, and socialization abilities. The test was designed to tap increases in social maturity and competence in the age range from birth to twenty-five years. The test manual stresses that the information obtained should reflect what the subject actually and habitually does in respect to each item and should provide details in regard to both quantity and quality of the behavior. The responses are scored to obtain an estimate of social age (SA) and social quotient (SQ). When the test is used with LD youngsters to evaluate competence in social perception and interpersonal interaction, the item category relating to socialization is relevant as part of an assessment battery.

Additional Tests

Other tests that may provide information relevant to the differentiation of potential bases for social interaction difficulties are projective tests employing pictorial techniques. Among these are (1) the *Children's Apperception Test* (Bellak & Bellak, 1954), (2) the *Blacky Pictures* (Blum, 1950), (3) *Make-A-Picture Story for Children* (MAPS) (Shneidman, 1960), and (4) *Symonds Picture Story Test* (Symonds, 1949). The interpretation of these projective tests of personality dynamics relies upon the training and experience of the examiner, the clinical psychologist. The psychologist must also assume the responsibility for translating the findings to the educator and determining their implications for the educational management of the learning disabled child.

Additional tests and measures that may assist in the identification and differentiation of social perceptual and social behavioral problems are (1) the *Rosenzweig Picture-Frustration Test* (Rosenzweig, Fleming, & Rosenzweig, 1948), (2) the *Rotter Incomplete Sentences Blank* (Rotter & Rafferty, 1950), (3) the *Mooney Problem Checking List* (College form) (Mooney & Gordon, 1950), and (4) the *Kohlberg Moral Development Measures* (Kohlberg, 1963, 1964).

Improving Social Perception and Nonverbal Communication

The perception and interpretation of the complex, dynamic nonverbal communication cues used in everyday life depend upon immediate perception of the visual-kinesic pattern, associated with a critical evaluation of the relationships among the individual components. Furthermore, the initial interpretation of the available nonverbal communication cues must be evaluated within the total social (nonverbal and verbal) context, compared with expectancy hypotheses, and revised on the basis of incongruencies. This process requires adequate visual analysis, synthesis, and concurrent processing at several (nonverbal-verbal; symbolic-nonsymbolic) levels. Serial processing, which may be the only available processing mode for some LD children, requires time. It is generally not available since the nonverbal communication cues change rapidly and may function in several relationships to verbal communication cues (Swensen, 1973).

Approaches to Intervention

Intervention models and strategies for deficits in social perception and interpersonal interactions have recently been described by Dupont (1969). Among the models for intervention presented are the *psychotherapeutic model* which focuses on anxiety removal, self-knowledge, and the development of acceptable outlets for emotions and drives (Morse, 1965; Redl, 1969). *Behavior modification* concentrates on changing the overt behaviors using operant conditioning principles (Hewitt, 1967a, 1967b). The *ecological approach* sets up environmental surrounds, events, and situations from which new experiences may be gained (Hobbs, 1973); On the other hand, the *psycho-educational model* stresses cognitive development, remedial techniques for specific deficits, and academic achievement (Fenichel, 1966; Hollister & Goldston, 1962).

The educator may choose a specific approach to intervention depending upon considerations of the learning disabled child's experiential background, age, and deficit modalities and areas. Other considerations may include the immediacy of the required behavioral change and the extent of the difficulties. Based on these considerations, behavior modification may be initially selected to modify socially unacceptable behaviors which are grossly maladaptive. After initial modification, the psycho-educational model may be selected for intervention in isolation or in association with psychotherapeutic strategies. The ecological model may be chosen at several stages during intervention in association with other approaches to remediation. Each model features unique methods and techniques, and each may result in general improvements.

Improving Perception of Body Language

Planning remediation for social imperception and difficulties in interpersonal interaction requires emphasis on kinesics (facial expression, gestures, body movement) and proxemics (distance and space), aspects not considered in the previously described approaches to intervention.

The significance of facial expressions in conveying emotions (Birdwhistell, 1952; Davitz, 1964; Ekman & Friesen, 1968) suggests that improving the perception and interpretation of facial expressions should receive major emphasis in intervention. Johnson and Myklebust (1967) suggest that LD children need initial practice in observing and interpreting the facial expressions of a single person. They indicate that direct experiences with and pictures of the person may facilitate the association between facial expressions and positive and negative emotions. They also suggest using a self-developing camera to record the child's facial expressions in various situations. In the later stages of training, the child is required to interpret how a person feels based on situational pictures. Picture stories and filmstrips are also used to develop the ability to follow and integrate a sequence of events and to perform simultaneous analysis-and-synthesis of various aspects of the nonverbal communication act. Another suggested activity is charades. The activities emphasize throughout that verbalizations and labeling must accompany perception and discrimination of the visual cues.

The general recommendations for remediation and intervention provided by Johnson and Myklebust (1967) may be expanded by widening the scope and suggesting general and specific strategies, procedures, and materials:

1. Discriminations among facial expressions, gestures, body movements, and spatial orientation and distance among persons should progress from simple to complex.

2. Techniques used to improve discrimination and differentiation of facial expressions may progress as follows: (a) matching of identical expressions, using pictures of a single person, (b) making same-different judgments of expressions made by one person, using direct experiences or pictures, (c) matching similar expressions made by different people, using direct experiences and pictures, (d) categorization and verbal labeling of positive-negative expressions, (e) verbal labeling of features signaling distinctions between various positive and negative expressions, and (f) verbal labeling of expressed emotions, using direct experience, pictures, films, and videotapes. Among materials which may be used to improve the perception and interpretation of facial expressions are (1) Developmental Learning Materials' Facial Expression Cards, Body Concept Spirit Masters, Body Concept Templates, Position in Space Posters, and People Puzzles, (2) Dial-a-Face by Ideal, (3) pictures of self and of family members, slides of family members and peers, and (4) silent movies and filmstrips.

3. Techniques designed to develop the perception and discrimination of gestures and body movement may progress in the same sequence from simple to difficult, using similar methods and materials. However, the focus should be expanded to develop the perception of the relationships among facial expressions, gestures, and body movements (Ekman & Friesen, 1968).

Materials presenting dynamic, sequential visual stimuli seem best suited for this training. Filmstrips and silent movies may be used to facilitate the perception and interpretation of the combined, nonverbal communication cues. A remedial paradigm suitable for improving social perception, using a filmstrip or movie, may proceed as follows:

a. The entire movie is shown initially.
b. After completion of the showing, the educator and the students review the contents of the story to determine the social and emotional context for further analysis.
c. The film is shown again, but it is now stopped at various points that display interpersonal interactions. The students are required to predict the subsequent actions of the persons displayed in the interactions.
d. The interpersonal interaction is replayed to verify or reject the expectancy hypothesis.
e. If the prediction proves incorrect, the educator and the students discuss and label the critical kinesic cues in the sequence and revise and restate the expectancy hypothesis.
f. The sequence is finally shown in its entirety for verification of the revised prediction.

In the selection of film materials, silent movies in which the kinesic cues may be overstated and unambiguous should be selected first. As the perception and interpretation of nonverbal communication cues improves, materials may be selected that contain ambiguities at the nonverbal level. It is possible to produce a series of short (two to four) slide sequences, in which kinesic ambiguities must be resolved. Such a series was developed for therapy with adult aphasics. One sequence portrays two adolescents facing each other with raised fists but with smiling faces; the second slide of the sequence shows them walking off with arms around each other's shoulders.

When these sequences are used with LD youngsters, they frequently focus on one aspect of the bodies, the faces or the fists, and fail to synthesize other aspects and resolve ambiguities. As a result, their predictions of consequences are random. Verbal labeling and resolution of the kinesic ambiguties appear to improve the perception and interpretation of nonverbal cues in direct experiences and in filmed materials. This observation concurs with findings reported by Johnson and Myklebust (1967).

Facilitating Social Perception

In addition to procedures emphasizing the perception and interpretation of body language, social perception may be facilitated using appropriate readings and reading programs. *The Triple "I" Series* (Franco, Kelley, & Whitman, 1970) introduces readings about, and associated pictures of, school-age children in social and moral situations. The materials are designed to elicit discussion and are familiar, interesting, and relevant. The series attempts to realistically reflect the lives of children and to provide reasons and ways for enhancing their social selves and their self-images. *Developing understanding of self and others: play kit and manual* (Dinkmeyer, 1970) and *The magic circle program* (Gerler, 1973) are other sources of materials for facilitating social perception.

Reid (1972) has provided references to literature appropriate for gaining insight into a diversity of human relations. These readings may serve as the basis for group discussions of social and interpersonal relations as they occur within community, group, and family settings; they are grouped by topic in the following sections: (1) patterns of family life, (2) community contrasts, (3) economic differences, (4) differences between generations, (5) adjustment to new places and situations, (6) how it feels to grow up, (7) belonging to groups, and (8) experience of acceptance and rejection. The educator may add current literature to the appropriate groupings.

The Social Contract Approach

Among approaches to improving social competence in learning disabled and emotionally disturbed children, the social contract approach has been proposed (Meisels, 1974). This approach introduces the alternative behavior model, using a social contract between educator and student to implement behavioral control. This psycho-educational model structures social situations in the classroom to make expectations clear and behavioral changes obvious. The social contract approach has two goals for each child: self-determination and self-actualization. The focus is on replacing inappropriate behaviors by alternative, adaptive behaviors, using stimulus-response reinforcement paradigms.

The social contract is described as similar to the academic contracts discussed by Homme (1972). Each social contract used three question areas
to resolve unsuccessful coping behavior:

1. In picture words, or concretely, what did you do that got you into trouble?
2. What was in it for you?
   What did you want to result?
3. How can you get what you want without getting into trouble? [Meisels,
   1974, p. 34]

Enhancing Interpersonal Communication

The implementation of the social contract has been outlined by Meisels
(1974) to include five sequential steps. The first step requires that the student
concretely define his inappropriate behavior. The second step requires that
the child defines the physical anxiety cue or cues leading to the inappropriate
behavior. In subsequent steps, the child must define the environmental stimulus that elicited the inappropriate behavior and choose an acceptable, alternative response that serves his needs and the needs of the group. The teacher
initially determines the possible alternative behaviors considered acceptable
to the group. In the last step, the child must make a choice between the alternatives and clarify the consequences of the decision, that is, predict the subsequent responses (positive reinforcement or punishment) he will receive
from the group. The author stresses that the success of the social contract depends upon the responsibilities accepted by both the child and the teacher
and upon administrative support.

A totally different approach to enhancing social perception and interpersonal communication is presented in *Let's Talk* (Sathre, Olson, &
Whitney, 1973). This text presents strategies and techniques for developing
both verbal and nonverbal interpersonal communication skills. The strategies
are described and developed in an easy-to-read text and in an activities supplement which may be used by both the educator and the student (Whitney,
Sathre, & Olson, 1973).

The text and the activities are designed according to these principles:

1. Lasting, rewarding interpersonal relationships are developed by *association* (interaction), *aspiration* (cooperation) and *appreciation* (feedback).
2. Each person can contribute uniquely to interpersonal interactions.
3. The full potential for interpersonal communication must be developed.
4. All relationships are limited by social, emotional, and physical constraints.
5. Interpersonal communication requires desire as well as skills.

The strategies and classroom-tested activities described cover a wide range
of approaches, from traditional, subject-oriented to initial encounter types.
The text and activities lend themselves well to intervention with LD adolescents with social imperception and interpersonal communication problems.
It presents an organized approach that can be used by the special educator.

Various points are illustrated with cartoons that seem to motivate learning disabled adolescents. Use of the text may have to be modified to account for reading and language comprehension deficits, a task relatively easy to accomplish.

Among sections appearing especially relevant to the LD youngster are those dealing with improving (1) openness and honesty in verbal interactions, (2) social listening skills, (3) self-perception, (4) group process through role playing, and (5) nonverbal communication abilities.

Grilli et al. (1975) provide suggestions for teachers, parents, counselors, educators, and other professionals for effecting social behavioral change in children. Their discussion focuses on programmed strategies that may be used in a variety of settings, and a variety of strategies to improve social perception and nonverbal communication in children are included.

Counseling

Clinical observation also suggests that the learning disabled child and adolescent with nonverbal communication deficits may benefit from counseling in association with other approaches to intervention. Counseling allows the child or adolescent to express feelings and reactions to specific deficits and problem situations. In the process he may gain insight into the bases for the difficulties he experiences in interpersonal communication and into the causes for emotional reactions and inappropriate behavioral responses. The youngster may also reveal specific questions regarding the nature and implications of his disabilities which have gone unanswered.

Experiences with counseling LD adolescents and young adults suggest that insight into the nature and implications of a nonverbal communication deficit improves motivation for intervention, facilitates compensation, and relieves anxieties often associated with the remediation process. Counseling experiences with school-age children with learning disabilities and interpersonal interaction and nonverbal communication problems suggest that it is equally important for the child to be allowed to express his feelings and gain insight into the problem. Often these children express frustrations reflecting conflicts in self-perception and in the development of the self, the ideal self, and the public self. Descriptions by the child that reflect how he believes himself to be (self-concept), how he wishes to be (ideal self), and how he wants others to perceive him (public self) may suggest discrepancies and conflicts which may need to be resolved. Self-acceptance seems essential to the outcome of intervention.

Direct intervention to improve social perception and nonverbal communication in learning disabilities appears most effective at or after puberty when the demands and the rewards for effective interpersonal communication have increased. Improved social perception and affective sensitivity have been observed to be associated with increased adaptive social behavior and improved self-actualization, and social, vocational, and professional potential.

References

Allport, G. W. *Pattern and growth in personality*. New York: Holt, Rinehart & Winston, 1961.

Argyle, M. *The psychology of interpersonal behavior*. Middlesex: Penguin Books, 1967.

Argyle, M. *Non-verbal communication in human social interaction*. Cambridge: Cambridge University Press, 1972.

Baker, H., & Leland, B. *Detroit tests of learning aptitude*. Indianapolis: Test Division of Bobbs-Merrill, 1959.

Bay, E. Aphasia and nonverbal disorders of language. *Brain*, 1962, **85**, 411-26.

Bellak, L., & Bellak, S. *Children's apperception test*. (Rev. ed.) (Manual) Larchmont, N.Y.: C.P.S., 1954.

Berman, A., & Siegal, A. Delinquents are disabled: an innovative approach to the prevention and treatment of juvenile delinquency. Paper presented at the Second International Scientific Conference on Learning Disabilities, Brussels, 1975.

Birdwhistell, R. L. *Introduction to kinesics*. Louisville: University of Louisville Press, 1952.

Birdwhistell, R. L. *Kinesics and context*. Philadelphia: University of Philadelphia Press, 1970.

Blum, G. *The Blacky pictures: a technique for the exploration of personality dynamics*. (Manual) New York: Psychological Corp., 1950.

Bruner, J. S. Personality dynamics and the process of perceiving. In R. R. Blake & G. V. Ramsey (Eds.), *Perception—an approach to personality*. New York: Ronald Press, 1951. Pp. 121-47.

Bryan, T. An observational analysis of classroom behaviors of children with learning disabilities. *Journal of Learning Disabilities*, 1974, **7**, 35-43.

Cohen, J. The factorial structure of the WISC at ages 7½, 10½, and 13½. *Journal of Consulting Psychology*, 1959, **23**, 285-99.

Cook, M. *Interpersonal perception*. Middlesex: Penguin Books, 1971.

Cooley, C. H. *Human nature and the social order*. Glencoe, Ill.: The Free Press, 1956.

Cowgill, M., Friedland, S., & Shapiro, R. Predicting learning disabilities from kindergarten reports. *Journal of Learning Disabilities*, 1973, **6**, 577-82.

Davitz, J. P. *The communication of emotional meaning*. New York: McGraw-Hill, 1964.

De Renzi, E., Faglioni, P., & Spinnler, H. Face recognition and brain damage. *Neurology*, 1966, **16**, 145-52.

Dinkmeyer, D. *Developing understanding of self and others: play kit and manual*. Circle Pines, Minn.: American Guidance Service, 1970.

Doll, E. A. *Vineland social maturity scale*. Circle Pines, Minn.: American Guidance Service, 1936.

Doll, E. A. *Vineland social maturity scale; manual of directions.* Circle Pines, Minn.: Educational Test Bureau, 1947. (a)

Doll, E. A. *Vineland social maturity scale.* Circle Pines, Minn.: Educational Test Bureau, 1947. (b)

Duncan, S. Nonverbal communication. *Psychological Bulletin,* 1969, **72,** 118-37.

Dupont, H. *Educating emotionally disturbed children.* New York: Holt, Rinehart & Winston, 1969.

Egolf, D. B., & Chester S. Nonverbal communication and the disorders of speech and language. *American Speech & Hearing Assn.,* 1973, **15,** 511-18.

Ekman, P., & Friesen, W. V. Nonverbal behavior in psychotherapy research. In J. M. Shlien (Ed.), *Research in psychotherapy* Vol. 3. Washington, D.C.: American Psychological Assn., 1968.

Exline, R., Gray, D., & Schuette, D. Visual behavior in a dyad as affected by interview content and sex of respondent. *Journal of Personality and Social Psychology,* 1965, **1,** 201-9.

Faglioni, P., Spinnler, H., & Vignolo, L. A. Contrasting behavior of right and left hemisphere-damaged patients on a discrimination task of auditory recognition. *Cortex,* 1969, **5,** 366-89.

Fenichel, C. Psycho-educational approaches for disturbed children in the classroom. In P. Knobloch (Ed.), *Intervention approaches in educating emotionally disturbed children.* Syracuse: Syracuse University Press, 1966.

Franco, J. M., Kelley, J. M., & Whitman, T. *Ideas, images, I. The triple "I" series.* Cincinnati, Ohio: American Book Co., 1970.

Fridja, N. H. Recognition of emotion. *Advances in Experimental Social Psychology,* 1969, **4,** 167-223.

Gerler, E. R. The magic circle program: how to involve teachers? *Elementary School Guidance and Counseling,* 1973, **8,** 86-91.

Giffen, M. The role of child psychiatry in learning disabilities. In H. R. Myklebust (Ed.), *Progress in learning disabilities.* New York: Grune & Stratton, 1968. Pp. 75-97.

Glasser, A. J., & Zimmerman, I. L. *Clinical interpretation of the Wechsler intelligence scale for children.* New York: Grune & Stratton, 1967.

Goldfarb, W. *Childhood schizophrenia.* Cambridge: Harvard University Press, 1961.

Grilli, R. W., Kalunian, P., Nickerson, E. T., & Semel, E. M. *Programmed strategies for behavior change in parents and children.* Dubuque, Iowa: Kendall-Hunt, 1975.

Haggard, E. A., & Isaacs, K. S. Micromomentary facial expressions as indicators of ego mechanism in psychotherapy. In L. A. Gottschalk & A. H. Auerbach (Eds.), *Methods of research in psycho-therapy.* New York: Meredith, 1966.

Hall, E. T. *The silent language.* New York: Fawcett, 1959.

Hall, E. T. *The hidden dimension.* New York: Doubleday, 1966.

Hewitt, F. The Tulare experimental class for educationally handicapped children. *California Education,* 1967, **33,** 459-67. (a)

Hewitt, F. Educational engineering with emotionally disturbed children. *Exceptional Children,* 1967, **33,** 459-67. (b)

Hobbs, N. Helping disturbed children: psychological and ecological strategies. In L. M. Dunn (Ed.), *Exceptional children in the schools.* New York: Holt, Rinehart & Winston, 1973. Pp. 279-80.

Hollister, W., & Goldston, S. Psychoeducational processes in classes for emotionally handicapped children. *Exceptional Children,* 1962, **28,** 351-56.

Homme, L. *How to use contingency contracting in the classroom.* Champaign, Ill.: Research Press, 1972.

Horenstein, S. Effect of cerebrovascular disease on personality and emotion. In A. L. Benton (Ed.), *Behavioral change in cerebrovascular disease.* New York: Harper & Row, 1970. Pp. 171-94.

Johnson, D. J., & Myklebust, H. R. *Learning disabilities: educational principles and practices.* New York: Grune & Stratton, 1967.

Kagan, N., & Krathwohl, D. R. *Studies in human interaction.* Lansing, Mich.: Educational Publication Service, 1967.

Kanner, L. *Child psychiatry.* (2nd ed.) Springfield, Ill.: Charles C Thomas, 1957.

Keogh, B. K., Tchir, C., & Windeguth-Behn, A. Teacher's perceptions of educationally high risk children. *Journal of Learning Disabilities,* 1974, **7**, 367-74.

Kohlberg, L. Moral development and education. In H. Stevenson (Ed.), *Child psychology. Sixty-second Yearbook of the National Society for Study of Education.* Chicago: University of Chicago Press, 1963. Pp. 277-332.

Kohlberg, L. Development of moral character and moral ideology. In M. L. Hoffman & L. W. Hoffman (Eds.), *Review of child development research.* Vol. 1. New York: Russell Sage Foundation, 1964. Pp. 383-431.

Koppitz, E. M. *The Bender Gestalt test for young children.* (Koppitz norms) New York: Psychological Corp., 1964.

Lerner, J. *Children with learning disabilities.* Boston: Houghton Mifflin Co., 1971.

Litz, P. J. Perception of nonverbal cues of emotions by stutterers. Unpublished master's thesis, Boston University, 1973.

Mahl, G. F. Gestures and body movements in interviews. In J. M. Shlien (Ed.), *Research in psychotherapy* Vol. 3. Washington, D.C.: American Psychological Association, 1968.

Mead, G. H. *Mind, self and society.* Chicago: University of Chicago Press, 1934.

Mehrabian, A. Significance of posture and position in the communication of attitude and status relationships. *Psychological Bulletin,* 1969, **71**, 359-72.

Mehrabian, A. A semantic space for nonverbal behavior. *Journal of Consulting and Clinical Psychology,* 1970, **35**, 248-57.

Meisels, L. The student's social contract: learning social competence in the classroom. *Teaching Exceptional Children,* 1974, **7**, 34-35.

Milgram, N. A. Cognitive and emphatetic factors in role taking by schizophrenic and brain-damaged patients. *Journal of Abnormal Social Psychology,* 1960, **60**, 219-24.

Mooney, R. L., & Gordon, L. V. *Mooney problem checking list.* (Rev. ed.) New York: Psychological Corp., 1950.

Morse, W. C. The crisis teacher. In L. Nicholas, W. C. Morse, & R. G. Newman (Eds.), *Conflict in the classroom.* Belmont, Calif.: Wadsworth Publishing Co., 1965. Pp. 251-254.

Myklebust, H. R. Learning disorders: psychoneurological disturbances in childhood. *Rehabilitation Literature,* 1964, **25**, 354-60.

Redl, F. Why life space interview? In H. Dupont (Ed.), *Educating emotionally disturbed children.* New York: Holt, Rinehart & Winston, 1969. Pp. 106-14.

Reid, V. M. (Ed.) *Reading ladders for human relations.* (5th ed.) Washington, D.C.: National Council of Teachers of English, 1972.

Rosenzweig, S., Fleming, E. E., & Rosenzweig, L. The children's form of the Rosenzweig picture-frustration study. *Journal of Psychology,* 1948, **26**, 141,91.

Rotter, J. B., & Rafferty, J. E. *The Rotter incomplete sentences blank.* New York: Psychological Corp., 1950.

Sathre, F. S., Olson, R. W., & Whitney, C. I. *Let's talk: an introduction to interpersonal communication*. Glenview, Ill.: Scott Foresman & Co., 1973.

Scheflen, A. E. On the structuring of human communication. *American Behavioral Scientist*, 1967, **10**, 8-12.

Shneidman, E. The MAPS test with children. In A. Rabin & M. Haworth (Eds.), *Projective techniques with children*. New York: Grune & Stratton, 1960. Pp. 130-48.

Sommer, R. Small group ecology. *Psychological Bulletin*, 1967, **67**, 145-52.

Sullivan, H. S. *The interpersonal theory of psychiatry*. New York: Norton, 1953.

Sullivan, H. S. *The psychiatric interview*. New York: Norton, 1954.

Sullivan, H. S. *The fusion of psychiatry and social science*. New York: Norton, 1964.

Swensen, C. H. *Introduction to interpersonal relations*. Glenview, Ill.: Scott Foresman & Co., 1973.

Symonds, P. M. *Adolescent phantasy*. New York: Columbia Press, 1949.

Tarnopol, L. Delinquency and minimal brain dysfunction. *Journal of Learning Disabilities*, 1970, **3**, 200-207.

Warrington, E. K., & James, M. Facial recognition in unilateral cerebral lesions. *Cortex*, 1967, **3**, 317.

Wechsler, D. *Manual for the WISC*. New York: Psychological Corp., 1949. (a)

Wechsler, D. *Wechsler intelligence scale for children*. New York: Psychological Corp., 1949. (b)

Wechsler, D. *Wechsler adult intelligence scale*. New York: Psychological Corp., 1955.

Wechsler, D. The measurement and appraisal of adult intelligence. Baltimore: Williams & Wilkins, 1958.

Whitney, C. I., Sathre, F. S., & Olson, R. W. *Let's talk: activities supplement*. Glenview, Ill.: Scott Foresman & Co., 1973.

Wiig, E. H., & Harris, S. P. Perception and interpretation of nonverbally expressed emotions by adolescents with learning disabilities. *Perceptual and Motor Skills*, 1974, **38**, 239-45.

Woodworth, R. S. *Experimental psychology*. New York: Holt, 1938.

Glossary

ADDITION: The process of introducing an element, phrase, or clause in sentence transformation.

AFFIX: A prefix or suffix that cannot be used alone since it does not have independent meaning.

ALLOMORPH: A variation of a morpheme which occurs in a specific environment. Examples are the allomorph *am* (a form of to *be*) which occurs in the environment of the personal pronoun *I*.

AMBIGUITY: Referring to the characteristic that the meaning is indefinite or that the spoken message may be understood in more than one way.

ANTONYM: A word with the exact opposite meaning of another word.

ANTONYM PAIR: Two words with exact opposite meanings.

APHASIA: Loss of ability to process and formulate language due to acquired brain damage.

ASPECT: The indication of whether the action expressed by a verb occurs habitually or momentarily or is of short or prolonged duration.

AUDIOLOGICAL: Refers to procedures and techniques employed in the assessment of hearing loss or in the rehabilitation of the hearing impaired.

AUDIOLOGIST: A professional trained in the identification and assessment of hearing loss and the rehabilitation of individuals with hearing impairments.

AUDIOLOGY: The study and science of normal and/or disordered hearing, encompassing the nature of hearing, identification of hearing loss, and rehabilitation of individuals with impaired hearing.

AUDITORY ACUITY: Sensitivity of the human ear to auditory stimuli such as noise, environmental sounds, speech, and so forth.

AUDITORY CLOSURE: The ability to perceive and reconstruct words when they are presented in spoken units and when one or more of the units (sounds or syllables) are missing.

AUDITORY FIGURE-GROUND SELECTION: The process of selectively attending to a significant auditory stimulus (the figure) in the presence of other auditory stimuli (the ground).

AUDITORY PERCEPTION: Meaningful awareness of external auditory stimuli such as environmental sounds, music, or speech.

AUDITORY-SYMBOLIC UNIT: The sound structure of a phoneme in spoken language.

AUDITORY-VISUAL INTEGRATION: The process of associating spoken sounds and words with their written representations.

AUXILIARY VERB: A verb form which has no complete meaning in itself and occurs in combination with a verb which has independent meaning to express mood, tense, or aspect.

BASE: The basic form of a word to which inflectional endings are added. A base may be a *root* (primary form of a word) or a *stem* (a root with a suffix).

BASE-STRUCTURE RULES: A set of rules that generate elemental and simple forms of sentences to which transformational rules may be applied to create more elaborate sentences.

BASE-STRUCTURE STRING: A simple sentence resulting from applying the base—structure rules.

BINAURAL SUMMATION: The process of fusing two parts of a message, each part delivered to one ear and each insufficient for understanding, into a meaningful whole.

CASE GRAMMAR: A set of rules that define the relationship between a sentence structure and the semantic roles played by the constituent structures (noun phrase, verb phrase, etc.).

CEILING: (1) Referring to the level on standardized tests at which the measured skill breaks down; generally expressed as the level at which more than 50% of the responses are incorrect. (2) Referring to the level at which a test becomes insensitive to further changes in performance.

CENTRAL INTEGRATION: Fusion at the subcortical level (first and second neuron) of two complementary parts of a message, delivered to each of the two ears separately.

CIRCUMLOCUTION: Use of an unnecessarily large number of words to express an idea.

CLASS INCLUSION: The process of perceiving that an object such as an *apple* can belong to a subclass as well as to a general class *(fruits)* and of apprehending that objects may belong simultaneously to two different level classes. The concept of inclusion is basic to the understanding of sentences such as "All apples are fruits. There are more fruits than there are apples."

CLAUSE: A subsection of a sentence that contains a separate subject and predicate combination.

CLOZE ITEM: A blank or pause in a narrative passage which signals that a deleted word must be replaced.

CLOZE PASSAGE: A stimulus narrative in which selected words are replaced by blanks. The narrative is usually a story with intact first and last sentences (Taylor, 1953).

CLOZE PROCEDURE: A teaching and/or testing technique in which students must provide responses to a narrative passage with word deletions (Taylor, 1953).

CLOZE RESPONSE: The replacement of a deleted word in a sentence or narrative passage.

COGNITION: The process of structuring and synthesizing the characteristics of previously perceived external stimuli (sensory data).

COGNITIVE PROCESSING OF AUDITORY-SYMBOLIC UNITS: The process of recognizing and differentiating the sound structure of the phonemes in spoken language.

COGNITIVE PROCESSING OF SEMANTIC CLASSES: The process of discerning relationships among two or more words or concepts based upon shared attributes or properties.

COGNITIVE PROCESSING OF SEMANTIC IMPLICATIONS: The process of discerning and interpreting cause-effect relationships and implied causes and effects expressed in language to form expectancies, anticipations, and predictions.

COGNITIVE PROCESSING OF SEMANTIC RELATIONS: The process of discerning and interpreting the logical relationships between words and concepts in sentences or in verbal analogies.

COGNITIVE PROCESSING OF SEMANTIC SYSTEMS: The process of discerning the logical structure that underlies a verbal problem.

COGNITIVE PROCESSING OF SEMANTIC TRANSFORMATIONS: The process of discerning and interpreting changes in the meaning, use, or function of words, concepts, phrases, and sentences.

COGNITIVE PROCESSING OF SEMANTIC UNITS: The process of interpreting the meaning of spoken words and concepts.

COGNITIVE-SEMANTIC PROCESSING OF LANGUAGE: The process of analyzing, structuring, and synthesizing the meaning conveyed in spoken language.

COMMUNICATION, NONVERBAL: The exchange of attitudes, affects, and intentions among individuals by using body language or other nonverbal cues.

COMMUNICATION PROCESS: The exchange of ideas, intentions, or information among individuals. This exchange may occur by verbal or nonverbal means.

COMMUNICATION, VERBAL: The exchange of ideas, intentions, or information by speakers using a common language.

COMPARATIVE: Form of an adjective or adverb denoting that one thing possesses more of a certain quality than another.

COMPOUNDING: The process of combining two words with independent meanings to form a new word.

COMPOUND WORD: A unit consisting of two or more parts or components. Examples are words such as "flashlight" and "bluebell."

CONCEPTUALIZATION: The process of transferring and applying skills to appropriate contexts and situations other than those in which the skill was initially acquired.

CONCRETE-OPERATIONAL STAGE OF DEVELOPMENT: According to Piaget, the period at which logical deduction begins and the concepts of conservation, reversibility, and compensation are acquired. Approximate age seven to eleven years.

CONJUNCTION: A word used to connect words or sentences; its use indicates a relationship between the connected elements.

CONJUNCTION DELETION: The process of omitting an element of a sentence when coordinating phrases, clauses, or sentences as in "Mary wants a red and an orange lollipop."

CONSENSUAL VALIDATION: Verification of a person's perception of self based on the perceived attitudes and reactions of others generally expressed nonverbally.

CONSERVATION: The process of perceiving and judging the equivalence of objects or of quantities of liquid. As an example, the concept of conservation is basic to understanding that two containers of different shapes may contain the same amount of liquid.

CONSERVING CHILDREN: Refers to children who have acquired the concept of conservation.

CONTRACTIBLE AUXILIARY: Forms of the auxiliary verb *be* which add little or nothing to the meaning of an utterance and are therefore contracted to 's or are deleted in early language.

CONTRACTIBLE COPULA: Forms of the copula which add little or nothing to the meaning of an utterance and are therefore contracted to 's or are deleted in early language.

CONVERGENT SEMANTIC PRODUCTION: The process of recalling or producing a specific word, word association, phrase, or sentence to fit the meaning of the stimulus.

COORDINATING CONJUNCTION: A word used to connect two words, phrases, or clauses which are of equal function or importance.

COPULA: Forms of the verb *to be* or its equivalent. Signifies a relationship between the subject and predicate of a sentence.

DELETION: The process of omitting an element, phrase, or clause in sentence transformations as in "John reads (something)."

DERIVATION: Formation of a new word by adding a prefix or suffix to an already existing word.

DICHOTIC LISTENING TASK: Simultaneous presentation of different sounds or messages to each of the ears via earphones. Under dichotic stimulation one of the two ears perceives the sound or message more easily than the other. Verbal stimuli are generally perceived most easily by the right ear, the ear contralateral to the left hemisphere of the brain. Nonverbal auditory stimuli are generally perceived most easily by the left ear, the ear contralateral to the right hemisphere.

DIRECT OBJECT: Person or thing directly affected by the action denoted by the verb.

DISTINCTIVE FEATURE: A significant acoustic or articulatory feature of a phoneme. Each phoneme is composed of a set of distinctive features.

DIVERGENT SEMANTIC PRODUCTION: The process of recalling and producing a variety of words and concepts, word associations, phrases, or sentences.

DYSNOMIA: Partial loss of or reduced ability to name objects or recall and retrieve words.

DYSPHASIA: Partial loss of ability to process and formulate language due to brain damage.

EMBEDDING: The process of placing a clause within a sentence as in the sentences "The boy who lives next door plays football" and "She told the neighbors that the boy plays football."

EMPHATIC: Form which conveys special emphasis, intensity, or stress.

EVALUATION: The process of comparing new information against past experiences with similar information using a set of criteria to decide if the criteria are met. In spoken language the information can be conveyed by words, phrases, sentences, or continuous discourse.

EVALUATION OF CONSISTENCY: The process of comparing new information (words, phrases, or sentences) against past experience to decide if the form or function is consistent with the rules of the language.

EVALUATION CRITERIA: A set of logical criteria employed in comparing new information with past experiences. Guilford (1967) proposes the following set of criteria: identity, similarity, and consistency.

EVAULATION OF IDENTITY: The process of comparing new information (words, phrases, or sentences) with past experiences to decide if they are identical in form or function in spite of their differences.

EVALUATION OF SIMILARITY: The process of comparing new information (words, phrases, or sentences) with past experiences to decide if they share characteristics in form or function in spite of their differences.

FORMAL-OPERATIONAL STAGE OF DEVELOPMENT: According to Piaget, the period during which the cognitive abilities for abstraction, implication, propositional logic, and hypothesis testing are developed. Approximate age eleven to fifteen years.

FREE-FIELD TESTING: Referring to the method of assessing hearing in which auditory stimuli are introduced into the testing environment by one or more loudspeakers.

FRICATIVE: A speech sound produced by forcing the air through a narrow opening between the lips and the teeth or between the tongue and the palate, resulting in high-frequency vibrations. Examples are *f* and voiced and unvoiced *th*.

FRONTAL LOBE: A part of either hemisphere of the brain which lies in front of the Rolandic fissure and above the Sylvian fissure.

GENDER: Grammatical categorization of words into *masculine, feminine,* and *neuter* genders.

GENERATIVE GRAMMAR: A finite set of explicit rules capable of generating a large number of grammatical utterances.

GLIDE: See semivowel.

HOMONYM: A word that sounds identical to another word in the language but expresses a different meaning.

Hz (Hertz): A unit of the frequency of sounds equal to one cycle per second.

IDIOM: Phrase or expression expressing a specific meaning of its own; often contrasts with the meaning of the individual words.

INDIRECT OBJECT: Person or thing *for* whom the action of the verb takes place.

INFINITIVAL COMPLEMENT: The use of an infinitive to complete the meaning of an utterance by expressing an action or a condition as in "George wants to fish."

INFLECTION: The process of modifying the meaning of a word by adding a suffix to express grammatical relationships, functions, and aspects.

INTERJECTION: An exclamation, often of stereotyped form, that expresses emtoion.

INTERROGATIVE SENTENCE: A sentence expressing a direct question.

INTERSENSORY FUNCTIONS: Referring to stimulus-response combinations that involve two different modalities such as auditory stimuli eliciting written responses or visual stimuli eliciting spoken responses.

INTONATION: Melodic pattern in speech.

INTRASENSORY FUNCTIONS: Referring to stimulus-response combinations that are within the same modality system such as auditory stimuli eliciting spoken responses and visual stimuli eliciting written responses.

KINESICS: The study of the role and function of body movements in interpersonal communication.

LANGUAGE PROCESSING: The act of receiving, perceiving, and interpreting spoken language.

LANGUAGE PRODUCTION: The process of formulating ideas into phrases and sentences in accordance with a set of grammatical and semantic rules.

LATERALIZATION: The process of comparing the loudness of sounds heard in both ears and recognizing in which ear the sound is loudest (localization of the intracranial position of sounds presented).

LEXICAL: Relating to the words, word combinations, and vocabulary of the language.

LINGUISTIC CONCEPTS: Words, word combinations, or sentences that express logical relationships between two or more words or concepts in a sentence. Examples are "if . . . then," " . . . all . . . except . . . ," "When . . . then," and comparative and passive sentences.

LINGUISTIC CONCEPTS; CONCEPTS OF EXCLUSION: Words or word combinations that express that one or more elements of a sentence do not belong to a group. Examples are "All . . . except," "All . . . but," " . . . not . . . any," and " . . . none."

LINGUISTIC CONCEPTS; CONCEPTS OF INCLUSION: Words or word combinations that express that one or more elements of a sentence belong to a group. Examples are " . . . all . . . ," " . . . many . . . ," and so forth.

LINGUISTIC LEVEL I: The stage during language acquisition when the semantic roles of and the syntactic relations among words are developed. This stage begins when two words are combined and ends when utterances of more than two words are used.

LINGUISTIC LEVEL II: The stage during language acquisition when more than two words are combined in utterances and when grammatical morphemes (articles, locative prepositions, present and past tense copula, forms of the auxiliary *be*, and inflectional morphemes) are developed and the meaning of words and phrases is modulated. Stage II ends when utterances contain more than seven morphemes.

LINGUISTIC LEVEL III: The stage during language acquisition when the average utterances contain more than two words and when the simple sentence structures developed during the previous stage are modified and elaborated upon.

LINGUISTIC LEVEL IV: The stage during language acquisition when the average utterances contain more than three words. Stage IV ends when utterances contain more than eleven morphemes.

LINGUISTIC LEVEL V: The stage during language acquisition when the average utterances contain four words. Stage V ends when utterances contain more than thirteen morphemes.

LINGUISTICS: The formal study of the form and function of language.

LOCALIZATION: The process of perceiving and identifying the source of a sound in the environment.

LOCATIVE PREPOSITION: A preposition used to denote a geographical or physical location of persons, objects, events, and so forth.

LOW-PASS FILTERED SPEECH: Speech which contains a range of frequencies extending from zero frequency to some critical cutoff frequency. Frequencies above the cutoff point are not transmitted, introducing distortion of the message.

MASKING: partial or complete obscuring of a tone or a sound by the simultaneous presence of one or more sounds in the environment.

MASS NOUN: A noun referring to an article or substance consisting of numerous small particles such as *rice* (a grain of rice) or *water* (a drop of water).

MEDIAL POSITION: The noninitial and nonfinal position of a speech sound or a cluster of speech sounds within a word or a word sequence.

METAPHOR: A figure of speech in which the meaning of a word is extended on the basis of a natural relationship between the primary and secondary application, for example, the *neck* of the bottle, the *arm* of the river.

MINIMAL PAIR: Word pair differing in only one phoneme such as *cat* and *hat*.

MOOD: The expression of the manner or form in which the action or state denoted by the verb occurs.

MORPHEME: The smallest meaningful grammatical unit in a language. Morphemes may be classified as *roots* or *affixes*.

MORPHOLOGICAL STRUCTURE: The combination of morphemes (roots and affixes) to form larger grammatical units (words and phrases).

MORPHOLOGY: The study of and the rules for the formation of words.

NARROW-BAND NOISE: A noise that contains a narrow range of frequencies, used for masking in testing hearing.

NASAL: A speech sound with nasal resonance. Examples are *m, n,* and *ng*.

NASALITY: A distinctive feature that results in change of a consonant by producing it while letting air escape through the nose.

NEAGATIVE, EXPLICIT: Sentence in which the negative aspect is conveyed by the addition of *not*.

NEGATIVE, INHERENT: Sentence in which the negative aspect is conveyed by a prefix as in *undiscovered* or by the word itself as in *absent*.

NESTING: The process of embedding two or more phrases or clauses within a sentence as in "The boy who sits on the grass in the center near the library next to the gas station is my brother."

NEUROPSYCHOLOGICAL MODEL FOR LANGUAGE PROCESSING: A model which proposes that the specific aspects of the process of perceiving and interpreting language depend upon the function of different parts of the brain (Luria, 1973).

NOMINAL-COMPOUND: The process of deriving a noun phrase which consists of two parts as in "The ice cream truck stopped outside." (The truck stopped outside. The truck contains ice cream.)

NOMINALIZATION: The process of forming a noun or nominal form describing an ongoing action or an event occurring at a specific time or place. Examples are "Mother went shopping all day Saturday" and "The parade was last Sunday on Fifth Avenue."

NONCONSERVING CHILDREN: Refers to children who have not yet acquired the concept of conservation.

OCCIPITAL LOBE: A part of either hemisphere which lies behind the occipito-parietal fissure in the back part of the brain.

PARADIGM: A model, pattern, or example.

PARADIGMATIC ASSOCIATION: A relationship between two words based on their membership in the same grammatical class. Examples are *dogs—cats, walk—run*.

PARALANGUAGE: A system of communication cues which serves to alter or modify the verbal messages.

PARALLEL PROCESSING MODEL: A model for language processing which proposes that the phonetic (speech-sound), lexical (vocabulary), syntactic (sentence structure), and semantic (meaning) characteristics are processed concurrently.

PARAPHASIA: Substitution of speech sounds, words, and/or phrases during spontaneous speech or while attempting to say something specific.

PARIETAL LOBE: A part of either hemisphere of the brain which lies in back of the Rolandic fissure and above the Sylvian fissure.

PERCEPTION: Meaningful awareness of external stimuli (objects, events, or relationships).

PERCEPTION OF SENSORY DATA: Meaningful awareness of external stimuli as a result of sensory stimulation.

PERCEPTUAL PROCESSING OF LANGUAGE: the act of attending to, recognizing, identifying, and discriminating among the speech sounds in spoken language.

PERMUTATION: the process of changing the sequence of elements or phrases in sentence transformation as in "The boy put his coat on" (The boy put on his coat).

PHONEME: A significant speech sound which when changed alters the meaning of a word. Each phoneme is composed of a set of distinctive features.

PHONEME DISCRIMINATION: The process of distinguishing between significant speech sounds (phonemes).

PHONETIC: Relating to the acoustic and articulatory characteristics of speech sounds.

PHONETIC MODELS: A pattern for the design of testing and/or training materials for speech-sound discrimination which accounts for the acoustic and articulatory features (distinctive features) of phonemes.

PHONOLOGICAL: Relating to the acoustic and articulatory characteristics of significant speech sounds in a language (phonemes).

PHONOLOGICAL CONDITIONING RULES: Limitations imposed on the selection of allomorphs of inflectional phonemes by the phonetic features of preceding sounds (phonemes). As an example, the plural allomorph /z/ occurs only after voiced sounds as in *beds,* /s/ occurs only after voiceless sounds as in *bets,* and /iz/ only after sibilants and affricates as in *churches.*

PHONOLOGICAL STRUCTURE: The combination of speech sounds (phonemes) according to rules to form larger speech units (syllables, words, phrases).

PHONOLOGY: The study of and the rules for the structure of speech sounds into larger units of speech.

PHRASE: A group of words in a grammatical pattern which relates meaning but which does not contain a subject-predicate structure.

PLOSIVE: A speech sound produced by building up air pressure which is suddenly released. Examples are *p, b, t,* and *d.*

PREDICATE: A word or word group that expresses the state, condition, or property of the subject of the sentence.

PREFIX: letter, syllable, or sequence of syllables without independent meaning that changes the meaning of a word when it is placed before and fused with it.

PREOPERATIONAL STAGE OF DEVELOPMENT: According to Piaget, the period when the sensorimotor schemata can be mentally activated. The mental operations are egocentric and irreversible and limited to concrete actions. Approximate age two to seven years.

PRODUCTIVE CONTROL OF LINGUISTIC STRUCTURE: Ability to formulate and produce grammatically acceptable phrases and sentences.

PRONOMINALIZATION: The process of replacing a noun by a pronoun.

PROSODIC FEATURES: Melodic features of phrases and sentences expressed by variations in pitch, intensity, and juncture.

PROXEMICS: The study of the role and function of spatial positioning in interpersonal communication.

PSYCHOLINGUISTICS: The formal study of the psycho-social and linguistic aspects of the communication process.

PURE-TONE: A sound of a single frequency (a pure sine wave without overtones).

QUESTION TRANSFORMATION: Deriving a question from an active declarative sentence by changing the syntactic structure.

REAUDITORIZATION: Internal auditory rehearsal of digits, words, or sentences.

REFERENTIAL MEANING: Containing or constituting a reference to objects, events, or relationships in the outside world.

REFLEXIVE PRONOUN: The forms of the personal pronouns which indicate that the agent and the object of the action are the same.

RELATIVE CLAUSES: An included clause functioning as a modifier, subject, or complement and introduced by a relative pronoun.

RELATIVE PRONOUN: A pronoun (who, whose, whom, which, what, that, when. where, whoever, whichever, whatever, etc.) that introduces a relative clause.

REVISUALIZATION: Internal, visual rehearsal of the perceptions of objects, events, and/or written materials.

REVISUALIZE: The process of reseeing objects, events, and/or written materials internally.

RHEMATIC: Referring to the information provided about the subject (theme) of an utterance.

RHEME: The information given about the subject (theme) of an utterance.

SALIENCE: Psychological prominence of concepts, ideas, thoughts, or intentions in a person's mind.

SEGMENTATION: The process of dividing words into smaller grammatical units (morphemes).

SELECTIONAL CONSTRAINTS: Restrictions in the choice of words imposed by the meaning of the context and of the ideas to be expressed.

SELECTIONAL RULES: Rules for the selection of words from the lexicon, given the restrictions imposed by the meaning of the context and of the ideas to be expressed.

SEMANTIC: Relating to the underlying meaning of words and grammatical forms and constructions in a language.

SEMANTIC CLASS: Two or more words or concepts that are related and can be grouped on the basis of meaning and/or association.

SEMANTIC CONSTRAINTS: Limitations in the selection of words or structures imposed by meaning or context.

SEMANTIC IMPLICATION: The causes, effects, and concomitant conditions implied by the content and structure of sentences.

SEMANTIC RELATION: A logical relationship between two or more words or concepts in a sentence as between "apple" and "watermelon" in the sentence "Watermelons are bigger than apples" or between the critical words in a verbal analogy such as "*People* have *feet; dogs* have *paws.*"

SEMANTIC SYSTEM: A verbal statement that presents a problem with an underlying logical structure.

SEMANTIC TRANSFORMATION: A change in the meaning, significance, and use of words and concepts, phrases and sentences.

SEMANTIC UNIT: The concept or meaning denoted by a word.

SEMANTICS: The formal study of the meaning expressed by words or by grammatical relationships between words.

SEMANTIC ASPECTS: Characteristics of the meaning of words, expressions, phrases, and sentences.

SEMIVOWEL: A speech sound which functions as a consonant, produced without stopping or impeding the airstream. Examples are *r* and *w*. Sometimes semivowels are called *glides*.

SENSATION: The process of receiving external stimuli through the sensory modalities.

SENSORIMOTOR STAGE OF DEVELOPMENT: According to Piaget, the period of development of sensorimotor schemata and acquisition of knowledge of actions and of object permanence. Approximate age birth to two years.

SENSORY INTEGRITY: Referring to adequate sensory abilities for hearing, vision, touch, olfaction, or proprioception.

SENSORY MODALITIES: Parts of the central nervous system (CNS) concerned with audition, vision, kinesthesis, or taction.

SENTENCE TRANSFORMATION: Deriving various sentence types, for example, passive, negative, interrogative, from an active declarative sentence by changing the syntactic structure.

SERIAL PROCESSING MODEL: A model for language processing which proposes that the phonetic (speech-sound), lexical (vocabulary), syntactic (sentence structure), and semantic (meaning) characteristics are processed sequentially.

SERIATION: The process of perceiving gradations in the physical attributes of objects such as in size, color, weight, and so forth, and of ordering objects correctly according to a single attribute (simple seriation) or to two or more attributes (seriation with multiple criteria).

SHADOWING: The process of imitating spoken language immediately upon hearing it.

SHADOWING LATENCIES: The time delays occurring in the process of imitating spoken language immediately upon hearing it.

SIBILANT: A speech sound produced by forcing air through a narrow opening between tongue and palate, resulting in a hissing sound. Examples are *s*, *z*, and *sh*.

SOCIAL PERCEPTION: Meaningful awareness of nonverbal communication cues that convey information of affect, attitudes, and intentions.

SOUND LOCALIZATION: The process of recognizing and identifying the location of an external sound source.

SPEECH PATHOLOGIST: A professional with specialized training in the evaluation and treatment of all aspects of functional and organic speech and language disorders.

STRUCTURE OF LANGUAGE, DEEP: The meaning structure of a spoken message. The same meaning structure may be conveyed by different surface structures. Deep structure is converted into surface structure according to grammatical rules.

STRUCTURE OF LANGUAGE, SURFACE: The structural characteristics of a spoken message.

SUFFIX: Letter, syllable, or syllable sequence without independent meaning which when added to an existing word can modify or change its meaning.

SUPERLATIVE: Form of an adjective or adverb which denotes that one thing among several possesses most of a certain quality.

SYLLABICATION: The process of dividing words into component syllables.

SYNDROME: A group of characteristic behaviors or responses which when combined constitute a specific deficit or disorder.

SYNONYM: Two or more different words in a language which share the same meaning.

SYNTACTIC: Relating to the grammatical forms and constructions of a language.

SYNTACTIC ASSOCIATION: A relationship between two words based on their frequent occurrence in sequence in a syntactic structure or sentence. Examples are: *dogs—bark, new—car, walk—slowly*.

SYNTACTIC CONSTRAINTS: Limitations in the selection of phrases or sentences imposed by grammatical rules.

TEMPORAL LOBE: A part of each hemisphere of the brain which lies below the Sylvian fissure and continues backwards to the occipital lobe.

TENSE: the expression of the time of an action denoted by a verb, as past, present, or future.

THEMATIC: Referring to the first part or subject of an utterance.

THEME: The first member of a sentence (the subject of an utterance).

UNCONTRACTIBLE AUXILIARY: Forms of the auxiliary verb *be (is, am,* and *are)* which add meaning to a relation and are therefore not deleted or contracted to *'s.*

UNCONTRACTIBLE COPULA: Forms of the copula, *is, am,* and *are,* which add meaning to a relation and are therefore not deleted or contracted to *'s.*

VERBAL PARAPHASIA: Substitution of an inappropriate word during spontaneous speech, while attempting to say something specific, or during reading.

VISUAL-MOTOR DEFICITS: Impairments in the process of perceiving and reproducing visual stimuli.

VOICING: a distinctive feature which results in change of a consonant by adding vibration of the vocal folds, for example, changing /p/ into /b/ by adding voicing.

WHITE NOISE: A noise which contains a wide range of audible frequencies, used for masking in testing hearing.

Name Index

332

Subject Index